# OSMOSIS

# RENAL PATHOLOGY

## Version 1.01

Fergus Baird, MA
Rishi Desai, MD, MPH
Tanner Marshall, MS
Kyle Slinn, RN, MEd
Vincent Waldman, PhD

2017

hi@osmosis.org

ISBN 978-1-947769-00-7

Osmosis
37 S. Ellwood Avenue
Baltimore, MD 21224
www.osmosis.org

Printed in the United States of America

Designed by Fergus Baird, Heidi Hildebrandt, Tanner Marshall, & Kyle Slinn
Copyedited by Fergus Baird & Andrea Day
Fonts: Roboto by Google Inc., Apache License, version 2.0
Written in Canada and United States of America
SCP 10 9 8 7 6 5 4 3 2 1

Edition: 1.0.1

We'd like to thank our Osmosis Prime members, our supporters, the hundreds of volunteers who double check our facts and translate our videos, and of course, our viewers on YouTube and Wikipedia. You all have played a huge part in helping us make the best learning experiences possible.

If you find any mistakes, let us know here:
https://goo.gl/forms/Djal70T3licqckpi1

## Osmosis Team

Lindsay Adelson, BS
John Bafford, BS
Fergus Baird, MA
Sarah Clifford, BMBS
Andrea Day, MA
Harry Delaney, MBChB
Rishi Desai, MD, MPH
Allison Dollar, BFA
Caleb Furnas, MA
Shiv Gaglani, MBA
Sam Gillespie, BSc
Ryan Haynes, PhD
Heidi Hildebrandt, MA

Thasin Jaigirdar, BA
Tanner Marshall, MS
Sam Miller, BA
Brandon Newton, BBA,
Brittany Norton, MFA
Viviana Popa
Vishal Punwani, MD
Kyle Slinn, RN, MEd
Diana Stanley, MBA
Sean Tackett, MD, MPH
Ashley Thompson, BSc
Vince Waldman, PhD
Yifan Xiao, MD

# AUTHORS

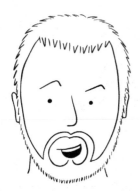

**Fergus Baird MA**

Fergus Baird is a copywriter and textbook designer at Osmosis, and he dabbles in a little scriptwriting for the YouTube channel as well.

Before moving to Canada, Fergus lived in a small village in Scotland. He earned his Master's degree in English literature at Concordia University in Montréal, writing his thesis on history and the graphic novel. Before joining Team Osmosis, Fergus worked as a gif curator, a movie subtitler, a meme master and a ghost writer, and spent a year teaching elementary school kids in Japan.

When he's not eating or cooking elaborate meals for his friends, Fergus spends his spare time playing video games and the theremin, drawing strange pictures, and consuming horror media in all its gruesome forms.

---

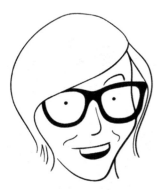

**Andrea Day MA**

Andrea is currently a content editor (and formerly a scriptwriter) at Osmosis, and she's responsible for making our educational copy as clear and accessible as possible. She's also wrapping up a PhD in English Literature.

During her studies, Andrea has worked as a course instructor, as a teaching assistant, and as a writing tutor in undergraduate and graduate writing centers. She's enjoying using her communication and teaching skills in a new environment, and the fact that she gets to work alongside her pals Kyle and Fergus is a pretty good bonus.

When she's not at work, Andrea can be found hugging her cat Mortimer, swimming, baking, or reading Victorian novels.

---

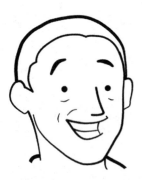

**Rishi Desai MD, MPH**

Rishi is a pediatric infectious disease physician at Stanford University and serves as the Chief Medical Officer at Osmosis. He recently led the Khan Academy Medicine team, which put together a collection of videos and questions for students entering the health sciences.

With the help of his parents and teachers, Rishi completed high school and received his BS in Microbiology from UCLA by the age of 18. He completed his medical training at UCSF, pediatric residency at Boston Children's Hospital, and did an infectious disease fellowship at Children's Hospital Los Angeles. He earned his MPH in epidemiology at UCLA, and then spent two years chasing down infectious disease outbreaks for the Centers for Disease Control and Prevention, before beginning his work in online medical education.

In his spare time, Rishi enjoys watching his son torment the family dog, while eating nature's finest fruit - the raspberry!

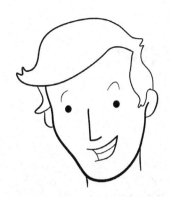

## Tanner Marshall
## MS

Tanner's the voice and illustrator behind the majority of Osmosis videos (as well as a few icons, graphics, and cartoons scattered around Osmosis). Tanner got both his undergrad and graduate degree in biomedical engineering from the University of Wisconsin-Madison (Go Badgers), before moving out to Portland, OR and starting his engineering career.

After working in the cardiac rhythm management business for bit, he stumbled upon the two goofballs Rishi and Kyle, and began working alongside (well, technically under, but who's counting!) them producing openly accessible videos for Khan Academy Medicine.

In addition to being an enthusiast for science education and being halfway-decent with a drawing tablet, he also takes pride in his diverse collection of hats (including both beanies and baseball caps), his skills on the ultimate frisbee field, and his vast knowledge of the *Star Wars* universe.

---

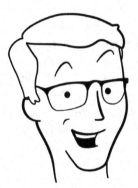

## Kyle Slinn
## RN, MEd

Kyle is a project manager and instructional designer at Osmosis. He wears many hats, such as managing volunteers and contractors, designing future projects, producing videos, leading internationalization efforts, and designing Osmosis's textbooks. A jack-of-all-trades. Before Osmosis, he worked as a project coordinator for Khan Academy Medicine, where he managed the creation of videos, questions, and text-based articles for MCAT and NCLEX-RN students.

Kyle also worked in the pediatric intensive care unit as a nurse at the Children's Hospital of Eastern Ontario, in Ottawa, Canada. He received his Bachelors of Science in Nursing from the University of Ottawa and holds a Masters of Education in Distance Education from Athabasca University.

With his free time, Kyle loves to go on adventures, hang out with friends, play board games, bake bread, and play musical instruments.

---

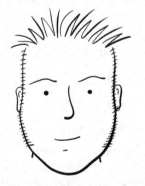

## Vince Waldman
## PhD

Vincent is the second video illustrator to join the Osmosis team. He received an undergraduate degree in chemistry from Coe College in Cedar Rapids, Iowa, then earned his PhD in biochemistry from Indiana, University in Bloomington, Indiana.

After performing a biophysics postdoc at Washington University in St. Louis, Missouri, Vince decided to follow his interests in photography, graphic design, writing and education, which ultimately led to his position as an Osmosis illustrator.

Vince currently lives in Lawrence, KS. In his free time he loves photography, gravel cycling, food, and road trips to nowhere in particular.

# ASSOCIATED AUTHORS

**Philip M. Boone MD, PhD**

Philip earned a B.S. in Biological Sciences from Stanford University and an MD and PhD in Molecular and Human Genetics from Baylor College of Medicine. He is currently a resident in pediatrics and a fellow in clinical genetics in Boston. Philip is a script writer for Osmosis educational videos and hosts his own YouTube channel, Quick Medical Genetics. His dream is to impart his love of genetics to learners around the world. In his spare time, he enjoys rock climbing and finding a balance between the KonMari method and the Boy Scout motto.

---

**Charles B. Davis BS**

Charlie writes content for Osmosis. He completed his BS in Biochemistry, Cell and Molecular Biology at Drake University. Next, he started a band and moved to New York City where he spent his days above ground as a research technician at Memorial Sloan Kettering Cancer Center, and his nights playing piano and ukulele in unfinished basements of Queens. He is currently a fourth-year medical student at the University of Kansas School of Medicine and will pursue a residency in radiology. Charlie believes that people are naturally curious and that it's the responsibility of educators to cultivate that curiosity with entertaining content presentations. In his free time, Charlie enjoys eating, reading science-fiction, and performing random acts of kindness.

---

**Amanda J. Grieco PhD**

Amanda writes content for Osmosis. Despite not being a super big fan of the cold, she completed her BS in Molecular Genetics at the University of Rochester, and even learned to love the snow! Next, she learned to navigate New York City while completing her MS and PhD at Albert Einstein College of Medicine in Biomedical Science. She has a background in teaching first year medical students and creating online medical education content for Khan Academy Medicine. Amanda is passionate about providing open access to quality scientific and medical resources to all. In her free time, she enjoys hiking, listening to podcasts, and crossing items off her bucket list.

---

**Kaitlyn Harper MA**

Kaitlyn received her BS in Biology from Pacific University, then received her MA in Urban Education while completing two years as a Teach For America corps member in Sacramento, California. After teaching high school science for three years, she decided to get nerdy again and went back to school for her MSc in Public Health at the University of British Columbia, where she studies intestinal disorders in children. Kaitlyn loves rollerblading, eating fresh figs from her yard, and playing ultimate frisbee (go T-Birds!)

## Maureen H. Richards PhD

Maureen edits scripts for Osmosis in collaboration with her work as an assistant professor at Rush University Medical College, Chicago, IL. Maureen complete her PhD in Immunology and Microbiology from Northwestern University. A native New Yorker, she settled in Chicago with her husband and son. When she is not editing for Osmosis, she researches the effects of chronic viral infections and inflammatory immune responses on the brain and teaches pre-clinical medical students. Maureen is committed to providing fun and quality scientific and medical content to all. In her free time, Maureen enjoys spending time with her husband and son, figure skating, and finding new restaurants.

---

## Thomas R. Shannon DVM, PhD

Thomas R. Shannon is a research scientist and teacher at Rush University, Chicago, IL. His research interests are in ionic channels, voltage gated ionic channels, fluorescence signal detection and electrophysiology, particularly as they relate to excitation-contraction coupling in striated muscle. Shannon uses multiple biochemical, biophysical and molecular approaches to study the control of the concentration of calcium in the storage organelle (the sarcoplasmic reticulum) of normal and abnormal cells of the heart. His teaching expertise is in the areas of cardiovascular, pulmonary, and renal biology and reproductive endocrinology.

---

## Maria Fernanda Villarreal MD

Maria is a content contributor for Osmosis. She completed her MD degree at the University of Monterrey. After her graduation, she performed a postdoctoral research fellowship in Medical Education, where she became enthusiastic about providing free articles and open-access resources to doctors around the world. In her free time, Maria enjoys watercolor painting, rock climbing, and chilaquiles.

And a special thanks to our other associated authors:

**Christa Morris**, BA
**Debal Sinharoy**, MBBS

# REVIEWERS

Creating accurate content is really hard. Thousands of eyeballs will look at our work for years to come and inevitably we'll have missed something, or something will go out of date. What's nice about our way of producing content is we get a lot of feedback really fast. Within 24 hours of releasing a video we've meticulously crafted and reviewed, we get thousands of views. In the rare instance there's a mistake, our audience is always quick to use the comment feature to point out where we went wrong. Yep, we're listening! We read every single comment across all of our videos. Whenever someone points out a factual inaccuracy, we update our video and rerelease it. Currently, YouTube doesn't allow editions of videos to exist. When we rerelease a video, we're effectively pulling the existing, well-established and easily searchable video out of circulation and putting a new, less searchable video in its place. There have been several times where our team has silently cried inside as we take down our most viewed video in the name of scientific accuracy. In the end, though, the result is that we can confidently say our videos (and textbooks) are factually accurate.

We'd like to thank the following people who have given us so much guidance as we've created our content.

**Jodi Berndt**, PhD

**Armando Hasudungan Faigl**, BBiomedSc

**Kristine Krafts**, MD

**Vanita Gaglani**, RPT

**Lisa Miklush**, PhD, RNC, CNS

**Thomas M. Schmid**, PhD

**Eric Strong**, MD

Our user interface designer has asked us not to say,
"This page is intentionally left blank."

# FOREWORD

It is our privilege to be able to introduce you to the Osmosis Renal Pathophysiology book that you hold in your hands. We started Osmosis while we were medical students at Johns Hopkins, back when only 118 of our classmates were using the platform. Fast forward a few years and the Osmosis audience has grown to more than 300,000 medical & health professional students around the globe. Our team now comprises more than two dozen incredibly passionate and smart people whose mission is to provide you the best education so that, ultimately, you can provide your future patients with the best care. We're proud of the work that the Osmosis content team has done to fulfill this mission - this book being the latest step on that path.

Given the crucial role the kidneys play in one's overall health, renal pathophysiology is one of the most interesting and important subjects for clinical medicine. We fondly remember learning about everything from Alport syndrome to Hyponatremia to Wilm's tumor in the lecture halls in Baltimore, MA. As biomedical engineers we share unique respect for the elegant structure and function of the kidneys, and it is our hope that this book will instill the same sense of awe within you. In the following 300+ pages you'll learn about more than 50 of the most common and clarifying renal pathophysiology conditions, which we explain with hundreds of high quality and visually appealing diagrams.

Finally, while you may not be able to sleep with your head on this textbook and "learn by Osmosis," you can use the powerful & comprehensive Osmosis learning platform to watch our renal pathophysiology videos and actively quiz yourself with tens of thousands of associated multiple choice questions & flashcards. We encourage you to visit www.osmosis.org to learn more.

Best wishes Osmosing!

Shiv Gaglani & Ryan Haynes
Co-founders of Osmosis

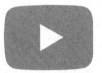

Watch our new videos every week:
www.youtube.com/osmosis

---

Follow us on Facebook:
www.facebook.com/osmoseit

---

Follow us on Twitter:
@osmoseit

---

Follow us on Instagram:
@osmosismed

---

Join our growing community on Reddit:
www.reddit.com/r/osmoseit

# CONTENTS

# Acute pyelonephritis

osmosis.org/learn/acute_pyelonephritis

**W**ith acute pyelonephritis, *pyelo-* means pelvis, and *neph-* refers to the kidney, so in this case it's the renal pelvis, which is the funnel-like structure of the kidney that drains urine into the ureter that's affected. *-Itis* means inflammation. So, acute pyelonephritis describes an inflamed kidney that develops relatively quickly, usually as a result of a bacterial infection **(Figure 1.1)**.

## PATHOLOGY

A urinary tract infection or UTI is any infection of the urinary tract which includes the upper portion of the tract (the kidneys and ureters) and the lower portion of the tract (the bladder and urethra). So, acute pyelonephritis is a type of upper urinary tract infection **(Figure 1.2)**.

Acute pyelonephritis is most often caused by ascending infection, meaning bacteria start by colonizing the urethra and bladder (which would be a lower urinary tract infection) and make their way up the ureters and kidney **(Figure 1.3)**. Therefore, upper UTI shares a lot of the same risk factors as lower UTI, like female sex, sexual intercourse, indwelling catheters, diabetes mellitus, and urinary tract obstruction.

One major factor that increases the risk of an upper UTI developing from a lower UTI spreading upward is vesicoureteral reflux, or VUR, which is where urine is allowed to move backward up the urinary tract, which can happen if the vesicourethral orifice fails **(Figure 1.4)**. The vesicourethral orifice is the one-way valve that allows urine to flow from each ureter into the bladder, but not in the reverse direction **(Figure 1.5)**.

VUR can be the result of a primary congenital defect or it can be caused by bladder outlet obstruction, which increases pressure in the bladder and distorts the valve. As kind of a double-whammy, obstruction also leads to urinary stasis, where urine stands still, which makes it easier for bacteria to adhere and colonize the urinary tract **(Figure 1.6; Figure 1.7)**.

So, for ascending infections that cause acute pyelonephritis, the most common organisms are *E coli*, *Proteus* species, and *Enterobacter* species, all of which are commonly found in the bowel flora. Now, it's also possible that kidneys can get infected via hematogenous infection,

**Figure 1.1**

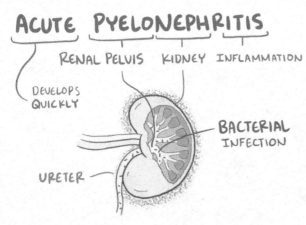

**Figure 1.2**

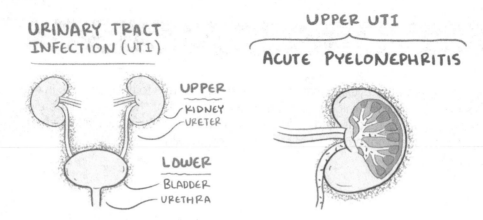

**Figure 1.3**

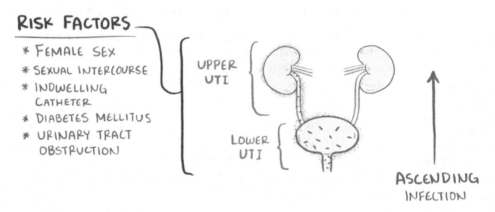

**Figure 1.4**

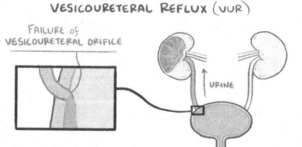

**Figure 1.5**

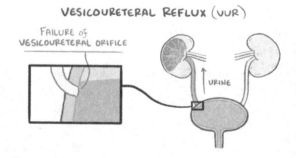

**Figure 1.6**

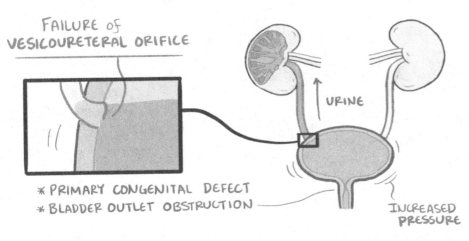

**Figure 1.7**

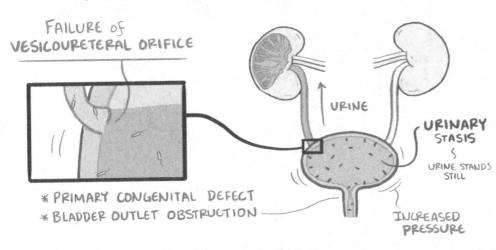

or spread through the bloodstream, although this is a lot less common. Usually pyelonephritis from hematogenous spread is a consequence of septicemia or bacteremia, which is bacteria in the blood, as well as infective endocarditis, an infection of the inner layer of the heart. In these situations, the most common organisms are *Staphylococcus* species and, again, *E. coli* (**Figure 1.8**).

Acute pyelonephritis is most often unilateral, meaning it affects just one kidney. When bacteria mount an attack, they usually start by adhering to the renal epithelium of the tubules, which triggers an inflammatory response. Chemokines attract neutrophils to the renal interstitium, but typically the glomeruli and vessels are spared. As neutrophils infiltrate and die off, they make their way through the urinary tract and are peed out, so people with acute pyelonephritis often have white blood cells in the urine (**Figure 1.9**). Sometimes the cells and the surrounding inflammatory protein debris are even "casted" into the shape of the tubule, which is then also peed out—this is called a white blood cell cast.

**Figure 1.8**

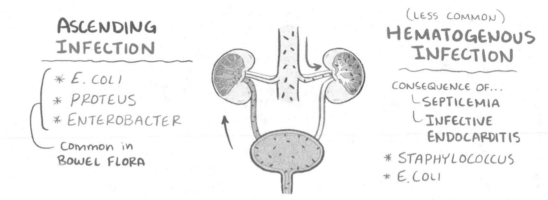

ASCENDING INFECTION

* E. COLI
* PROTEUS
* ENTEROBACTER

Common in BOWEL FLORA

(LESS COMMON)
HEMATOGENOUS INFECTION

CONSEQUENCE OF...
└ SEPTICEMIA
└ INFECTIVE ENDOCARDITIS

* STAPHYLOCOCCUS
* E. COLI

**Figure 1.9**

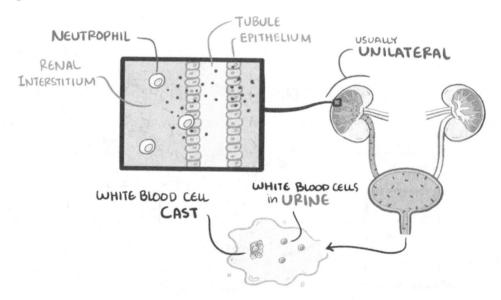

NEUTROPHIL

RENAL INTERSTITIUM

TUBULE EPITHELIUM

USUALLY UNILATERAL

WHITE BLOOD CELL CAST

WHITE BLOOD CELLS in URINE

**Figure 1.10**

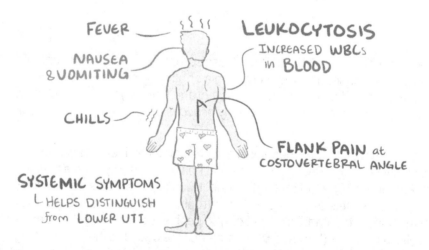

FEVER

NAUSEA & VOMITING

CHILLS

LEUKOCYTOSIS
INCREASED WBCs in BLOOD

FLANK PAIN at COSTOVERTEBRAL ANGLE

SYSTEMIC SYMPTOMS
└ HELPS DISTINGUISH from LOWER UTI

**Figure 1.11**

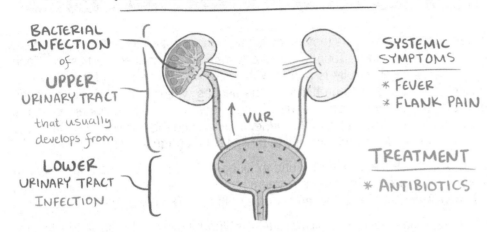

ACUTE PYELONEPHRITIS

BACTERIAL INFECTION of UPPER URINARY TRACT

that usually develops from

LOWER URINARY TRACT INFECTION

VUR

SYSTEMIC SYMPTOMS
* FEVER
* FLANK PAIN

TREATMENT
* ANTIBIOTICS

Patients also can present with increased white blood cells in their blood, in a condition called leukocytosis, and, as a result of the inflammatory immune response, patients can also develop fevers, chills, nausea and vomiting, as well as flank pain at the costovertebral angle (**Figure 1.10**). These systemic symptoms are what often distinguish acute pyelonephritis from a lower urinary tract infection.

## TREATMENT

Treatment is typically antibiotics and making sure that the individual stays well-hydrated. Like most bacterial infections, there is also the possibility of a renal abscess that can form as a complication. Also, if there are recurrent infections, which can be the case in people that have an anatomical problem that allows bacteria to easily cause infections, this can lead to chronic pyelonephritis as well as papillary necrosis, which means death of the renal papillae tissue. This has a much worse prognosis because it can affect the kidney's overall ability to function (**Figure 1.11**).

## SUMMARY

All right, as a quick recap: acute pyelonephritis is typically a bacterial infection of the upper urinary tract, which usually develops from a lower urinary tract infection, especially in individuals with vesicoureteral reflux. The infection causes systemic symptoms like fevers and flank pain at the costovertebral angle and is treated with antibiotics.

# Alport syndrome

osmosis.org/learn/alport_syndrome

Collagens are a family of proteins that are collectively the most abundant form of protein in the body, and they can be found throughout the various connective tissues. Each member of the collagen family is named with a Roman numeral, and if collagen is mutated or absent, this can lead to problems in the tissues where that particular collagen is found. Alport syndrome occurs as a result of mutations in Type IV collagen, which is particularly important in the glomerulus of the kidney, the eye, and the cochlea, and that's why the symptoms of Alport syndrome are specific to those tissues **(Figure 2.1)**.

Type IV collagen is a sheet-like structure found in all basement membranes and serves to support cells and form barriers. The three basement membrane layers are the lamina lucida, lamina densa (where Type IV collagen is), and lamina reticularis **(Figure 2.2)**.

Now, within the kidneys there are glomeruli that filter the blood; a glomerulus and a tubule form a nephron. These glomeruli happen to have a basement membrane, called the glomerular basement membrane, or GBM. That GBM, along with the fenestrated (meaning "has pores") capillary endothelium and the podocyte slit diaphragm, forms a selective filter. This means that water and certain other plasma components can escape the capillary and form the filtrate that will become urine, but red blood cells and most proteins stay in the glomerular capillary **(Figure 2.3)**.

## CAUSES

In Alport syndrome, kidney function is normal through early childhood, but over time, the missing or nonfunctional Type IV collagen causes the GBM to become thin and overly porous **(Figure 2.4)**. This allows red blood cells to pass right through from the capillary to the urinary filtrate, leading to microscopic hematuria, which is where red blood cells are seen in the urine under a microscope; this might eventually lead to gross hematuria, where the red blood cells can be seen with the naked eye. Over time, excessive amounts of protein start to get through the filter, resulting in proteinuria, or protein in the urine. Finally, this excessive protein loss and other factors cause the GBM to undergo sclerosis **(Figure 2.5)**.

**Figure 2.1**

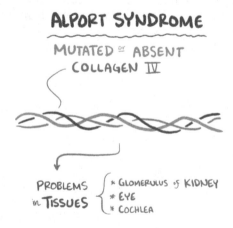

**Figure 2.2**

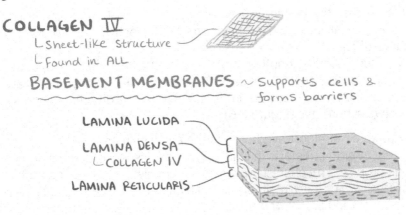

COLLAGEN IV
  └ Sheet-like structure
  └ Found in ALL

BASEMENT MEMBRANES ~ supports cells &
                      forms barriers

LAMINA LUCIDA
LAMINA DENSA
  └ COLLAGEN IV
LAMINA RETICULARIS

**Figure 2.3**

KIDNEY

**Figure 2.4**

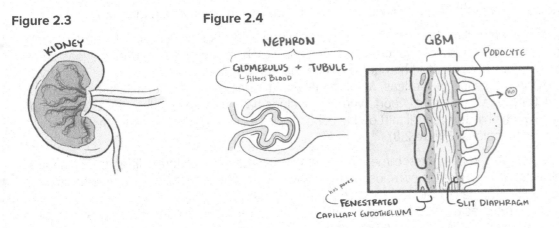

NEPHRON

GLOMERULUS + TUBULE
  └ filters Blood

GBM                PODOCYTE

H₂O

has pores
FENESTRATED          SLIT DIAPHRAGM
CAPILLARY ENDOTHELIUM

**Figure 2.5**

ALPORT SYNDROME
  └ CHILDHOOD ~ KIDNEYS NORMAL

[GBM] ┌ MISSING or NONFUNCTIONAL
           COLLAGEN IV

SCLEROSIS

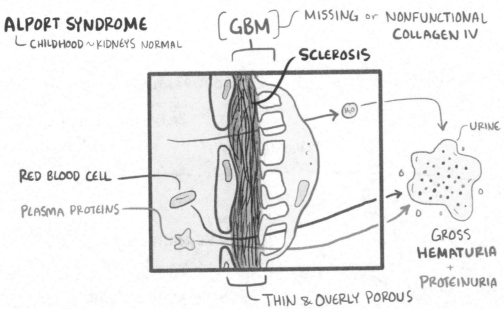

H₂O

URINE

RED BLOOD CELL

PLASMA PROTEINS

GROSS
HEMATURIA
+
PROTEINURIA

THIN & OVERLY POROUS

# PATHOLOGY

As there are fewer and fewer healthy glomeruli, somebody with Alport syndrome might develop renal insufficiency or even failure, which can lead to renovascular hypertension as well. Together, hematuria, renal insufficiency, and hypertension contribute to the categorization of Alport syndrome as a glomerulonephritis. Another kind of glomerulonephritis, Goodpasture syndrome, is caused by autoantibodies against the basement membrane in the glomeruli and the alveoli. So, although abnormality in the basement membrane is from a different cause, the results are similar in these two syndromes (Figure 2.6).

Another part of the body affected in Alport syndrome is the ear, which can lead to hearing loss. Usually this isn't present at birth but starts in childhood or adolescence, and the precise mechanism is unclear. One proposed mechanism involves the cochlea or inner ear structure that contains the Organ of Corti, which has a really small, but highly specialized set of hair cells that are attached to a basement membrane. Abnormal Type IV collagen might prevent those hair cells from generating normal nerve signals in response to sound vibrations. Because it's an inner ear problem, this is a type of sensorineural hearing loss, as opposed to middle ear and outer ear problems, which would lead to conductive hearing loss (Figure 2.7).

Some patients with Alport syndrome also have eye findings, which are also not typically present at birth. These include anterior lenticonus, where the center part of the lens starts to push into the anterior chamber because the anterior lens capsule lacks the integrity to maintain the shape of the lens. Myopia (nearsightedness) and lens opacities can result as well. Other eye changes in Alport syndrome include having white or yellow flecks around the macula, which is the central part of the retina, as well as having problems with the cornea, like recurrent erosions (Figure 2.8).

Type IV collagen is a heterotrimer, meaning that it's made up of three different polypeptide subunits, which are each composed of an alpha chain, fitting together in a triple helix. Each alpha chain has a very long repetitive amino acid sequence, with glycine followed by two variable amino acids, repeated over and over. Just remember that this is a repeat of amino acids, not a DNA triplet repeat (Figure 2.9).

Now, glycine is the smallest amino acid, which allows it to fit tightly into the triple helix of collagen. If a mutation causes a larger amino acid to get put in place of glycine, then that regular helix can't be packed as tightly and might get degraded.

Figure 2.6

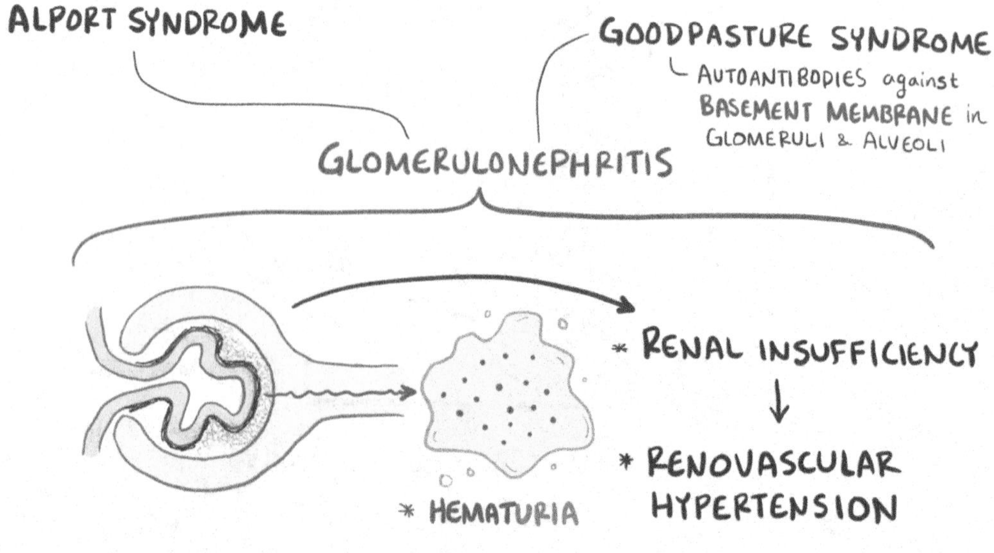

**Figure 2.7**

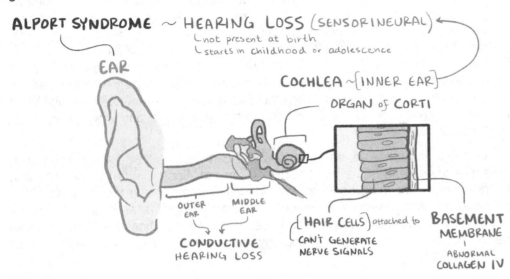

ALPORT SYNDROME ~ HEARING LOSS (SENSORINEURAL)
└ not present at birth
└ starts in childhood or adolescence

EAR

COCHLEA ~ [INNER EAR]
ORGAN of CORTI

OUTER EAR  MIDDLE EAR

CONDUCTIVE HEARING LOSS

[HAIR CELLS] attached to
CAN'T GENERATE NERVE SIGNALS

BASEMENT MEMBRANE
│
ABNORMAL COLLAGEN IV

**Figure 2.8**

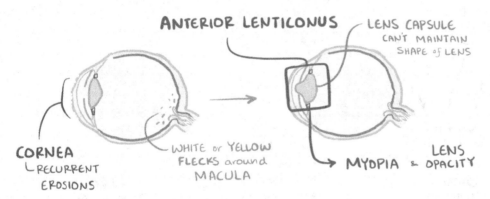

ALPORT SYNDROME ~ EYE FINDINGS
└ not present at birth

ANTERIOR LENTICONUS

LENS CAPSULE
CAN'T MAINTAIN SHAPE of LENS

CORNEA
└ RECURRENT EROSIONS

WHITE or YELLOW FLECKS around MACULA

MYOPIA

LENS & OPACITY

**Figure 2.9**

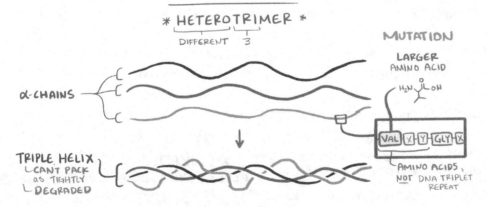

TYPE IV COLLAGEN

* HETEROTRIMER *
DIFFERENT  3

MUTATION
LARGER AMINO ACID
$H_2N$ OH

α-CHAINS

VAL X Y GLY X

AMINO ACIDS,
NOT DNA TRIPLET REPEAT

TRIPLE HELIX
└ CAN'T PACK as TIGHTLY
└ DEGRADED

Now, there are six similar alpha chains to choose from when building a collagen IV trimer. These are encoded by six genes with names that start with COL4, for collagen IV, then an A, since they code for alpha chains, and a number from 1-6 to designate *which* alpha chain. One version of Type IV collagen combines the alpha-3, alpha-4, and alpha-5 chains; another combines two alpha-1s with an alpha-2; a third version has two alpha-5s and an alpha-6. The alpha-1/alpha-1/alpha-2 collagen IV is present in basement membranes at birth, but during infancy it gets replaced by the alpha-3/alpha-4/alpha-5 collagen IV, particularly in the glomerulus, inner ear, and the eyes. When there's a mutation in the COL4A3, COL4A4, or COL4A5 genes, the alpha-3/alpha-4/alpha-5 heterotrimer is affected, and this causes Alport syndrome **(Figure 2.10)**.

COL4A5 is on the X-chromosome, so mutations in it can cause X-linked Alport syndrome, which presents early on and is the most common form of Alport syndrome. COL4A3 and A4 are on autosomes, meaning non-sex chromosomes; mutations in these cause either autosomal recessive Alport syndrome, which is also early onset, or autosomal dominant Alport syndrome, which causes late onset disease. Also, mild mutations in COL4A3 and A4 can cause thin basement membrane nephropathy, where microscopic hematuria is the only symptom **(Figure 2.11)**.

**Figure 2.10**

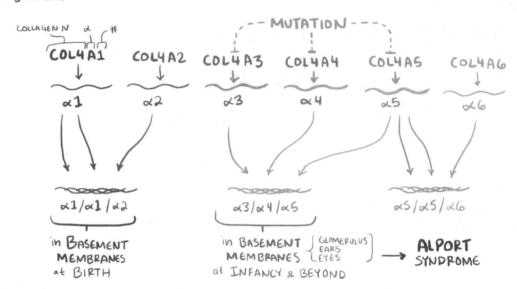

**Figure 2.11**

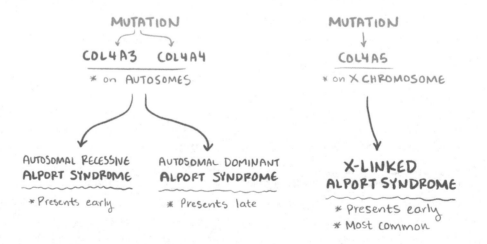

## DIAGNOSIS

Alport syndrome is typically suspected when there are clinical signs like gross hematuria or if there are vision or hearing problems, or if there's microscopic hematuria with no apparent cause. A family history of Alport syndrome is also a good clue, but it also might be absent in cases of recessive Alport syndrome or new spontaneous mutations.

To confirm the diagnosis, a kidney or skin biopsy is often analyzed by immunohistochemistry, meaning a labelled antibody is applied to a biopsy sample on a slide. Since misfolded collagen tends to get degraded, absent staining for collagen alpha chains suggests Alport syndrome. Skin is easier to biopsy, and although it contains the alpha-5/alpha-5/alpha-6 form of Type IV collagen, it doesn't have any alpha-3 or alpha-4 chains, so it can only be used to detect alpha-5 chain mutations. Alternatively, the biopsy can be looked at under an electron microscope, which early in the disease would show GBM thinning, while later in the disease, it would show a GBM with both thin and thick, abnormal segments and a lamina densa that appears split, with strands that look like a woven basket. Finally some people might have gene testing for the COL4A genes.

## TREATMENT

The treatment for Alport syndrome usually focuses on the symptoms. Proteinuria is treated with angiotensin converting enzyme inhibitors and/or angiotensin receptor blockers because there is evidence that this prevents progression to kidney failure. Anterior lenticonus can be treated with a replacement lens, and kidney failure necessitates dialysis or even kidney transplant.

## SUMMARY

Okay, as a quick recap: Alport syndrome is due to a mutation in genes COL4A 3, 4, and 5, which encode for Type IV collagen alpha subunits 3, 4, and 5. This causes kidney problems like hematuria and eventually glomerulonephritis, inner ear problems like sensorineural hearing loss, and eye problems like anterior lenticonus (**Figure 2.12**).

**Figure 2.12**

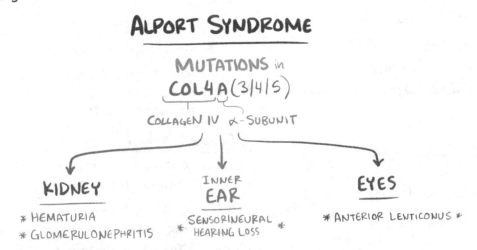

# Angiomyolipoma

Angiomyolipomas are the most common benign tumors found in the kidneys, although they can also be found in other tissues, like the liver, and, on rare occasions, in some reproductive structures as well. If we break down the word, we see that they are tumors that are comprised of blood vessels (*angio-*), smooth muscle (*-myo*), and adipose, or fat tissue (*-lipo*). Angiomyolipomas are often described as hamartomas, which means that they are focal, abnormal growths of cells which are normally found at that site but are disorganized. It's a bit like a house with a front door that can't be reached: it's the right part for the structure, but it's not organized in the right way. Angiomyolipomas also belong to the perivascular epithelioid cell tumor family, or PEComa family, meaning that they are made of epithelial-like cells that are found around blood vessels. Now, it's worth mentioning that normally there are no perivascular epithelioid cells that exist; the name just refers to the way that the tumor cells look under the microscope. The actual cell type from which PEComas, including angiomyolipomas arise, is not known **(Figure 3.1)**.

## CAUSES

The majority of angiomyolipomas will pop up sporadically (which means they are not a part of a syndrome) as isolated lesions. Interestingly, the tumors develop more often in the right kidney than the in left. However, these tumors are also strongly associated with tuberous sclerosis, a genetic disease that causes benign tumors to develop in various parts of the body. Individuals with tuberous sclerosis often have multiple angiomyolipomas along the surface of both kidneys, which can be larger in size than the sporadic ones **(Figure 3.2)**.

Figure 3.1

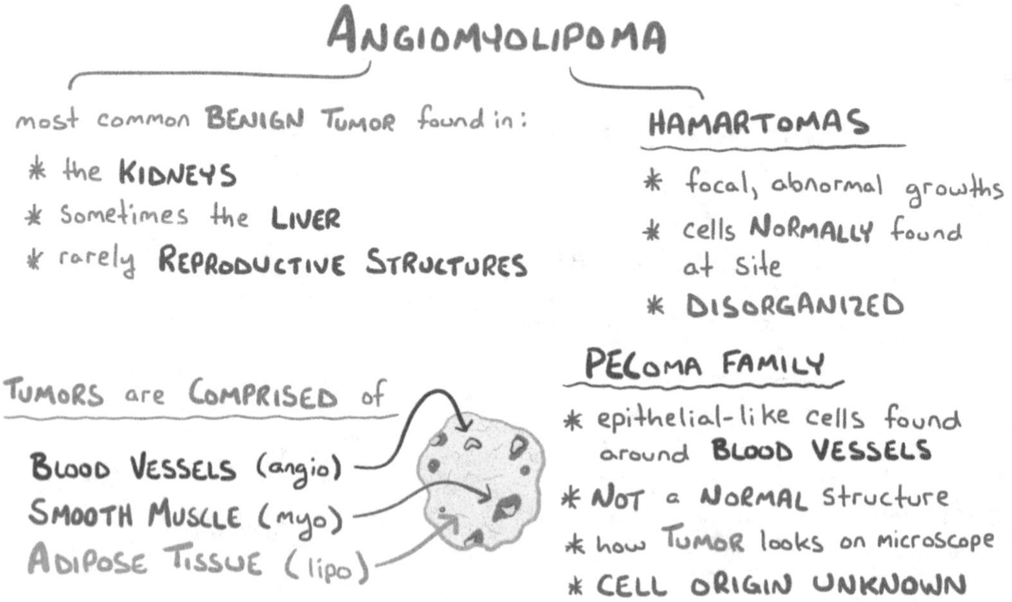

ANGIOMYOLIPOMA

most common BENIGN TUMOR found in:

* the KIDNEYS
* Sometimes the LIVER
* rarely REPRODUCTIVE STRUCTURES

TUMORS are COMPRISED of

BLOOD VESSELS (angio)
SMOOTH MUSCLE (myo)
ADIPOSE TISSUE (lipo)

HAMARTOMAS

* focal, abnormal growths
* cells NORMALLY found at site
* DISORGANIZED

PECOMA FAMILY

* epithelial-like cells found around BLOOD VESSELS
* NOT a NORMAL structure
* how TUMOR looks on microscope
* CELL ORIGIN UNKNOWN

**Figure 3.2**

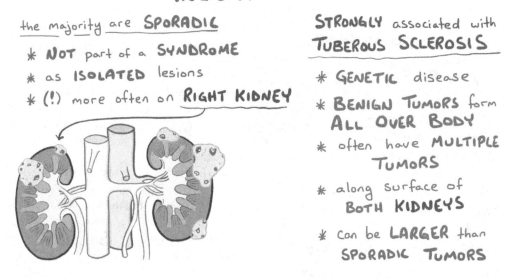

ANGIOMYOLIPOMA

the majority are **SPORADIC**
 * **NOT** part of a **SYNDROME**
 * as **ISOLATED** lesions
 * (!) more often on **RIGHT KIDNEY**

**STRONGLY** associated with
**TUBEROUS SCLEROSIS**

 * **GENETIC** disease
 * **BENIGN TUMORS** form
   **ALL OVER BODY**
 * often have **MULTIPLE**
   **TUMORS**
 * along surface of
   **BOTH KIDNEYS**
 * can be **LARGER** than
   **SPORADIC TUMORS**

**Figure 3.3**

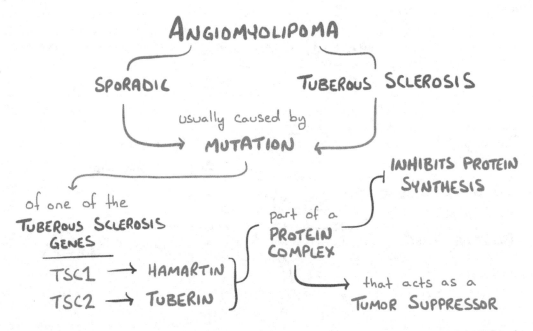

ANGIOMYOLIPOMA

SPORADIC          TUBEROUS SCLEROSIS

usually caused by
**MUTATION**

of one of the
**TUBEROUS SCLEROSIS**
**GENES**

TSC1 ⟶ HAMARTIN
TSC2 ⟶ TUBERIN

part of a
**PROTEIN**
**COMPLEX**

**INHIBITS PROTEIN**
**SYNTHESIS**

that acts as a
**TUMOR SUPPRESSOR**

## PATHOLOGY

Regardless of whether the angiomyolipoma occurs sporadically or as a consequence of tuberous sclerosis, there is usually an underlying mutation in one of the tuberous sclerosis genes (TSC1 or TSC2) which code for the tuberous sclerosis complex proteins hamartin and tuberin, respectively. These proteins are part of a protein complex that acts as a tumor suppressor by inhibiting protein synthesis, which is why mutations in the complex promote uncontrolled cellular growth and proliferation **(Figure 3.3)**.

**Figure 3.4**

# ANGIOMYOLIPOMA

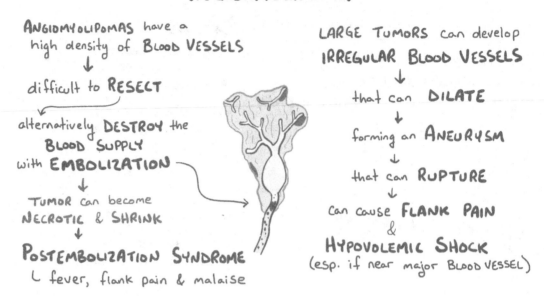

ANGIOMYOLIPOMAS have a
high density of BLOOD VESSELS
↓
difficult to RESECT

alternatively DESTROY the
BLOOD SUPPLY
with EMBOLIZATION
↓
TUMOR can become
NECROTIC & SHRINK
↓
POSTEMBOLIZATION SYNDROME
└ fever, flank pain & malaise

LARGE TUMORS can develop
IRREGULAR BLOOD VESSELS
↓
that can DILATE
↓
forming an ANEURYSM
↓
that can RUPTURE
↓
can cause FLANK PAIN
&
HYPOVOLEMIC SHOCK
(esp. if near major BLOOD VESSEL)

**Figure 3.5**

# ANGIOMYOLIPOMA

## BENIGN TUMORS

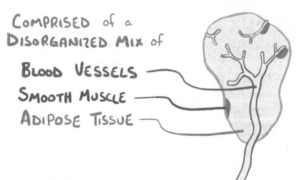

COMPRISED of a
DISORGANIZED MIX of

BLOOD VESSELS
SMOOTH MUSCLE
ADIPOSE TISSUE

COMMONLY
ARISE in the KIDNEYS

are STRONGLY ASSOCIATED with
TUBEROUS SCLEROSIS

## TREATMENT

If they are small, angiomyolipomas are usually harmless and don't require treatment, but if the angiomyolipoma is large, it may start to have a mass effect, pushing on healthy tissue of the kidney and impairing its function, ultimately leading to chronic kidney disease. In rare instances, this could eventually lead to end-stage renal disease and the need for dialysis. These large tumors can also develop irregular blood vessels that can steadily dilate and form an aneurysm that could rupture. A ruptured aneurysm would cause sudden flank pain, and would have the dangerous potential of causing hypovolemic shock, especially if the angiomyolipoma involves a major blood vessel like the renal artery **(Figure 3.4)**.

Because these angiomyolipomas often have a high density of blood vessels, they can be difficult to surgically resect. An alternative treatment that can help to preserve healthy kidney function is destroying the blood supply of large angiomyolipomas using a procedure called embolization. Destroying the disorganized blood vessels that help to supply the other disorganized tissue in the angiomyolipoma can make the angiomyolipoma become necrotic, which shrinks the lesion and reduces the risk of hemorrhage. Embolization can cause significant inflammation, causing postembolization syndrome, which is characterized by symptoms like fever, flank pain, and malaise for a few days after the procedure.

## SUMMARY

All right, to recap: angiomyolipomas are benign tumors comprised of a disorganized mix of blood vessels, smooth muscle, and adipose tissue. These tumors most commonly arise in the kidneys and are strongly associated with tuberous sclerosis **(Figure 3.5)**.

# Bladder exstrophy

osmosis.org/learn/bladder_exstrophy

**B**ladder exstrophy is a congenital abnormality that results in an "inside-out" bladder, where the bladder protrudes out of the abdomen, leaving the inside of the bladder exposed to the outside environment **(Figure 4.1)**.

Normally, in the first trimester, endoderm in the hindgut expands to form the cloaca, which is a temporary structure that connects the urinary, digestive, and reproductive tracts. Separately, the ectoderm forms the anterior abdominal wall. At around eight weeks of development, three important things happen. First, the anterior abdominal wall matures and forms the muscles and connective tissue of the lower abdomen. Second, the cloaca splits to form the rectum and the urogenital sinus, which later goes on to become the urinary and genital ducts, as well as the urinary bladder. And third, the cloacal membrane opens up to the outside of the body, creating openings for the urogenital tract and anus **(Figure 4.2)**.

## CAUSES

All right, so bladder exstrophy occurs when the developing bladder and urethra herniate anteriorly, and this causes some problems. First, it prevents the normal development of the lower abdominal wall, leaving it open. Second, it prevents fusion of the pelvis, leaving a wide split at the symphysis pubis **(Figure 4.3)**.

Most cases of bladder exstrophy involve epispadias, which is where the urethra exits the top of the penis. However, the opposite is not true: not all cases of epispadias involve bladder exstrophy **(Figure 4.4)**.

One way to think about the final result of bladder exstrophy is to imagine the bladder and urethra and make a cut through the top of the urethra and bladder. Then, imagine that the cut goes *up* through the symphysis pubis as well as the abdominal wall **(Figure 4.5)**.

After that, imagine pushing on the bladder from the bottom until it's inside out. This is essentially is what the final defect in bladder exstrophy looks like: the bladder pushes through the abdominal wall into the outside world.

**Figure 4.1**

### BLADDER EXSTROPHY
* CONGENITAL ABNORMALITY *

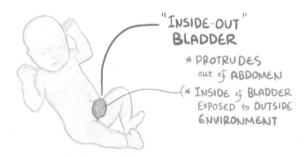

"INSIDE-OUT" BLADDER

* PROTRUDES out of ABDOMEN
(* INSIDE of BLADDER EXPOSED to OUTSIDE ENVIRONMENT

**Figure 4.2**

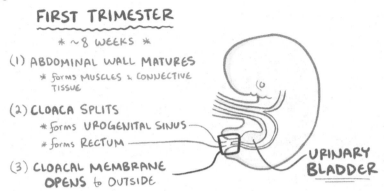

FIRST TRIMESTER

* ~8 WEEKS *

(1) ABDOMINAL WALL MATURES
* forms MUSCLES & CONNECTIVE TISSUE

(2) CLOACA SPLITS
* forms UROGENITAL SINUS
* forms RECTUM

(3) CLOACAL MEMBRANE OPENS to OUTSIDE

URINARY BLADDER

**Figure 4.3**

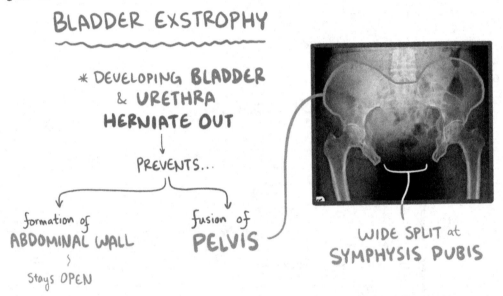

BLADDER EXSTROPHY

* DEVELOPING BLADDER & URETHRA HERNIATE OUT

↓

PREVENTS...

formation of ABDOMINAL WALL
↳ Stays OPEN

fusion of PELVIS

WIDE SPLIT at SYMPHYSIS PUBIS

**Figure 4.4**

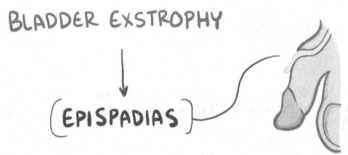

BLADDER EXSTROPHY

↓

(EPISPADIAS)

## PATHOLOGY

In addition to this, bladder exstrophy causes other changes as well. For example, the anus is usually more anteriorly located. Also, in boys the anterior part of the penis is shortened, and in girls, the vagina is wider, shorter and more vertically oriented.

The exact reason that bladder exstrophy happens in some infants is unknown, but one theory is that the mesenchymal cells fail to migrate between the endoderm of the cloaca and the ectoderm of the anterior abdominal wall.

**Figure 4.5**

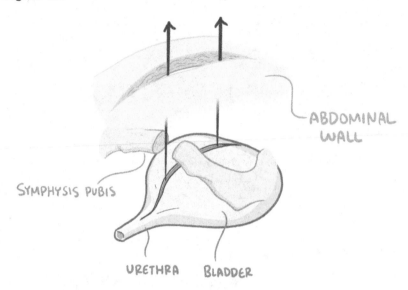

ABDOMINAL WALL

SYMPHYSIS PUBIS

URETHRA    BLADDER

**Figure 4.6**

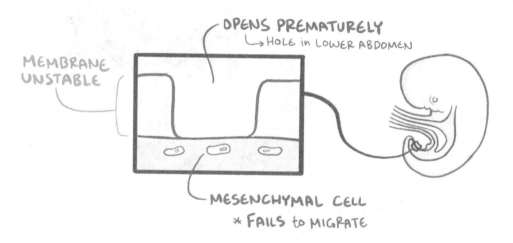

CAUSE ~ UNKNOWN

OPENS PREMATURELY
↳ HOLE in LOWER ABDOMEN

MEMBRANE UNSTABLE

MESENCHYMAL CELL
* FAILS to MIGRATE

Without mesenchymal support, the cloacal membrane becomes unstable and opens to the outside prematurely. This creates a hole in the lower abdominal wall, exposing the internal structures to the outside **(Figure 4.6)**.

## TREATMENT

Having a bladder and urethra exposed to the outside environment can lead to complications like incontinence as well as an increased risk of urinary tract infections. As far as diagnosis, goes, the defect is clinically obvious when a baby is born, but can also be diagnosed earlier on a prenatal ultrasound. Generally, within the first few weeks of life, the bladder and urethral defect are surgically closed, but sometimes staged surgeries are needed over months, or even years.

# SUMMARY

All right, as a quick recap: bladder exstrophy is a congenital problem where the bladder protrudes through the front of the abdominal wall, and it's often accompanied by epispadias. It can cause incontinence and increase the risk of urinary tract infections, and it requires early surgical correction.

# Chronic kidney disease

## osmosis.org/learn/chronic_kidney_disease

**C**hronic kidney disease is a broad term that includes subtle decreases in kidney function that develop over a minimum of three months. In contrast, acute kidney injury refers to any deterioration in kidney function that happens in less than three months **(Figure 5.1)**.

## PHYSIOLOGY

Now, the kidneys' job is to regulate what's in the blood, so they remove waste, make sure electrolyte levels are steady, regulate the overall amount of water in the blood, and even make hormones **(Figure 5.2)**. Blood enters the kidney through the renal artery; once inside, it goes into tiny clumps of arterioles called glomeruli where it's initially filtered. Then, the filtrate, which is the stuff that gets filtered out, moves into the renal tubule **(Figure 5.3)**. The rate at which this filtration takes place is known as glomerular filtration rate, or GFR. In a normal healthy person, this is somewhere around 100-120 milliliters of fluid filtered per minute per 1.73 m² of body surface area. The value is usually slightly less in women than in men, and it decreases slowly in all of us as we grow older **(Figure 5.4)**.

**Figure 5.1**

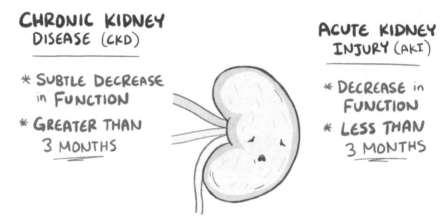

**Figure 5.2**

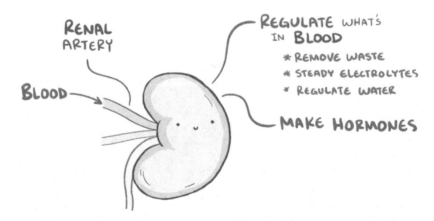

**Figure 5.3**

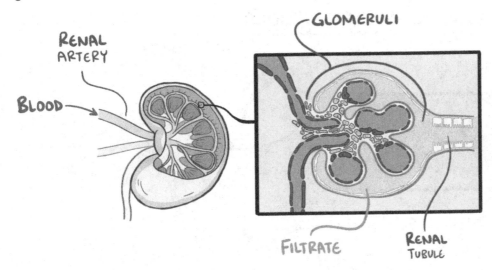

**Figure 5.4**

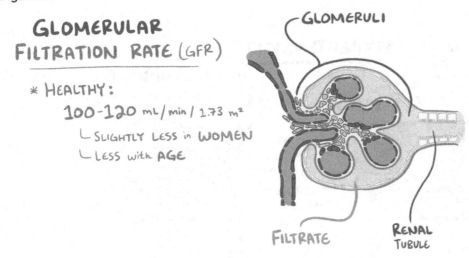

# GLOMERULAR
## FILTRATION RATE (GFR)

* HEALTHY:

  100-120 mL/min/1.73 m²
  └ SLIGHTLY LESS in WOMEN
  └ LESS with AGE

**Figure 5.5**

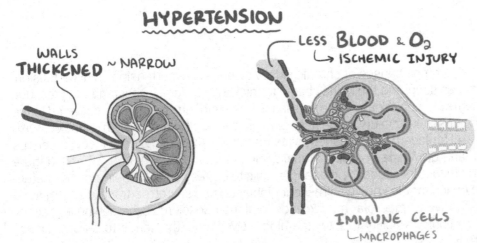

**Figure 5.6**

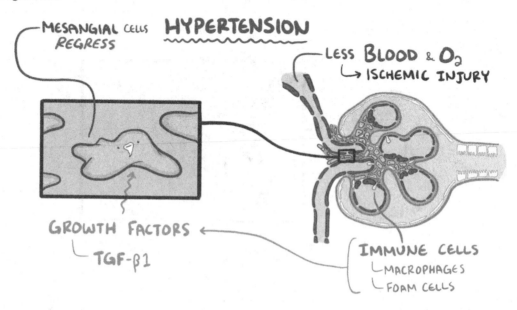

**Figure 5.7**

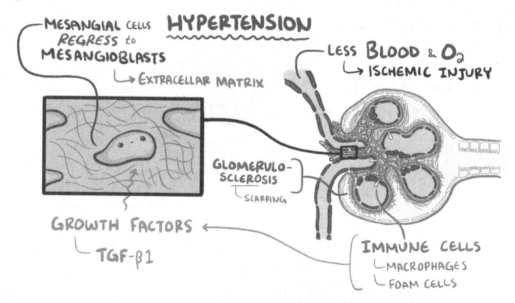

## CAUSES

One of the most common causes of chronic kidney disease is hypertension. In hypertension, the walls of arteries supplying the kidney begin to thicken in order to withstand the pressure, resulting in a narrow lumen. A narrow lumen means less blood and oxygen are delivered to the kidney, resulting in ischemic injury to the nephron's glomerulus **(Figure 5.5)**. Immune cells like macrophages and fat-laden macrophages called foam cells slip into the damaged glomerulus and start secreting growth factors like Transforming Growth Factor ß1, or TGF-ß1 **(Figure 5.6)**. These growth factors cause the mesangial cells to regress back to their more immature stem cell state (when they're known as mesoangioblasts) and secrete extracellular structural matrix. This excessive extracellular matrix leads to glomerulosclerosis, hardening and scars, diminishing the nephron's ability to filter the blood. Over time, this leads to chronic kidney disease **(Figure 5.7)**.

**Figure 5.8**

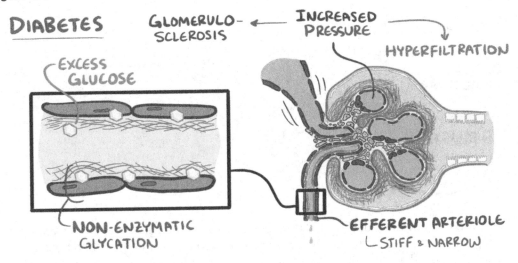

DIABETES

GLOMERULO-SCLEROSIS ← INCREASED PRESSURE → HYPERFILTRATION

EXCESS GLUCOSE

NON-ENZYMATIC GLYCATION

EFFERENT ARTERIOLE
└ STIFF & NARROW

**Figure 5.9**

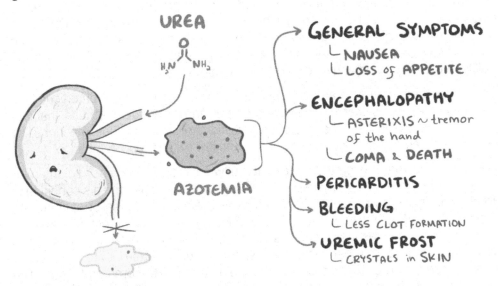

UREA

AZOTEMIA

GENERAL SYMPTOMS
└ NAUSEA
└ LOSS of APPETITE

ENCEPHALOPATHY
└ ASTERIXIS ~ tremor of the hand
└ COMA & DEATH

PERICARDITIS

BLEEDING
└ LESS CLOT FORMATION

UREMIC FROST
└ CRYSTALS in SKIN

**Figure 5.10**

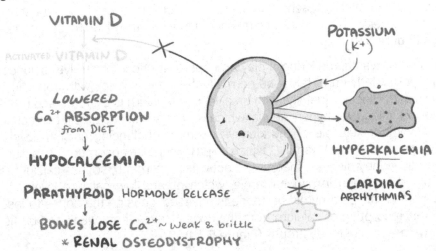

VITAMIN D

ACTIVATED VITAMIN D

LOWERED Ca²⁺ ABSORPTION from DIET

HYPOCALCEMIA

PARATHYROID HORMONE RELEASE

BONES LOSE Ca²⁺ ~ weak & brittle
* RENAL OSTEODYSTROPHY

POTASSIUM (K⁺)

HYPERKALEMIA

CARDIAC ARRHYTHMIAS

**Figure 5.11**

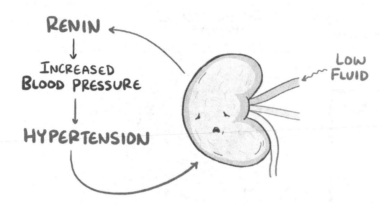

The second most common cause of CKD is diabetes. Here, excess glucose in the blood starts sticking to proteins in the blood. This process is called non-enzymatic glycation because no enzymes are involved. This glycation particularly affects the efferent arteriole and causes it to become stiff and more narrow; this process is called hyaline arteriosclerosis **(Figure 5.8)**. This creates an obstruction that makes it difficult for blood to leave the glomerulus and increases pressure within the glomerulus, leading to *hyper*filtration. In response to this high-pressure state, the supportive mesangial cells secrete more and more structural matrix, expanding the size of the glomerulus. Over many years, this process of glomerulosclerosis diminishes the nephron's ability to filter the blood and leads to chronic kidney disease.

Although diabetes and hypertension are responsible for the vast majority of chronic kidney disease cases, there are other systemic diseases, like lupus and rheumatoid arthritis, that can also cause glomerulosclerosis. Other causes of chronic kidney disease include infections like HIV, long-term use of medications like NSAIDs, and toxins like those found in tobacco.

Now, normally urea in the body is excreted in the urine, but when there's a decreased glomerular filtration rate, less urea is filtered out; therefore, it accumulates in the blood. This condition is called azotemia, and it can cause general symptoms like nausea and loss of appetite. As the toxin levels really build up, they can affect the functioning of the central nervous system, causing encephalopathy. This results in asterixis, a tremor of the hand that kind of resembles a bird flapping its wings, and it's most easily seen when the person attempts to extend their wrists. Further accumulation of these toxins in the brain can lead to coma and death. The buildup of toxins can also cause pericarditis, which is inflammation of the lining of the heart. In addition, there can be an increased likelihood of bleeding, since excess urea in the blood makes platelets less likely to stick to each other, lessening clot formation. Finally, in some cases, uremic frost can develop, where urea crystals can deposit in the skin—these look like powdery snowflakes **(Figure 5.9)**.

In addition to getting rid of waste, the kidneys play an important role in electrolyte balance. Potassium levels are particularly important, and normally the kidneys helps with potassium excretion. In chronic kidney disease, just like with urea, less potassium is excreted and more builds up in the blood. This leads to hyperkalemia, which is worrisome because it can cause cardiac arrhythmias. Another key role of the kidneys relates to balancing calcium levels. Normally, the kidney helps to activate Vitamin D, which helps to increase absorption of calcium from the diet. In chronic kidney disease, there's less activated Vitamin D, so less calcium is absorbed into the blood, resulting in hypocalcemia, which means low calcium levels. As calcium levels in the blood fall, parathyroid hormone is released, causing the bones to lose calcium. Over time, this resorption of calcium from the bones leaves them weak and brittle; this condition is known as renal osteodystrophy **(Figure 5.10)**.

**Figure 5.12**

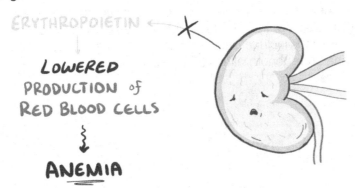

The kidneys also release key hormones. For example, normally when the kidneys start sensing a lower than normal amount of fluid being filtered, they respond by releasing the hormone renin to increase the blood pressure. In chronic kidney disease, the falling glomerular filtration rate leads to more and more renin secretion, which in turn leads to hypertension. Now, remember that hypertension itself is a cause of chronic kidney disease, so this creates quite the vicious cycle **(Figure 5.11)**.

The kidneys also secrete the hormone erythropoietin, which stimulates the production of red blood cells from the bone marrow. In chronic kidney disease erythropoietin levels fall, leading to lowered production of red blood cells and, ultimately, anemia **(Figure 5.12)**.

## DIAGNOSIS

The diagnosis of chronic kidney disease comes down to looking at changes in the glomerular filtration rate over time. Chronic kidney disease might be suspected with a GFR of less than 90 ml/min/1.73 m$^2$ , and irreversible kidney damage might happen with a GFR below 60 ml/min/1.73 m$^2$. To confirm the diagnosis, a kidney biopsy can identify changes like glomerulosclerosis. Treatment for chronic kidney disease often involves managing the underlying cause. In severe situations, dialysis or a kidney transplant might be needed.

**Figure 5.13**

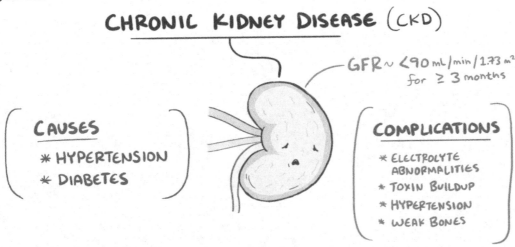

## SUMMARY

All right, as a quick recap: chronic kidney disease is when the glomerular filtration rate falls below 90 ml/min/1.73 m² over at least three months. Chronic kidney disease is mainly caused by diabetes and hypertension. Complications include electrolyte abnormalities, accumulation of toxins in the body, hypertension, and bone abnormalities **(Figure 5.13)**.

# Chronic pyelonephritis

osmosis.org/learn/pyelonephritis

**W**ith chronic pyelonephritis, *pyelo-* means pelvis, and *neph-* refers to the kidneys, so in this case it's the renal pelvis, the funnel-like structure of the kidney that drains urine into the ureter, that's affected. *-Itis* means inflammation. This inflammation is usually caused by bacterial infection of the kidney, known as *acute* pyelonephritis. When somebody has recurrent episodes of acute pyelonephritis, the kidney becomes visibly scarred, at which point it's referred to as *chronic* pyelonephritis **(Figure 6.1)**.

A urinary tract infection or UTI is any infection of the urinary tract which includes the upper portion of the tract (the kidneys and ureters) and the lower portion of the tract (the bladder and urethra). So, acute and chronic pyelonephritis are types of upper urinary tract infections. Acute pyelonephritis often clears up without much complication. Certain people, though, are predisposed to recurring episodes of acute pyelonephritis, which eventually leads to chronic pyelonephritis and permanent scarring of the renal tissue **(Figure 6.2)**.

**Figure 6.1**

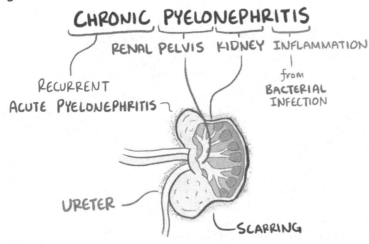

**Figure 6.2**

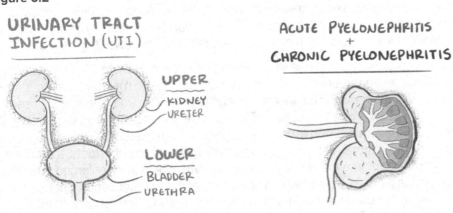

**Figure 6.3**

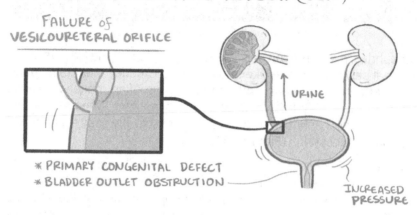

VESICOURETERAL REFLUX (VUR)

FAILURE of
VESICOURETERAL ORIFICE

URINE

\* PRIMARY CONGENITAL DEFECT
\* BLADDER OUTLET OBSTRUCTION

INCREASED PRESSURE

**Figure 6.4**

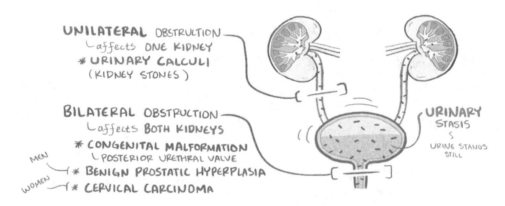

CHRONIC OBSTRUCTION

UNILATERAL OBSTRUCTION
└ affects ONE KIDNEY
\* URINARY CALCULI
(KIDNEY STONES)

BILATERAL OBSTRUCTION
└ affects BOTH KIDNEYS
\* CONGENITAL MALFORMATION
└ POSTERIOR URETHRAL VALVE
MEN ─┤\* BENIGN PROSTATIC HYPERPLASIA
WOMEN ─┤\* CERVICAL CARCINOMA

URINARY
STASIS
└ URINE STANDS STILL

## CAUSES

The most common risk factor for recurrent acute pyelonephritis and therefore chronic pyelonephritis, is vesicoureteral reflux, or VUR, where urine is allowed to move backward up the urinary tract if the vesicourethral orifice fails. The vesicourethral orifice is the one-way valve that allows urine to flow from each ureter *into* the bladder, but not in the reverse direction. VUR can be the result of a primary congenital defect, or it can be caused by bladder outlet obstruction, which increases pressure in the bladder and distorts the valve (**Figure 6.3**).

That being said, chronic obstruction is its own independent risk factor for chronic pyelonephritis. Obstructions in the urinary tract causes urinary stasis, meaning they tends to cause urine to stand still. This makes it easier for bacteria to adhere to and colonize the tissue, making lower UTIs more likely; therefore, upper UTIs are more likely to follow as well. Bilateral obstruction increases pressure in the bladder and therefore affects both kidneys. Causes include: congenital malformations, like posterior urethral valve, which obstructs the flow of urine through the urethra; benign prostatic hyperplasia in men, which is an enlarged prostate; and cervical carcinoma in women, both of which can compress the urethra shut. Obstructions can be unilateral as well, meaning they would be a little higher and affect only one kidney, as in the case of urinary calculi or kidney stones (**Figure 6.4**).

Figure 6.5

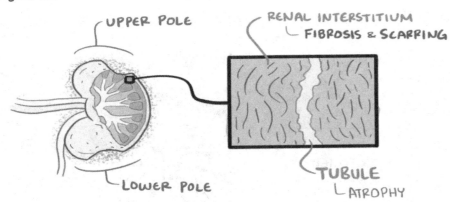

Figure 6.6

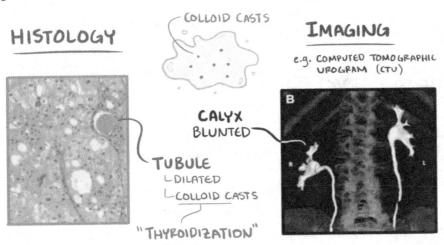

## PATHOLOGY

Although one episode of inflammation might not lead to any permanent damage, recurrent episodes eventually lead the renal interstitium to undergo fibrosis and scarring, and the tubules atrophy. These changes are generally found on the upper and lower poles of the kidney (**Figure 6.5**).

Also, on imaging studies like, for example, a computed tomographic urogram or CTU, the renal calyces become "blunted" or flattened. On histology, some tubules might be dilated and full of glassy-looking proteinaceous material called colloid, which forms as a result of the chronic inflammation. This material ends up being shaped like the tubules having formed what are known as colloid casts. Since this material happens to look a little like thyroid tissue, this process is sometimes referred to as *thyroidization* of the kidney. Those colloid casts can then get peed out, so they show up in the urine (**Figure 6.6**).

A rare type of chronic pyelonephritis is xanthogranulomatous pyelonephritis, or just XGP, which happens when an infected kidney stone causes chronic obstruction. The combination of infection and the increased pressure creates granulomatous tissue, which is full of foamy or fat-laden macrophages; this can easily be confused for a kidney tumor on imaging (**Figure 6.7**).

**Figure 6.7**

# XANTHOGRANULOMATOUS PYELONEPHRITIS (XGP)

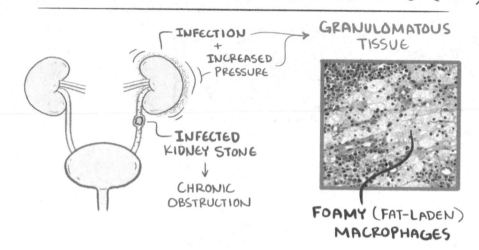

INFECTION + INCREASED PRESSURE → GRANULOMATOUS TISSUE

INFECTED KIDNEY STONE ↓ CHRONIC OBSTRUCTION

FOAMY (FAT-LADEN) MACROPHAGES

**Figure 6.8**

# CHRONIC PYELONEPHRITIS

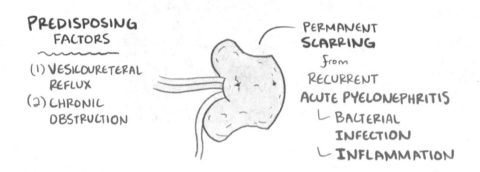

PREDISPOSING FACTORS
(1) VESICOURETERAL REFLUX
(2) CHRONIC OBSTRUCTION

PERMANENT SCARRING from RECURRENT ACUTE PYELONEPHRITIS
└ BACTERIAL INFECTION
└ INFLAMMATION

## TREATMENT

Treatment for chronic pyelonephritis involves correcting the underlying cause of the recurrent infection. This could include surgery to correct congenital structural causes, or to remove obstructions like kidney stones. In some cases, though, dialysis or nephrectomy (the removal of some or all of a kidney) might be needed.

## SUMMARY

All right, as a quick recap: chronic pyelonephritis is where the kidney develops permanent scarring as a result of recurring bouts of acute pyelonephritis, bacterial infection and inflammation of the kidney. The two major predisposing factors to developing chronic pyelonephritis are vesicoureteral reflux and chronic obstruction (**Figure 6.8**).

# Cystitis
# (Lower urinary tract infection)

**osmosis.org/learn/cystitis**

With cystitis, *cyst-* refers to the bladder, and *-itis* refers to inflammation. Therefore, cystitis describes an inflamed bladder, which is usually the result of a bacterial infection, but it can also result from fungal infections, chemical irritants, foreign bodies like kidney stones, or physical trauma **(Figure 7.1)**.

## PHYSIOLOGY

A urinary tract infection or UTI is any infection of the urinary tract which includes the upper portion of the tract (the kidneys and ureters) and the lower portion of the tract (the bladder and urethra). So cystitis, when caused by an infection, is a type of lower UTI **(Figure 7.2)**.

## CAUSES

Lower UTIs are almost always caused by an *ascending* infection, where bacteria move from the rectal area to the urethra and then migrate up the urethra and into the bladder. On rare occasions, a *descending* infection can happen when bacteria start in the blood or lymph and then go to the kidney and make their way down to the bladder and urethra **(Figure 7.3)**.

**Figure 7.1**

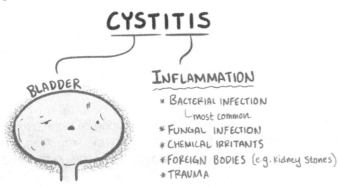

**Figure 7.2**

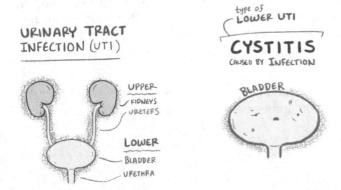

**Figure 7.3**

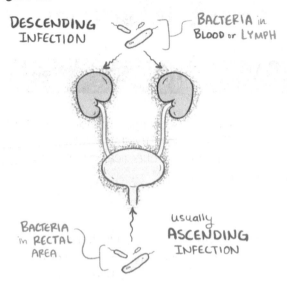

**Figure 7.4**

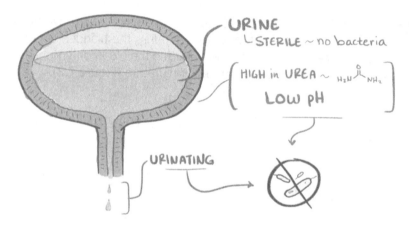

Normally, urine is *sterile*, meaning bacteria don't live there; the composition of urine, which has a high urea concentration and low pH, helps keep bacteria from setting up camp. Also, the unidirectional flow in the act of urinating helps to keep bacteria from invading the urethra and bladder **(Figure 7.4)**.

Some bacteria, though, are better surviving in and resisting these conditions, and can stick to and colonize the bladder mucosa. *E. coli* accounts for the vast majority of UTIs, though other gram negative bacteria that can infect the bladder include *Klebsiella*, *Proteus*, *Enterobacter*, and *Citrobacter* species. On the other hand, gram-positive bacteria can also cause problems, like *Enterococcus* species and *Staphylococcus saprophyticus*, which is actually the second most common cause after *E. coli*; this particularly affects young, sexually active women **(Figure 7.5)**.

That said, as far as risk factors go, sexual intercourse is a major risk factor, because bacteria can be introduced into the urethra; this is sometimes even somewhat romantically referred to as "honeymoon cystitis" **(Figure 7.6)**.

**Figure 7.5**

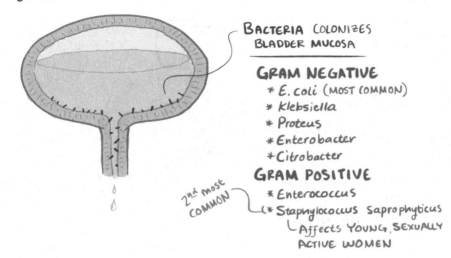

BACTERIA COLONIZES BLADDER MUCOSA

**GRAM NEGATIVE**
* E. coli (MOST COMMON)
* Klebsiella
* Proteus
* Enterobacter
* Citrobacter

**GRAM POSITIVE**
* Enterococcus
* Staphylococcus saprophyticus
 └ Affects YOUNG, SEXUALLY ACTIVE WOMEN

2nd most COMMON

**Figure 7.6**

# RISK FACTORS

* SEXUAL INTERCOURSE
 └ BACTERIA → Urethra
 └ "HONEYMOON CYSTITIS"
* FEMALE GENDER
 └ SHORTER URETHRA ~ shorter distance for ASCENDING BACTERIA
 └→ POST-MENOPAUSE
  └ DECREASED ESTROGEN → LOSS of PROTECTIVE VAGINAL FLORA
* FOLEY CATHETER

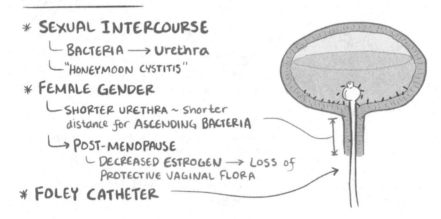

## PATHOLOGY

In general, women are at higher risk for cystitis than men due to women's having a shorter urethra. This is because bacteria ascending up the urethra don't have to travel as far. Also, in postmenopausal women, there is a decrease in estrogen levels, which causes the normal protective vaginal flora to be lost, increasing the risk of a UTI. Other risk factors include presence of a Foley catheter in the urethra, which can introduce pathogens. Another risk factor is having diabetes mellitus, since people with diabetes tend to have hyperglycemia or high blood glucose. Normally with an infection, neutrophils move out of the circulatory system toward the infection, called diapedesis, as well as carry out phagocytosis, but hyperglycemia inhibits these processes, making those neutrophils less effective at killing invaders. Also, infant boys with foreskin around their penis have a slightly higher risk of a UTI compared to infant boys who've have had a circumcision. A final important risk factor is impaired bladder emptying causing urinary stasis, which means urine tends to sit still, allowing bacteria the chance to adhere and colonize in the bladder **(Figure 7.7)**.

**Figure 7.7**

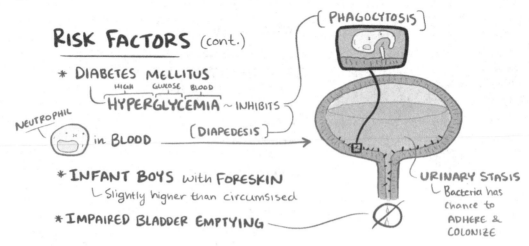

## RISK FACTORS (cont.)

* DIABETES MELLITUS
  HIGH · GLUCOSE · BLOOD
  HYPERGLYCEMIA ~ INHIBITS

NEUTROPHIL in BLOOD [DIAPEDESIS]

[PHAGOCYTOSIS]

* INFANT BOYS with FORESKIN
  └ Slightly higher than circumsised
* IMPAIRED BLADDER EMPTYING

URINARY STASIS
└ Bacteria has chance to ADHERE & COLONIZE

**Figure 7.8**

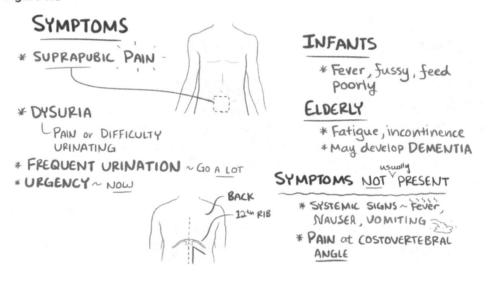

## SYMPTOMS

* SUPRAPUBIC PAIN
* DYSURIA
  └ PAIN or DIFFICULTY URINATING
* FREQUENT URINATION ~ GO A LOT
* URGENCY ~ NOW

BACK
12th RIB

### INFANTS
* Fever, fussy, feed poorly

### ELDERLY
* Fatigue, incontinence
* May develop DEMENTIA

### SYMPTOMS NOT usually PRESENT
* SYSTEMIC SIGNS ~ Fever, NAUSEA, VOMITING
* PAIN at COSTOVERTEBRAL ANGLE

**Figure 7.9**

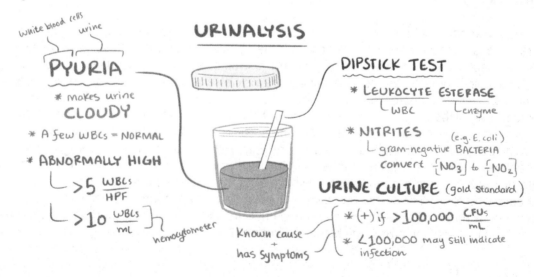

## URINALYSIS

white blood cells   urine

### PYURIA
* makes urine CLOUDY
* A few WBCs = NORMAL
* ABNORMALLY HIGH
  └ $>5 \frac{WBCs}{HPF}$
  └ $>10 \frac{WBCs}{mL}$

hemocytometer

Known cause + has symptoms

### DIPSTICK TEST
* LEUKOCYTE ESTERASE
  └ WBC  └ enzyme
* NITRITES (e.g. E. coli)
  └ gram-negative BACTERIA convert $[NO_3]$ to $[NO_2]$

### URINE CULTURE (gold standard)
* (+) if $>100,000 \frac{CFUs}{mL}$
* $<100,000$ may still indicate infection

**Figure 7.10**

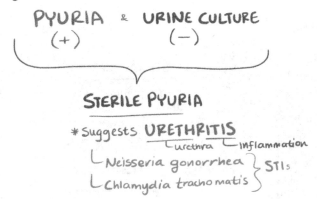

## SYMPTOMS

Symptoms of cystitis include: suprapubic pain, which is pain in the lower abdomen; dysuria, which is painful or difficulty urinating; and frequent urination and urgency, meaning you have to go a lot and you have to go *now*—typically, the urine voids are small in volume. Having said that, symptoms can differ by age: infants might have a fever, become fussy, and feed poorly, whereas elderly patients might feel fatigue, become incontinent, or even develop dementia. Symptoms that are *not* typically present with lower UTIs are systemic signs like fevers and nausea or vomiting, as well as pain at the costovertebral angle, which is the angle formed on either side of the back between the twelfth rib and the vertebral column. If they do present, this might suggest an upper urinary tract infection, which includes an infection of the kidneys themselves **(Figure 7.8)**.

## DIAGNOSIS

If a urinalysis is done, there may be signs of inflammation like pyuria, the presence of white blood cells in the urine, which can make the urine appear cloudy. Having a couple white blood cells in the urine can be normal, but it'd be considered abnormally high if there are more than 5 white blood cells per high powered field on microscopy, or more than 10 white blood cells per mL on a hemocytometer. Similarly, a dipstick test that shows the presence of leukocyte esterase, which is an enzyme created by leukocytes, or white blood cells. It might also be positive for nitrites, since gram negative organisms like *E coli*. convert nitrates in the urine to nitrites, but it's worth remembering that not all uropathogens are able to do that. Finally, a urine culture is the gold standard for diagnosis, and it's considered positive if it shows more than 100,000 colony-forming units per mL from a clean catch urine sample, although a lower number of colony-forming units per mL might still indicate an infection depending on the source of the specimen and the specifics of the clinical scenario. Remember, this test assumes the bacteria that grows is a known bacterial cause of UTIs and that the patient has clinical symptoms **(Figure 7.9)**.

Now, if there is pyuria but the urine culture doesn't reveal a bacteria, this is known as *sterile pyuria*, and it suggests urethritis, inflammation of just the urethra, as opposed to cystitis. Isolated urethritis is most commonly caused by *Neisseria gonorrhoeae* and *Chlamydia trachomatis*, both of which are sexually transmitted infections **(Figure 7.10)**.

For a UTI, imaging studies can also be helpful. For example, a renal ultrasound can be used for children who may have a kidney malformation that could contribute to developing a UTI. In addition, a voiding cystourethrogram or VCUG might be used, which is where an individual is given a radiocontrast liquid and fluoroscop (which are like real-time X-rays) and then

**Figure 7.11**

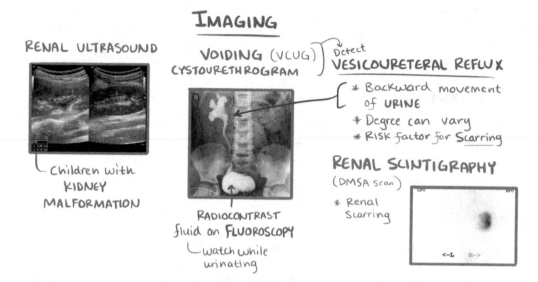

IMAGING

RENAL ULTRASOUND

VOIDING (VCUG)
CYSTOURETHROGRAM

Detect
VESICOURETERAL REFLUX
* Backward movement of URINE
* Degree can vary
* Risk factor for Scarring

Children with
KIDNEY
MALFORMATION

RADIOCONTRAST
fluid on FLUOROSCOPY
watch while urinating

RENAL SCINTIGRAPHY
(DMSA scan)
* Renal Scarring

**Figure 7.12**

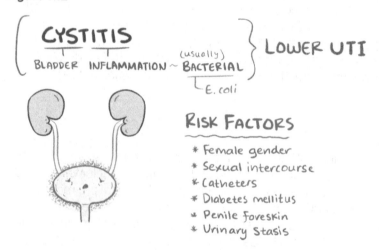

CYSTITIS
BLADDER  INFLAMMATION ~ (usually) BACTERIAL
E. coli

LOWER UTI

RISK FACTORS
* Female gender
* Sexual intercourse
* Catheters
* Diabetes mellitus
* Penile foreskin
* Urinary stasis

healthcare professionals watch how the fluid is urinated out. This is particularly helpful in children with severe or recurrent UTIs to detect evidence of vesicoureteral reflux, which is the retrograde movement of urine from the bladder back up into the ureters and kidneys. The degree of vesicoureteral reflux can vary, and it is an important risk factor for kidney scarring with a UTI. Finally, in some situations, renal scintigraphy using DMSA or DMSA scan, which is a radionuclide, can be used to detect evidence of kidney scarring **(Figure 7.11)**.

## TREATMENT

Treatment for a lower UTI usually involves antibiotics targeted to the bacterial cause. Symptoms usually clear up within a few days as the urine becomes sterile; at the same time, pain medication may also sometimes be administered. Preventing UTIs mainly involves drinking lots of fluids to help flush out bacteria that may try to ascend the urethra, and emptying the bladder as often as possible, which is especially relevant for women after sexual activity. Finally, maintaining good hygiene like wiping from the urethra to the rectum is a good way to prevent fecal bacteria from making it up the urethra.

# SUMMARY

All right, as a quick recap: cystitis is inflammation of the bladder usually caused by bacterial infection, which makes it a type of lower urinary tract infection. *E. coli.* is by far the most common culprit. Other risk factors include female gender, sexual intercourse, having catheters, diabetes mellitus, having penile foreskin in infant boys, and urinary stasis **(Figure 7.12)**.

# Diabetic nephropathy

osmosis.org/learn/diabetic_nephropathy

**D**iabetic nephropathy refers to the kidney damage caused by both Type I and Type II diabetes. Due to the growing number of people affected by diabetes, diabetic nephropathy is currently the leading cause of end-stage renal disease in high-income countries.

## PHYSIOLOGY

Each kidney has millions of nephrons, each of which is served by a tiny capillary bed called a glomerulus. The tiny arteriole that approaches the glomerulus is called the afferent arteriole, which you can remember by thinking, "*a for approaching,*" and the arteriole that exits the glomerulus is called the efferent arteriole, so just remember "*e for exits*" **(Figure 8.1)**. The glomeruli are tiny clusters of capillaries that are physically supported by mesangial cells. So, when blood is filtered, it moves through the endothelium lining the capillary, then through the basement membrane, then through the epithelium lining the nephron, and finally into the nephron itself; at this point it's called filtrate. The endothelium has pores that keep cells from entering the filtrate, and the basement membrane is negatively charged and repels other negatively charged molecules and proteins, like the protein albumin.

The epithelium has a special type of cell called a podocyte. This looks like an octopus because it has foot processes that wrap around the basement membrane, leaving tiny gaps between its octopus-like projections, which are called filtration slits **(Figure 8.2)**.

## CAUSES

In diabetes mellitus, there's an excess of glucose in the blood because it can't get into the cells. When blood is filtered through the kidneys, some of that excess glucose starts to spill into the urine; this is called glycosuria. When there's a lot of glucose in the blood, it also starts sticking to proteins in the blood; this process is called non-enzymatic glycation because no enzymes are involved **(Figure 8.3)**.

Figure 8.1

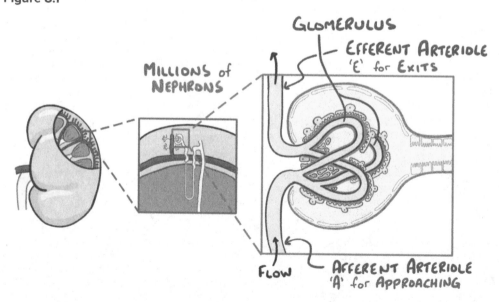

**Figure 8.2**

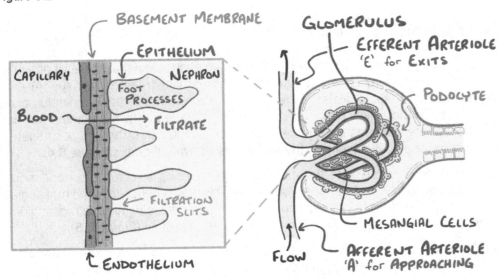

**Figure 8.3**

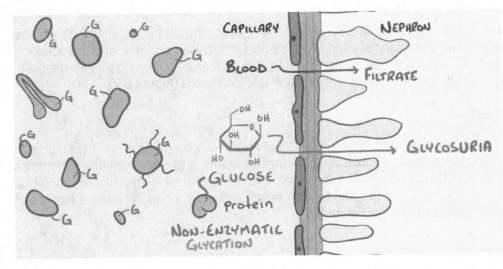

**Figure 8.4**

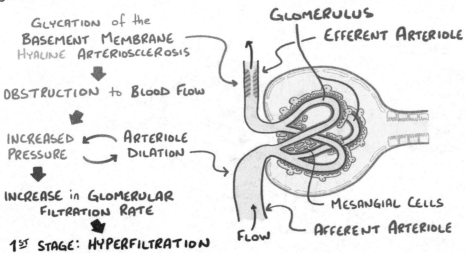

## PATHOLOGY

Because glucose can get through the endothelium, this process of glycation can also affect the basement membrane of small blood vessels by causing them thicken. This particularly affects the efferent arteriole by causing it to get stiffer and narrower; this process is called hyaline arteriosclerosis. Hyaline arteriosclerosis creates an obstruction that makes it difficult for blood to leave the glomerulus, which increases pressure within the glomerulus. At the same time, the afferent arteriole dilates, allowing more blood flow into the glomerulus and increasing pressure further. High pressure in the glomerulus leads to an increase in the glomerular filtration rate, which is simply the amount of blood filtered through per minute. This is the first stage of diabetic nephropathy, and it's called hyperfiltration (**Figure 8.4**).

In response to this high-pressure state, the supportive mesangial cells secrete more and more structural matrix, expanding the size of the glomerulus. This matrix deposition and mesangial expansion can happen uniformly, or they can result in little nodules within the mesangium called Kimmelstiel-Wilson nodules, which are tiny little balls of protein (**Figure 8.5**).

The thickening of the basement membrane counterintuitively makes it *more* permeable, allowing proteins like albumin through that otherwise would have been filtered out. It makes sense if you think about our octopus friend once more: as the glomerulus expands, the legs of the octopus naturally have larger gaps between them. In other words, the filtration slits widen, making it easier for substances to slip through (**Figure 8.6**).

So, in the end, the key abnormalities in diabetic nephropathy are a thickened glomerular basement membrane, mesangial expansion, Kimmelstiel-Wilson nodules, and disruption of the podocytes. Eventually, these changes damage the glomerulus so much that it's unable to filter blood normally, and the glomerular filtration rate decreases (**Figure 8.7**).

## SYMPTOMS

Typically, diabetic nephropathy starts quietly. There are no symptoms during the hyperfiltration phase, but, over time, more and more of the nephrons are affected. The kidney becomes less and less effective at filtering the blood into the urine, and the glomerular filtration rate decreases dramatically . Once the kidneys no longer can do their job of filtering the blood, end stage renal disease is the result (**Figure 8.8**).

**Figure 8.5**

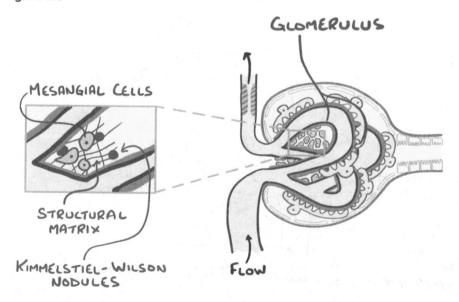

**Figure 8.6**

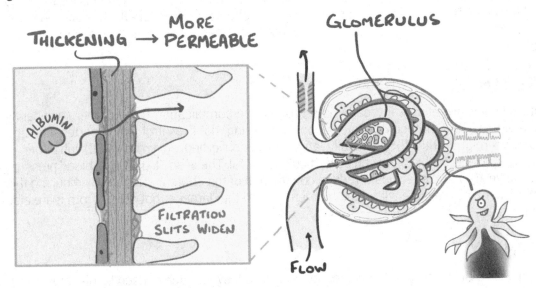

THICKENING → MORE PERMEABLE

GLOMERULUS

ALBUMIN

FILTRATION SLITS WIDEN

FLOW

**Figure 8.7**

DIABETIC NEPHROPATHY

* THICKENED GLOMERULAR BASEMENT MEMBRANE

* MESANGIAL EXPANSION

* KIMMELSTIEL-WILSON NODULES

* DISRUPTION of PODOCYTES

EVENTUALLY the DAMAGE DECREASES the GLOMERULAR FILTRATION RATE

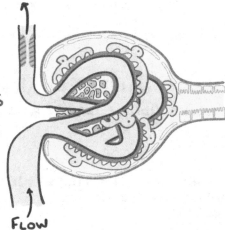

FLOW

**Figure 8.8**

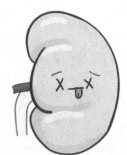

SYMPTOMS

typically NO SYMPTOMS during HYPERFILTRATION

BUT... as MORE NEPHRONS are AFFECTED the GLOMERULAR FILTRATION RATE DECREASES

WHEN the KIDNEYS can NO LONGER FILTER BLOOD

END STAGE RENAL DISEASE

Because there are no overt symptoms of diabetic nephropathy, regularly screening the urine of individuals with diabetes is super important. Microalbuminuria (which means excreting 30 to 300 mg of albumin in a day) is a reliable signal that diabetic nephropathy has started to set in. Excreting above 300 mg per day is considered macroalbuminuria, and it's a sure sign of a problem.

## TREATMENT

Unfortunately, diabetic nephropathy is a progressive complication that can be significantly slowed down but not completely stopped. Keeping tight control on hypertension and hyperglycemia is critical. Specifically, angiotensin-converting enzymes (ACE) inhibitors or angiotensin receptor blockers can be particularly useful. These don't just lower blood pressure as a whole; they also specifically reduce constriction of the efferent arteriole. By reducing this constriction, the pressure within the glomerulus and the damage that stems from it are also reduced.

## SUMMARY

All right, as a quick recap: diabetic nephropathy is kidney damage caused by diabetes, and it results in glomerular basement membrane thickening, mesangial expansion, and sclerosis. An initial phase of increased glomerular filtration rate is followed by progressive albuminuria, then a gradual decline in glomerular filtration rate, and, finally, renal failure **(Figure 8.9)**. This progression can be slowed by tight control of blood sugar and blood pressure and the use of ACE-inhibitors or angiotensin receptor blockers to decrease pressure specifically within the glomerulus.

**Figure 8.9**

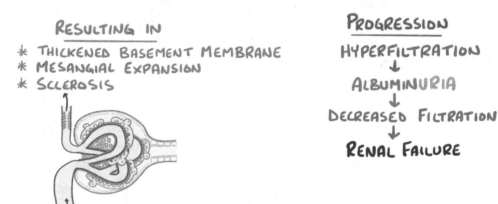

DIABETIC NEPHROPATHY
KIDNEY DAMAGE from DIABETES

RESULTING IN
* THICKENED BASEMENT MEMBRANE
* MESANGIAL EXPANSION
* SCLEROSIS

PROGRESSION
HYPERFILTRATION
↓
ALBUMINURIA
↓
DECREASED FILTRATION
↓
RENAL FAILURE

FLOW

# Focal segmental glomerulosclerosis

osmosis.org/learn/focal_segmental_glomerulosclerosis

Focal segmental glomerulosclerosis, sometimes known as focal glomerular sclerosis or sometimes as just FSGS, is a type of kidney disease that affects the kidney's glomeruli, which is where small molecules are first filtered out of the blood and into the urine.

## PHYSIOLOGY

The word *glomerulosclerosis* indicates sclerosis, or scar tissue, forming in the glomeruli. Segmental means that only a segment, or part, of the glomeruli is affected, and focal means that among all those glomeruli in the kidney, only some are affected. Those glomeruli that are affected, though, allow proteins to filter through into the urine, and ultimately people with FSGS develop nephrotic syndrome **(Figure 9.1; Figure 9.2)**.

**Figure 9.1**

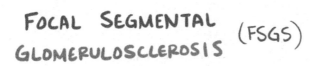

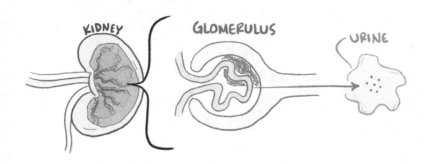

**Figure 9.2**

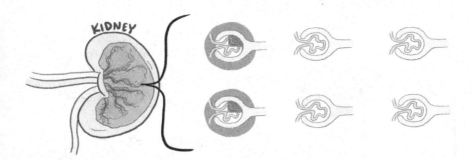

**Figure 9.3**

# FOCAL SEGMENTAL GLOMERULOSCLEROSIS (FSGS)

### * NEPHROTIC SYNDROME *

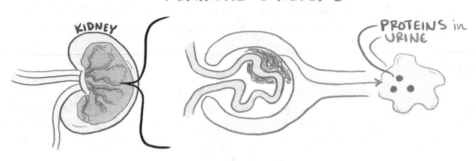

**Figure 9.4**

### * NEPHROTIC SYNDROME *

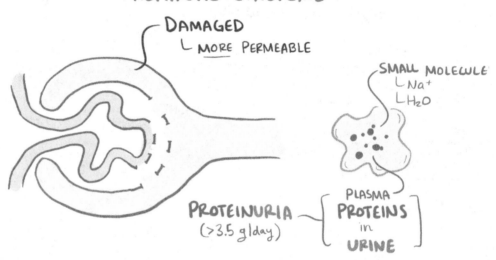

**Figure 9.5**

### * NEPHROTIC SYNDROME *

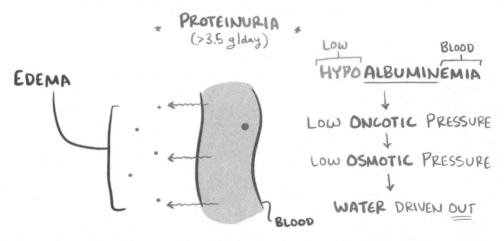

# PATHOLOGY

But what exactly is nephrotic syndrome? Well, usually the glomerulus only lets small molecules, like sodium and water, move from the blood into the kidney nephron, where it eventually makes its way into the urine. But with nephrotic syndromes, the glomeruli are damaged and they become more permeable, so they start letting plasma proteins come across from the blood to the nephron and then into the urine, which causes proteinuria, which typically means greater than 3.5 grams of protein in the urine per day **(Figure 9.3; Figure 9.4)**.

An important protein in the blood is albumin, and when it starts leaving the blood, people get hypoalbuminemia, which means low albumin in the blood. With less protein in the blood, the oncotic pressure falls, which lowers the overall osmotic pressure and drives water out of the blood vessels and into the tissues, causing a condition called edema.

Finally, it's thought that as a result of either losing albumin or losing some protein or proteins that inhibit the synthesis of lipids, or fat, you get increased levels of lipids in the blood, called hyperlipidemia.

Just like the proteins, these lipids can also get into the urine, causing lipiduria. And those are the hallmarks of nephrotic syndrome: proteinuria, hypoalbuminemia, edema, hyperlipidemia, and lipiduria **(Figure 9.5)**.

# CAUSES

So, focal segmental glomerulosclerosis is a type of nephrotic syndrome, that's helpful, but why does the glomerulus develop segmental sclerosis in the first place? Well, primary FSGS is when it's idiopathic, or there's no clear underlying cause **(Figure 9.6)**. What is known, though, is that the podocytes, which are the cells that have these long tentacle-like projections, called foot processes, that wrap around the capillaries in the glomeruli, are damaged. These damaged podocytes allow some plasma proteins and lipids to sneak by, which then get into the urine.

Over time, some of these proteins and lipids get trapped and build up in the glomerulus, resulting in hyalinosis, where the tissue has a hyaline or glassy appearance on histology, and it's thought that over time these areas develop sclerosis, or scar tissue **(Figure 9.7)**.

Some research suggests that these changes in FSGS are a continuation of another nephrotic syndrome called minimal change disease which is also characterized by podocyte injury, Other research suggests that minimal change disease and FSGS have different mechanisms of podocyte injury.

# SYMPTOMS

Fundamentally, FSGS is a histopathologic description, which basically what it looks like under a microscope, and this could be the end result of a number of different pathophysiologic mechanisms.

As opposed to primary FSGS, secondary FSGS is when there's a clear underlying cause, and there are several important conditions that can be associated with it. Sickle cell disease, where blood cells are sickle-shaped due to a structurally abnormal hemoglobin protein that can cause tissue ischemia, has been linked to FSGS. HIV, a retrovirus that infects various human cell types, can lead to FSGS and is called HIV-associated nephropathy. Heroin abuse has also been linked to FSGS, which is called heroin nephropathy. Also, other conditions, like kidney hyperperfusion, increased perfusion of blood, and increased pressure in the glomerular capillaries, have been linked to FSGS as well **(Figure 9.8)**.

**Figure 9.6**

# PRIMARY FSGS

IDIOPATHIC ~ no clear cause

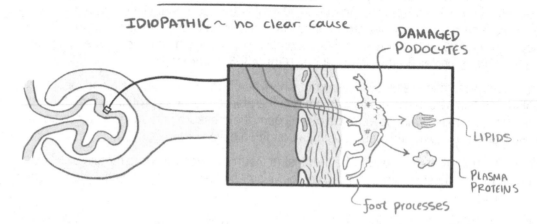

**Figure 9.7**

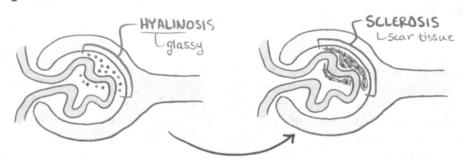

**Figure 9.8**

# SECONDARY FSGS

\* CLEAR UNDERLYING CAUSE \*

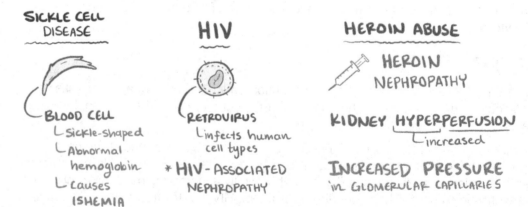

**Figure 9.10**

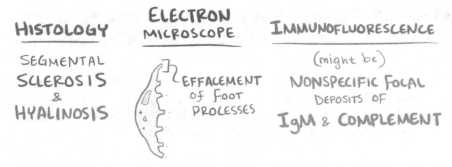

HISTOLOGY

ELECTRON MICROSCOPE

IMMUNOFLUORESCENCE

SEGMENTAL SCLEROSIS & HYALINOSIS

EFFACEMENT of FOOT PROCESSES

(might be)
NONSPECIFIC FOCAL DEPOSITS OF IgM & COMPLEMENT

## DIAGNOSIS

On histology, there'll be segmental sclerosis and hyalinosis of the glomeruli, and under electron microscope, there's effacement of the foot processes of the podocytes. On immunofluorescence, there might be nonspecific focal deposits of IgM and complement proteins, and these get trapped in the areas of hyalinosis, but this isn't always seen **(Figure 9.9)**.

## TREATMENT

FSGS is the most common cause of nephrotic syndrome in African-Americans and Hispanics, and it can affect both children and adults. FSGS is usually treated with steroids, although it has an inconsistent response, and for that reason, and especially in adults, FSGS can involve more and more segments of the kidney's glomeruli to the point where it causes chronic renal failure.

## SUMMARY

All right, as a quick recap: focal segmental glomerulosclerosis is a nephrotic syndrome characterized by sclerosis and hyalinosis in some, but not all, glomeruli, and it usually only affects part of these glomeruli **(Figure 9.10)**.

**Figure 9.9**

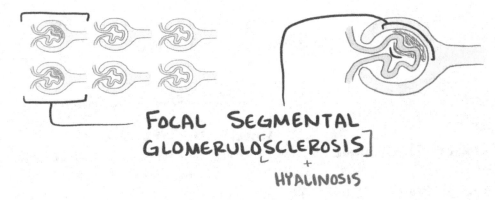

FOCAL SEGMENTAL GLOMERULOSCLEROSIS + HYALINOSIS

# Goodpasture syndrome

osmosis.org/learn/goodpasture_syndrome

**G**oodpasture syndrome is an autoimmune disease that primarily affects the lungs and the kidneys. It causes inflammation and eventually bleeding in the lungs, leading to hemoptysis, or coughing up of blood, and hematuria, or blood in the urine. This pattern was first recognized by the pathologist Dr. Ernest Goodpasture (**Figure 10.1**).

**Figure 10.1**

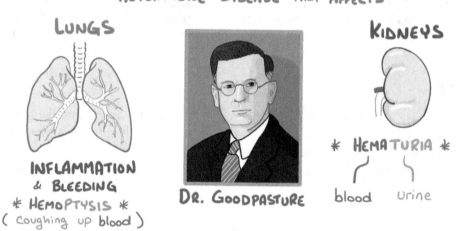

GOODPASTURE SYNDROME
an AUTOIMMUNE DISEASE that AFFECTS

LUNGS

INFLAMMATION & BLEEDING
* HEMOPTYSIS *
( coughing up blood )

DR. GOODPASTURE

KIDNEYS

* HEMATURIA *
blood    urine

**Figure 10.2**

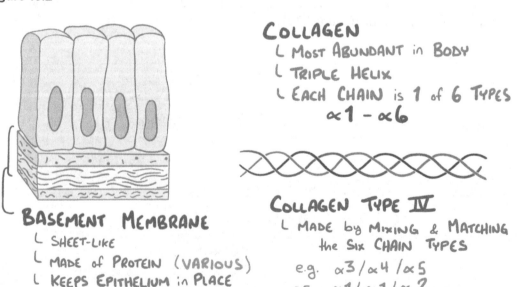

BASEMENT MEMBRANE
L SHEET-LIKE
L MADE of PROTEIN (VARIOUS)
L KEEPS EPITHELIUM in PLACE
L in EVERY ORGAN SYSTEM

COLLAGEN
L MOST ABUNDANT in BODY
L TRIPLE HELIX
L EACH CHAIN is 1 of 6 TYPES
$\alpha 1 - \alpha 6$

COLLAGEN TYPE IV
L MADE by MIXING & MATCHING
the SIX CHAIN TYPES
e.g. $\alpha 3 / \alpha 4 / \alpha 5$
or $\alpha 1 / \alpha 1 / \alpha 2$
or $\alpha 5 / \alpha 5 / \alpha 6$ etc...

Figure 10.3

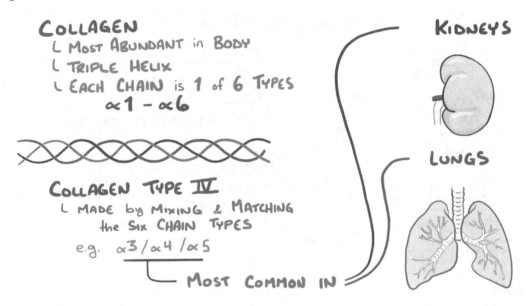

Figure 10.4

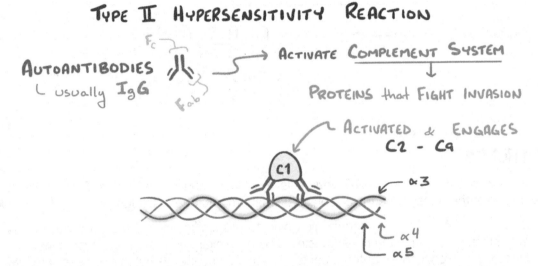

# PHYSIOLOGY

To understand Goodpasture syndrome, let's start by thinking about the basement membrane, which is a thin, sheet-like layer of tissue made of protein that keeps the epithelium stuck firmly to the actual organ. It's kind of like double-sided tape that keeps wrapping paper stuck to a gift **(Figure 10.2)**. The basement membrane is made up of various proteins, but the major one is collagen, and since basement membrane exists throughout every organ system, it's no wonder that collagen is the most abundant protein in the human body **(Figure 10.3)**. As far as proteins go, collagen is a pretty sweet looking one, with a triple-helix structure composed of three separate chains that are intertwined like braided hair. Each of the chains can be one of six Types, named α1 through α6, and the most common form of collagen found in the basement membrane is collagen Type IV, which is made by mixing and matching these six α-chains. One version of Type IV collagen combines the α3, α4, and α5 chains. Another combines two α1s and an α2, and a third version has two α5s and an α6. This list of combinations goes on.

Figure 10.5

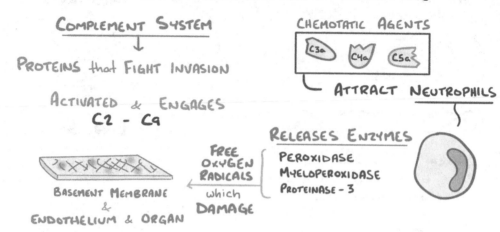

## TYPE II HYPERSENSITIVITY REACTION

**COMPLEMENT SYSTEM**

PROTEINS that FIGHT INVASION

ACTIVATED & ENGAGES
**C2 - C9**

**CHEMOTATIC AGENTS**

C3a  C4a  C5a

ATTRACT NEUTROPHILS

RELEASES ENZYMES
PEROXIDASE
MYELOPEROXIDASE
PROTEINASE-3

FREE OXYGEN RADICALS which DAMAGE

BASEMENT MEMBRANE & ENDOTHELIUM & ORGAN

Figure 10.6

## RISK FACTORS

GENETIC: GENES that CODE for HLA-DR15

IDENTIFIES & BINDS to FOREIGN MOLECULES

## PATHOLOGY

So, it turns out that the α3/α4/α5 variant is most common in the glomerular basement membrane of the kidneys and the alveolar basement membrane of the lungs.

In Goodpasture syndrome, autoantibodies bind to a specific part of the α3 chain that is usually hidden deep within the folded chains. This is an example of a Type II hypersensitivity reaction, because once these autoantibodies, which are usually IgG but in rare cases are IgM or IgA, bind to the the α3 chain, they activate the complement system. Now, the complement system is a series of small proteins present in the blood that acts like an enzymatic cascade to fight off bacterial and other pathogenic invasions. When the $F_{ab}$ portion of the IgG molecule inappropriately binds to the α3 chain, C1, which is the first of the complement proteins, binds to the $F_c$ portion of the IgG. This bound C1 is now activated and it starts engaging other members of the complement family from C2 through C9 (**Figure 10.4**).

Some of these are activated by being cleaved or chopped by an enzyme. The cleaved fragments C3a, C4a, and C5a act as chemotactic agents, meaning they attract certain cells like neutrophils. Once neutrophils join the party, they dump a bunch of enzymes like peroxidase, myeloperoxidase, and proteinase-3, all of which cause free oxygen radicals to form, damaging the basement membrane as well as the nearby endothelium and the underlying organ itself (**Figure 10.5**).

**Figure 10.7**

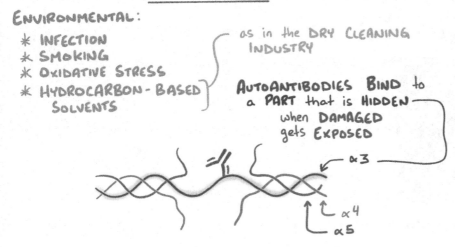

RISK FACTORS

ENVIRONMENTAL:
* INFECTION
* SMOKING
* OXIDATIVE STRESS
* HYDROCARBON-BASED SOLVENTS

as in the DRY CLEANING INDUSTRY

AUTOANTIBODIES BIND to a PART that is HIDDEN when DAMAGED gets EXPOSED

α3
α4
α5

**Figure 10.8**

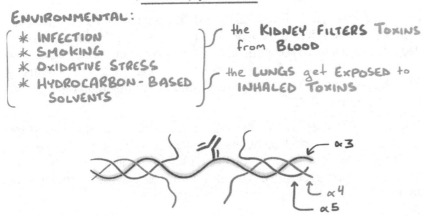

RISK FACTORS

ENVIRONMENTAL:
* INFECTION
* SMOKING
* OXIDATIVE STRESS
* HYDROCARBON-BASED SOLVENTS

the KIDNEY FILTERS TOXINS from BLOOD

the LUNGS get EXPOSED to INHALED TOXINS

α3
α4
α5

**Figure 10.9**

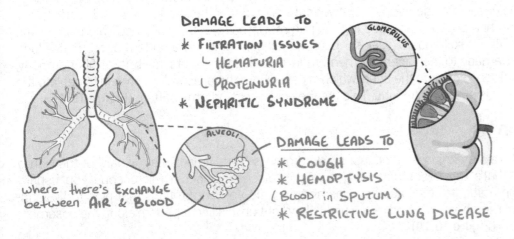

LUNG SYMPTOMS USUALLY COME BEFORE KIDNEY SYMPTOMS

DAMAGE LEADS TO
* FILTRATION ISSUES
 └ HEMATURIA
 └ PROTEINURIA
* NEPHRITIC SYNDROME

GLOMERULUS

ALVEOLI

DAMAGE LEADS TO
* COUGH
* HEMOPTYSIS (BLOOD in SPUTUM)
* RESTRICTIVE LUNG DISEASE

where there's EXCHANGE between AIR & BLOOD

**Figure 10.10**

DIAGNOSIS

DONE with BIOPSY, usually
of the KIDNEY

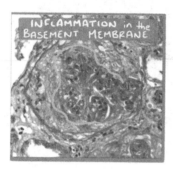

## CAUSES

Genetic risk factors for Goodpasture syndrome include having genes that encode a specific type of immune molecule called HLA-DR15 that's used to identify and bind to foreign molecules **(Figure 10.6)**.

Environmental risk factors also play a role. This relates back to the fact that the autoantibodies bind to a specific part of the α3 chain that is usually hidden deep within the folded chains. When the collagen molecules are damaged by infection, smoking, oxidative stress, or some hydrocarbon-based solvents, as in the case of people who work in the dry-cleaning industry, these antigenic regions on the α3 chain are exposed to the antibodies present in the blood of genetically susceptible people **(Figure 10.7)**.

This also helps explain why Goodpasture syndrome specifically affects the kidney and the lungs. The kidney filters toxins from the blood, so as these toxins pass through the basement membrane of the kidney, they likely expose parts of the α3 chain. Similarly, the lungs are exposed to various inhaled toxic substances, like cigarette smoke, once again exposing the parts of the α3 chain that lead to Goodpasture syndrome **(Figure 10.8)**.

## SYMPTOMS

In Goodpasture syndrome, lung symptoms usually precede kidney symptoms. Damage to the lungs' basement membranes causes widespread damage to the alveoli, the small air sacs where the gas exchange happens between the air we breathe in and the blood, leading to a cough and hemoptysis, or blood in the sputum. Damage to the alveoli can also impair the lungs' ability to exchange oxygen for carbon dioxide, leading to a pattern of restrictive lung disease. Damage to the basement membrane in the kidney affects its ability to filter properly, allowing blood to get into the urine, which is called hematuria, as well as protein to get into the urine, which is called proteinuria. This fits the nephritic syndrome pattern **(Figure 10.9)**.

## DIAGNOSIS

The best way to diagnose Goodpasture syndrome is by doing a biopsy, usually of the kidney because that's the best-studied organ in this disease. Under a microscope you usually see inflammation of the basement membrane; if fluorescent proteins that bind to the anti-basement membrane antibodies are used, they light up in a linear pattern along the basement membrane **(Figure 10.10)**.

## TREATMENT

In the past Goodpasture syndrome was usually fatal, but aggressive treatment with corticosteroids and immunosuppressive agents as well as plasmapheresis, which involves filtering out the fluid part of blood or plasma, has improved the prognosis with fewer individuals developing chronic renal failure and needing dialysis.

## SUMMARY

All right: as a quick recap, Goodpasture syndrome is an autoimmune disease in which the immune system attacks the α3 chain of Type IV collagen that's present in basement membrane. The specific spot that gets affected is usually well hidden, but it gets exposed by various toxins, which is why the disease predominantly affects the lungs and kidneys and causes symptoms like hemoptysis and hematuria **(Figure 10.11)**.

**Figure 10.11**

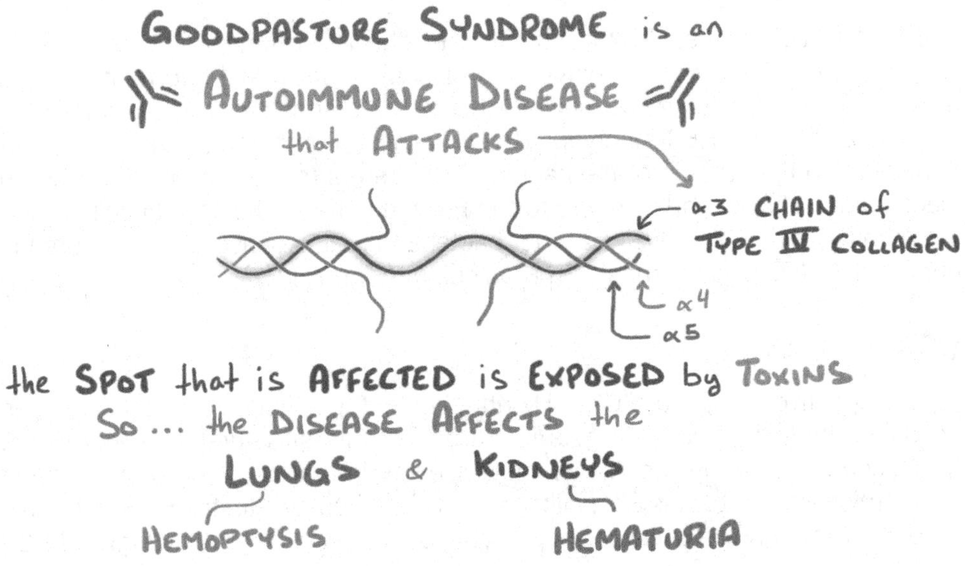

# Hemolytic-uremic syndrome

osmosis.org/learn/hemolytic-uremic_syndrome

With hemolytic uremic syndrome, *hemo-* refers to the blood, *-lytic* refers to breaking down, and uremic refers to increased urea levels in the blood. This helps explain hemolytic uremic syndrome: its two main effects are the destruction of red blood cells and the declining function of the kidney, which causes uremia. These effects are both caused by tiny blood clots that form in tiny blood vessels, predominantly in the kidneys.

## CAUSES

Classically, especially in children, hemolytic uremic syndrome is triggered by a bout of bloody diarrhea. When that happens, it's called diarrhea-positive or D positive hemolytic syndrome, which is sometimes shortened to HUS or *typical* HUS (**Figure 11.1**).

*Escherichia coli*, or *E. coli*, is usually the culprit, and children often pick it up through contaminated food or drink, like contaminated beef or unpasteurised milk from an infected cow. The particular strain of *E.coli* responsible for hemolytic uremic syndrome is known as enterohemorrhagic *E. coli*, or EHEC serotype O157:H7. These numbers and letters refer to the specific antigens on the surface of the bacteria. '157' refers to the O-antigen present in the lipopolysaccharide cell wall and '7' refers to the H-antigen located on the flagella of the bacteria. Other strains of E. coli as well as other bacteria can also cause hemolytic uremic syndrome, but E. coli O157:H7 is the most common culprit (**Figure 11.2**).

## PATHOLOGY

After entering the digestive tract, *E. coli* O157:H7 attaches to the intestinal wall and secretes a toxin called Shiga-like toxin. The toxin gets its name from its structural similarity to the shiga toxin produced by *Shigella dysenteriae*, another bacteria that causes bloody diarrhea and hemolytic uremic syndrome. This Shiga-like toxin is absorbed by intestinal blood vessels and then picked up by immune cells like eosinophils, basophils, and neutrophils (**Figure 11.3**).

**Figure 11.1**

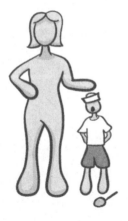

HEMOLYTIC UREMIC SYNDROME

CLASSICALLY
ESPECIALLY in CHILDREN
└ TRIGGERED by BLOODY DIARRHEA
└ CALLED
    — DIARRHEA-POSITIVE HUS
    — D+ HUS
    — TYPICAL HUS

**Figure 11.2**

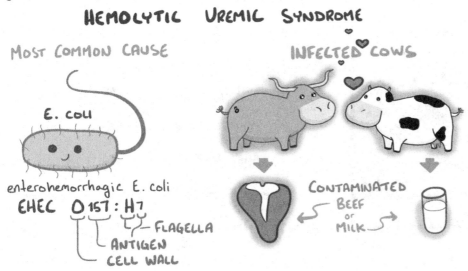

HEMOLYTIC UREMIC SYNDROME

MOST COMMON CAUSE

E. COLI

enterohemorrhagic E. coli
EHEC O 157 : H7
└─ FLAGELLA
└─ ANTIGEN
└─ CELL WALL

INFECTED COWS

CONTAMINATED BEEF or MILK

**Figure 11.3**

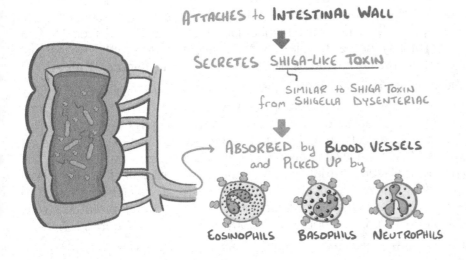

ATTACHES to INTESTINAL WALL
↓
SECRETES SHIGA-LIKE TOXIN
SIMILAR to SHIGA TOXIN from SHIGELLA DYSENTERIAE
↓
ABSORBED by BLOOD VESSELS and PICKED UP by

EOSINOPHILS    BASOPHILS    NEUTROPHILS

**Figure 11.4**

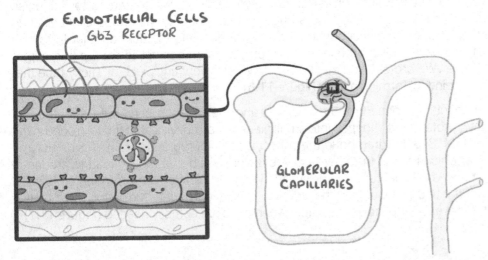

ENDOTHELIAL CELLS
Gb3 RECEPTOR

GLOMERULAR CAPILLARIES

**Figure 11.5**

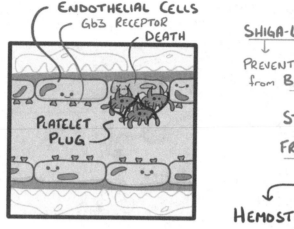

## PHYSIOLOGY

From there, the toxin is carried on the surface of these cells to the site of blood filtration, which is the glomerular capillaries of the kidney. Endothelial cells lining these glomerular capillaries express a glycolipid receptor called globotriaosylceramide, or Gb3-receptor, that has an incredibly strong affinity for the shiga-like toxin: the receptor is like a little magnet that can simply snatch the toxin away from a white blood cell as it drifts by **(Figure 11.4)**.

Once the toxin binds to the Gb3-receptor, it's engulfed by the endothelial cell; once it's inside, the toxin wreaks havoc on the cell. The toxin prevents aminoacyl-tRNA, which is the little molecule that carries the amino acids to make proteins, from binding to the ribosome. This stops all protein synthesis in the cell. In addition to this, preventing this bonding also leads to fragmentation of the DNA that activates apoptotic, or cell-suicide, pathways, causing the endothelial cell to die. Normally, any disruption to the endothelial cell lining of a blood vessel is immediately repaired by primary hemostasis, which is where a platelet plug forms to prevent more bleeding. That means that when large numbers of kidney endothelial cells start undergoing apoptosis, lots of tiny blood clots start to form in the kidneys **(Figure 11.5)**.

Another way that clots form is through a condition called thrombotic thrombocytopenic purpura, or TTP. In TTP, clots start to form inappropriately, and the underlying reason for this has to do with a molecule called von Willebrand factor, or vWF, which named for a Finnish doctor called Erik von Willebrand. vWF is a huge protein made by the endothelial cells and platelets, and this protein is released when it's time for platelets to stick together to form a clot. Now, platelets have a glycoprotein receptor on their surfaces called the Gp-Ib receptor that binds with the vWF protein. You can think of vWF as a very tiny piece of sticky tape that multiple platelets bind to, forming a clot **(Figure 11.6)**.

Under normal conditions, once time has passed and the clot has served its role, the von Willebrand factor protein gets chopped into small pieces by an enzyme that floats around in the blood called ADAMTS13. In thrombotic thrombocytopenic purpura, the ADAMTS13 enzyme is not as active, which means that there is excess von Willebrand factor floating around in the blood, and that von Willebrand factor starts binding to platelets and forming clots willy-nilly throughout the body, including in the kidneys. This inappropriate formation of clots also means that there are fewer platelets available when clots are actually needed **(Figure 11.7)**.

**Figure 11.6**

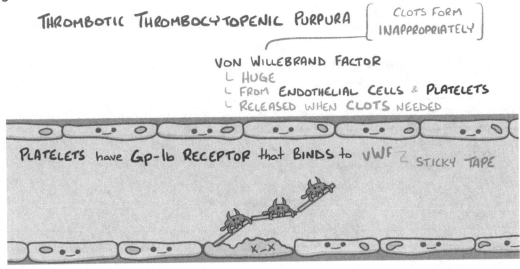

THROMBOTIC THROMBOCYTOPENIC PURPURA [ CLOTS FORM INAPPROPRIATELY ]

VON WILLEBRAND FACTOR
└ HUGE
└ FROM ENDOTHELIAL CELLS & PLATELETS
└ RELEASED WHEN CLOTS NEEDED

PLATELETS have Gp-1b RECEPTOR that BINDS to vWF ← STICKY TAPE

**Figure 11.7**

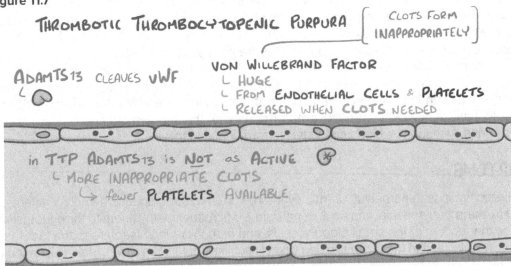

THROMBOTIC THROMBOCYTOPENIC PURPURA [ CLOTS FORM INAPPROPRIATELY ]

ADAMTS13 CLEAVES vWF
└

VON WILLEBRAND FACTOR
└ HUGE
└ FROM ENDOTHELIAL CELLS & PLATELETS
└ RELEASED WHEN CLOTS NEEDED

in TTP ADAMTS13 is NOT as ACTIVE
└ MORE INAPPROPRIATE CLOTS
└→ fewer PLATELETS AVAILABLE

**Figure 11.8**

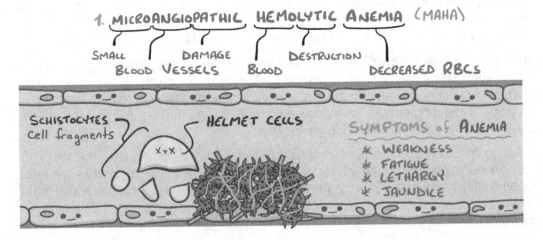

TRIAD of FINDINGS in HUS

1. MICROANGIOPATHIC HEMOLYTIC ANEMIA (MAHA)

SMALL          DAMAGE          DESTRUCTION
BLOOD VESSELS          BLOOD          DECREASED RBCS

SCHISTOCYTES          HELMET CELLS
Cell fragments

SYMPTOMS of ANEMIA
* WEAKNESS
* FATIGUE
* LETHARGY
* JAUNDICE

**Figure 11.9**

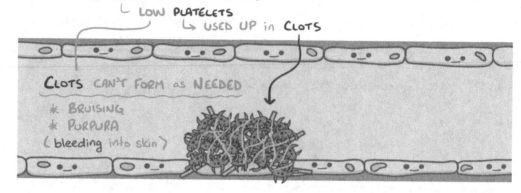

TRIAD of FINDINGS in HUS

1. MICROANGIOPATHIC HEMOLYTIC ANEMIA (MAHA)
2. THROMBOCYTOPENIA
   └ LOW PLATELETS
        ↳ USED UP in CLOTS

CLOTS CAN'T FORM as NEEDED

* BRUISING
* PURPURA
( bleeding into skin )

Now, there are other relatively rare ways for abnormal clots to start forming, and these are lumped together and called *atypical* hemolytic uremic syndrome. In atypical hemolytic uremic syndrome, there is no preceding diarrhea, so it's also known as D- hemolytic uremic syndrome. In this type, there is often damage to the endothelial cells lining the glomerular capillaries. That damage can come from infectious causes that are not associated with diarrhea, as well as from certain medications, and autoimmune causes. There are also familial forms of atypical hemolytic uremic syndrome, where genetic mutations seem to relate to a predisposition for damage to these endothelial cells. Regardless of the cause, the end result follows a pattern similar to typical hemolytic uremic syndrome, where the glomerular endothelium gets damaged and, in response, blood clots start to form in the kidneys.

## SYMPTOMS

The classic findings in hemolytic uremic syndrome are microangiopathic hemolytic anemia, or MAHA, thrombocytopenia, and acute renal failure. *Microangiopathy* refers to the endothelial damage that occurs in the small blood vessels, and *hemolytic anemia* refers to the fact that the clots forming within these small blood vessels act like boulders in a river, making it difficult for red blood cells to flow through without getting damaged and destroyed. Unlucky red blood cells can get smacked up against a blood clot and break, forming schistocytes, which are cell fragments, or "helmet" cells; they're called this because they look like little red helmets with pointed ends after a bit of the cell broke off. Ultimately, this destruction of red blood cells leads to fewer normal functioning red blood cells in the blood, also known as hemolytic anemia. This results in the usual symptoms of anemia like weakness, fatigue, and lethargy, but it can also cause jaundice as well because of the destruction of red blood cells **(Figure 11.8)**.

The thrombocytopenia, or low number of platelets, happens because they're used up in clot formation. This means that clots can't form when they need to, which causes easy bruising and purpura, which is bleeding into the skin. Finally, severe ongoing damage to the capillary endothelium of the glomeruli in the kidney can result in renal failure, and that can lead to uremia, or excess urea in the blood **(Figure 11.9)**.

In addition to the classic symptoms of hemolytic uremic syndrome, individuals with thrombotic thrombocytopenic purpura typically have neurologic findings because blood clots can affect the blood supply to the brain. This might result in visual disturbances, altered mental status and even seizures and stroke, which can lead to death. People suffering from TTP usually also have a fever.

# DIAGNOSIS

Hemolytic uremic syndrome is diagnosed by evaluating the urine for signs of kidney damage, like proteinuria, which is excess protein in the urine, and hematuria, which is the presence of blood in the urine. There may also be elevated amounts of waste products, like urea and creatinine, in the urine. On a blood smear, there may be evidence of schistocytes or helmet cells, and in cases where there is a history of bloody diarrhea, the stool can be cultured to look for the culprit bacteria. Finally, in suspected TTP-HUS, ADAMTS13 activity in plasma can be measured.

# TREATMENT

Treatment of typical or D+ hemolytic uremic syndrome is mainly supportive as the Shiga-like toxin gradually clears out of the body over a matter of days to weeks. It's thought that killing bacteria with antibiotics can potentially result in the increased release of toxin from dead bacteria, which can worsen the problem, so antibiotics are not typically recommended. In TTP-HUS, a key treatment option is plasmapheresis, where the patient's plasma is exchanged with plasma that has a normal amount of ADAMTS13 and lacks the antibodies that might be destroying it. Of the various types, atypical hemolytic-uremic syndrome usually has the worst prognosis and treatment usually involves identifying and addressing the underlying cause.

# SUMMARY

All right, as a quick recap: hemolytic uremic syndrome is a disease characterised by microangiopathic hemolytic anemia, thrombocytopenia, and renal failure. Typical hemolytic uremic syndrome is caused by bacteria like *E. coli* O157:H7, but it is also associated with thrombotic thrombocytopenic purpura as well as atypical causes. The diagnosis is made by analyzing the blood or urine, and the treatment for typical hemolytic uremic syndrome is supportive **(Figure 11.10)**.

**Figure 11.10**

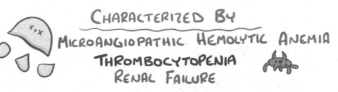

HEMOLYTIC UREMIC SYNDROME

CHARACTERIZED BY
MICROANGIOPATHIC HEMOLYTIC ANEMIA
THROMBOCYTOPENIA
RENAL FAILURE

CAUSED BY
TYPICAL HUS → E.COLI O157:H7
THROMBOTIC THROMBOCYTOPENIC PURPURA
ATYPICAL CAUSES

DIAGNOSED WITH
BLOOD & URINE ANALYSIS

TREATMENT
SUPPORTIVE

# Horseshoe kidney

osmosis.org/learn/horseshoe_kidney

**H**orseshoe kidney, sometimes called renal fusion, is a congenital disorder where the two kidneys fuse together during fetal development, resulting in one large, horseshoe-shaped kidney **(Figure 12.1)**.

## PHYSIOLOGY

Normally during fetal development, the kidneys develop in the pelvis, and they progress through a series of phases called pronephros, mesonephros, and metanephros before finally migrating upward into the abdomen and becoming everyone's favorite organ duo.

**Figure 12.1**

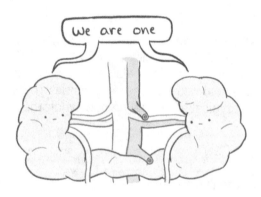

(RENAL FUSION)
## HORSESHOE KIDNEY

we are one

**Figure 12.2**

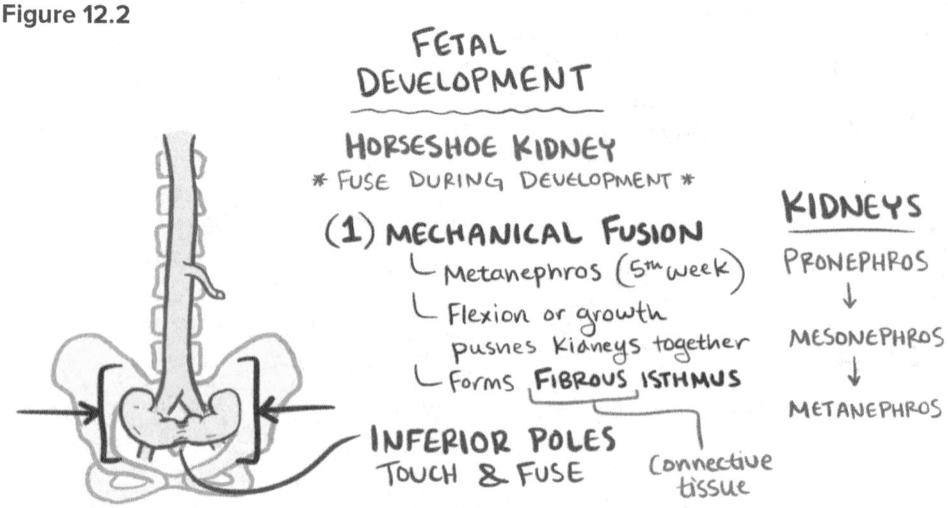

FETAL DEVELOPMENT

HORSESHOE KIDNEY
* FUSE DURING DEVELOPMENT *

(1) MECHANICAL FUSION
└ Metanephros (5th week)
└ Flexion or growth pushes kidneys together
└ Forms FIBROUS ISTHMUS

INFERIOR POLES
TOUCH & FUSE    Connective tissue

KIDNEYS
PRONEPHROS
↓
MESONEPHROS
↓
METANEPHROS

**Figure 12.3**

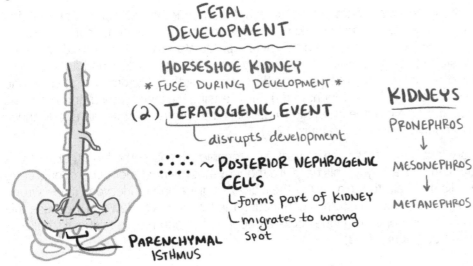

FETAL DEVELOPMENT

HORSESHOE KIDNEY
* FUSE DURING DEVELOPMENT *
(2) TERATOGENIC EVENT
└ disrupts development
∴ ~ POSTERIOR NEPHROGENIC CELLS
└ forms part of KIDNEY
└ migrates to wrong spot
PARENCHYMAL ISTHMUS

KIDNEYS
PRONEPHROS
↓
MESONEPHROS
↓
METANEPHROS

**Figure 12.4**

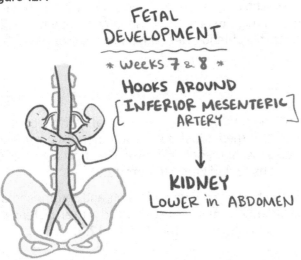

FETAL DEVELOPMENT
* weeks 7 & 8 *
HOOKS AROUND
[INFERIOR MESENTERIC] ARTERY
↓
KIDNEY
LOWER in ABDOMEN

**Figure 12.5**

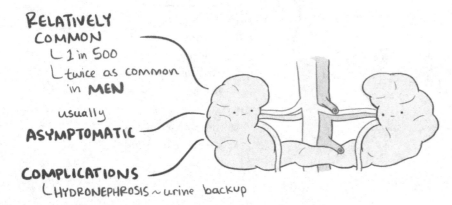

RELATIVELY COMMON
└ 1 in 500
└ twice as common in MEN

usually ASYMPTOMATIC

COMPLICATIONS
└ HYDRONEPHROSIS ~ urine backup

## CAUSES

For people with horseshoe kidney, their kidneys fused together at some point during development, and there are two main working theories on how this might happen. The first is mechanical fusion, which happens during the metanephros stage, which is around about the fifth week of gestation. At this point, the two kidneys are still in the pelvis, and are therefore pretty close together, so it's thought that some flexion or growth of the developing spine and pelvic organs essentially pushes the kidneys together, causing the lower or inferior poles of the kidneys to touch and fuse together, forming what's called a *fibrous* isthmus (fibrous because it's composed of connective tissue) **(Figure 12.2)**.

The other theory involves a *teratogenic event*. Teratogenic means something that disrupts fetal development in some way. In this case, it's thought that the posterior nephrogenic cells, which are the cells that help to form part of the kidney, migrate and rendezvous in the wrong spot, therefore again forming an isthmus connecting the two kidneys. However, because this time the isthmus is composed of kidney cells as opposed to connective tissue, it's called a *parenchymal* isthmus **(Figure 12.3)**.

## PATHOLOGY

Whichever one happens, now you've got this single, horseshoe-shaped kidney in the pelvis. During the seventh and eighth weeks, it tries to migrate up into the abdomen, but it hits a bit of a roadblock and hooks around the inferior mesenteric artery, which keeps it lower in the abdomen than normal **(Figure 12.4)**.

## SYMPTOMS

Horseshoe kidney is actually a relatively common congenital disorder, affecting about 1 in 500 people, and is about twice as common in men. Most people with horseshoe kidney are asymptomatic, although it does predispose someone to certain complications like hydronephrosis, or backup of urine, due to an obstructed ureter **(Figure 12.5)**.

Also, having a horseshoe kidney is associated with kidney stones, infection, and chromosomal disorders like Turner syndrome, trisomy 13, 18, and 21. Finally, it's associated with an increased risk of kidney cancer, especially Wilms' tumor and carcinoid tumor **(Figure 12.6)**.

Figure 12.6

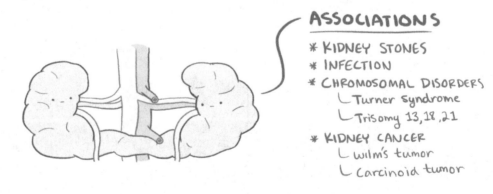

ASSOCIATIONS
* KIDNEY STONES
* INFECTION
* CHROMOSOMAL DISORDERS
    └ Turner syndrome
    └ Trisomy 13, 18, 21
* KIDNEY CANCER
    └ Wilm's tumor
    └ Carcinoid tumor

## TREATMENT

People with horseshoe kidney alone typically don't need treatment and have a normal lifespan, although it's important to keep in mind the abnormal structure of the horseshoe kidney if surgical intervention is needed for one of the complications or for some other abdominal procedure.

## SUMMARY

All right, as quick recap: horseshoe kidney is a congenital disorder where the kidneys fuse sometime during development, and as it migrates, it gets hooked around the inferior mesenteric artery, keeping it lower in the abdomen **(Figure 12.7)**.

**Figure 12.7**

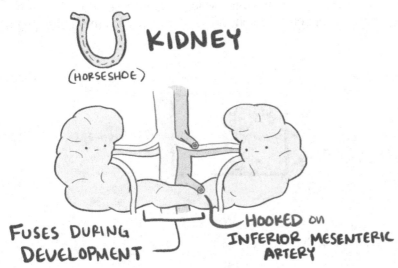

# Hydronephrosis

osmosis.org/learn/hydronephrosis

**W**ith hydronephrosis, *hydro-* means water, *nephro-* means kidneys, and *-osis* refers to a disease state, so hydronephrosis refers a disease or condition where excessive amounts of water, in the form of urine, causes the kidneys to dilate.

## PHYSIOLOGY

Now, normally inside the kidneys, urine forms in the nephron and then drains through the papilla, which is an inverted cone-shaped pyramid. Like a shower head, it pours urine into the calyces, which get their name from the Latin calix, which means large cup, like a Roman chalice. From there, it enters the renal pelvis, which funnels the urine into the ureter **(Figure 13.1)**.

**Figure 13.1**

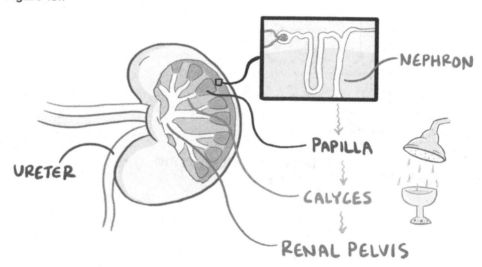

**Figure 13.2**

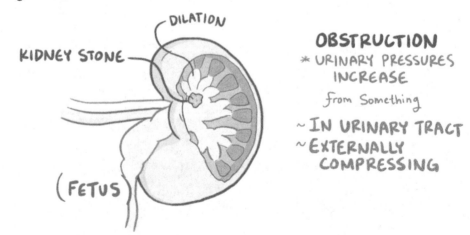

**Figure 13.3**

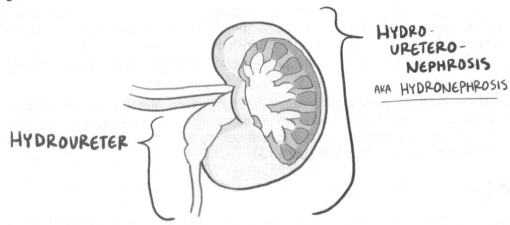

HYDRO-
URETERO-
NEPHROSIS
AKA HYDRONEPHROSIS

HYDROURETER

**Figure 13.4**

CAUSES of HYDRONEPHROSIS in CHILDREN

* CONGENITAL MALFORMATION
    └ URETEROCELE
        * SAC of TISSUE
          OBSTRUCTS FLOW
          of URINE
    └ POSTERIOR
      URETHRAL VALVES
        * FLAPS of TISSUE
          OBSTRUCT FLOW
          of URINE

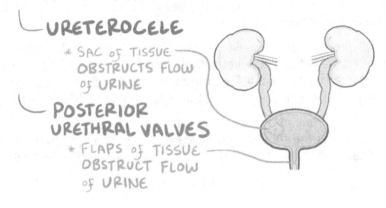

**Figure 13.5**

CAUSES of HYDRONEPHROSIS in ADULTS

* RESULT of ACQUIRED
  DISEASE
    └ KIDNEY STONES
    └ PROSTATIC
      HYPERPLASIA
      (ENLARGED PROSTATE)

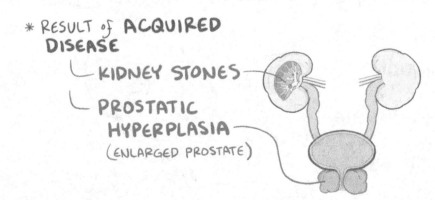

## PATHOLOGY

If there's an obstruction to this normal flow of urine, then it can cause urinary pressures to increase and push out on the walls of these structures, making them dilate. This might happen because of something within the urinary tract, like a kidney stone, or from external compression, like when a fetus pushes up against the urinary tract during pregnancy **(Figure 13.2)**.

Typically, the dilation starts closest to the site of the problem and then slowly continues back up towards the kidneys. Now, if there's dilation of just the ureter, it's called hydroureter, but if there's dilation of the ureter, renal pelvis, and the calyces, it's called hydroureteronephrosis, or more commonly, just hydronephrosis **(Figure 13.3)**.

## CAUSES

The causes of hydronephrosis differ by age group. Hydronephrosis in the fetus is called antenatal hydronephrosis, and sometimes the cause here is unknown. Sometimes it develops and disappears on its own, so it may be a variation of normal development. But if hydronephrosis progresses through fetal development into the third trimester, then there may be an actual underlying pathology. For example, there's congenital ureteropelvic junction obstruction, which is where the ureteropelvic junction, which connects the ureter to the kidney, fails to canalize during development, which can obstruct the flow of urine. Another cause is vesicoureteral reflux, which is where urine is allowed to backflow from the bladder into the ureters and, eventually, the kidneys.

In young children, hydronephrosis usually results from a congenital malformation like a ureterocele, a sac of tissue in the distal ureter, that also obstructs the flow of urine from the ureter into the bladder, as well as posterior urethral valves, which is a malformation of the posterior urethra where flaps of tissue obstruct the outflow of urine **(Figure 13.4)**.

In contrast, adults with hydronephrosis usually develop it as a result of an acquired disease, like kidney stones, which is the most common cause, as well as prostatic hyperplasia, or enlarged prostate, which blocks the flow of urine out of the bladder **(Figure 13.5)**.

**Figure 13.6**

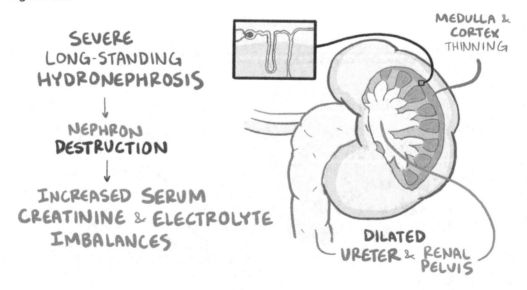

**Figure 13.7**

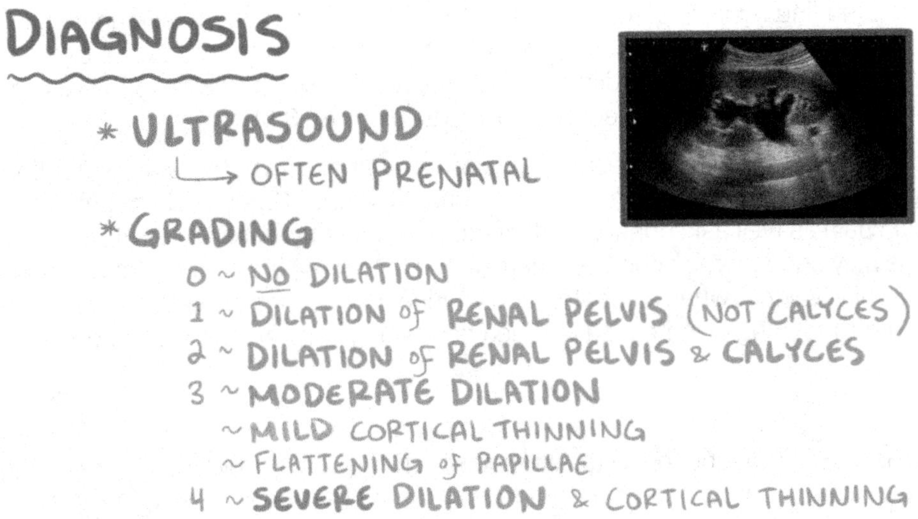

# DIAGNOSIS

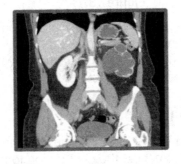

* ULTRASOUND
  └→ OFTEN PRENATAL

* GRADING
  - 0 ~ NO DILATION
  - 1 ~ DILATION of RENAL PELVIS (NOT CALYCES)
  - 2 ~ DILATION of RENAL PELVIS & CALYCES
  - 3 ~ MODERATE DILATION
    - ~ MILD CORTICAL THINNING
    - ~ FLATTENING of PAPILLAE
  - 4 ~ **SEVERE DILATION** & CORTICAL THINNING

**Figure 13.8**

# DIAGNOSIS

* INTRAVENOUS UROGRAPHY
  or PYELOGRAPHY
  └ OFTEN USED for CHILDREN

* CT SCAN
  └ OFTEN USED for ADULTS
  └ USEFUL for finding KIDNEY STONES

**Figure 13.9**

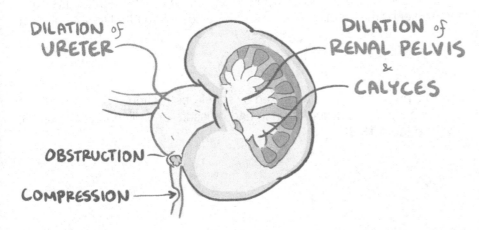

HYDRONEPHROSIS

DILATION of URETER

DILATION of RENAL PELVIS & CALYCES

OBSTRUCTION

COMPRESSION

## SYMPTOMS

Now, severe long-standing hydronephrosis can lead to nephron destruction and can result in an increase in serum creatinine, as well as electrolyte imbalances. When this sort of damage has happened, the kidney can develop a dilated ureter and renal pelvis, as well as compression atrophy, which is thinning of the renal medulla and cortex **(Figure 13.6)**.

Symptoms and complications of hydronephrosis are often related to symptoms of obstruction, since that's the context in which hydronephrosis is usually found. Obstruction might cause flank pain or groin pain as well as a urinary tract infection, and the hydronephrosis itself might cause symptoms only once there's serious damage to the kidneys. A worrisome complication is postrenal azotemia, which is when an obstruction to urine flow causes the kidney to increase reabsorption of urea, resulting in increased nitrogen-containing compounds in the blood.

## DIAGNOSIS

Hydronephrosis is usually diagnosed with ultrasound, often prenatal ultrasound, meaning during pregnancy. Hydronephrosis is given a grade from 0 to IV based on the severity. Grade 0 means there's no dilation. Grade 1 is when there is a dilation of the renal pelvis but the calyces remain normal. Grade 2 is when there is a dilation of the renal pelvis and calyces. Grade 3 is when there is a moderate dilation of the renal pelvis and calyces in addition to mild cortical thinning and flattening of the papillae. Lastly, Grade 4 is when there is a severe renal dilation and cortical thinning **(Figure 13.7)**.

In children, intravenous urography or pyelography is also commonly used to assess for congenital pelviureteric junction obstruction. In adults, a CT scan is commonly done because it can be helpful in identifying kidney stones, which are the most common underlying cause of the hydronephrosis **(Figure 13.8)**.

## TREATMENT

Hydronephrosis treatment focuses on relieving the obstruction and allowing the urine that may have accumulated behind the obstruction to flow out normally. Acutely, a nephrostomy tube can be used, which is this plastic tube inserted through the skin into the renal pelvis, and this allows the accumulated urine to drain out. Chronically, somebody could have a ureteric stent, which pops the ureter open or a pyeloplasty, which is a surgical remake of the renal pelvis. Lower urinary tract obstructions, like prostatic hyperplasia, can be treated with the insertion of a urinary catheter that keeps the urethra open or a suprapubic catheter that causes bladder decompression.

## SUMMARY

All right, to recap: hydronephrosis is typically caused by either obstruction in or compression of the urinary tract, which leads to buildup of urine and pressure and dilation of the ureter, renal pelvis and calyces **(Figure 13.9)**.

# Hypercalcemia

**W**ith hypercalcemia, *hyper-* means over, *calc-* refers to calcium, and *-emia* refers to the blood, so hypercalcemia means higher than normal calcium levels in the blood, so generally over 10.5 mg/dL **(Figure 14.1)**.

## PHYSIOLOGY

Now, calcium, or Ca2+, exists as an ion with a double positive charge, and it's the most abundant metal in the human body. So, I know what you're thinking; yeah, we're all pretty much cyborgs. Anyway, about 99% of that calcium is in our bones in the form of calcium phosphate, also called hydroxyapatite. The last 1% is split so that the majority, about 0.99%, is extracellular, which means in the blood and in the interstitial space between cells, and 0.01% is intracellular **(Figure 14.2)**.

**Figure 14.1**

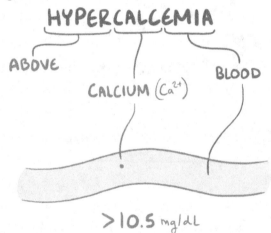

**Figure 14.2**

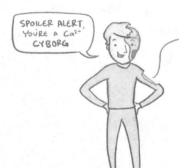

**Figure 14.3**

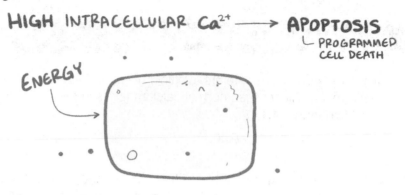

HIGH INTRACELLULAR Ca²⁺ → **APOPTOSIS**
└ PROGRAMMED CELL DEATH

ENERGY

**Figure 14.4**

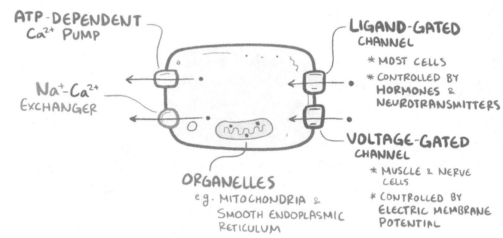

ATP-DEPENDENT Ca²⁺ PUMP

Na⁺-Ca²⁺ EXCHANGER

ORGANELLES
e.g. MITOCHONDRIA & SMOOTH ENDOPLASMIC RETICULUM

LIGAND-GATED CHANNEL
* MOST CELLS
* CONTROLLED BY HORMONES & NEUROTRANSMITTERS

VOLTAGE-GATED CHANNEL
* MUSCLE & NERVE CELLS
* CONTROLLED BY ELECTRIC MEMBRANE POTENTIAL

**Figure 14.5**

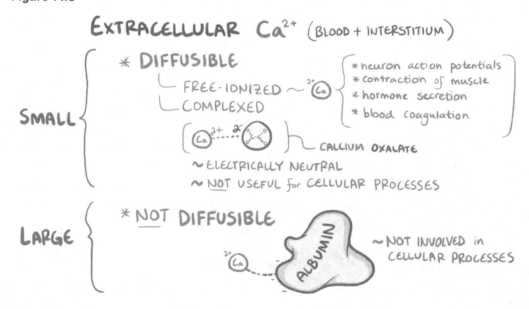

EXTRACELLULAR Ca²⁺ (BLOOD + INTERSTITIUM)

SMALL
* DIFFUSIBLE
  └ FREE-IONIZED ~ Ca²⁺
  └ COMPLEXED

  * neuron action potentials
  * contraction of muscle
  * hormone secretion
  * blood coagulation

  Ca²⁺ ⋯ ²⁻
  CALCIUM OXALATE
  ~ ELECTRICALLY NEUTRAL
  ~ NOT USEFUL for CELLULAR PROCESSES

LARGE
* NOT DIFFUSIBLE
  Ca²⁺ ⋯ ALBUMIN
  ~ NOT INVOLVED in CELLULAR PROCESSES

High levels of intracellular calcium cause cells to die. In fact, that's exactly what happens during apoptosis, which is also known as programmed cell death. For that reason, cells end up using a ton of energy just by keeping their intracellular calcium levels low **(Figure 14.3)**. Now, calcium gets into the cell through two types of channels, or cell doors, within the cell membrane. The first type are ligand-gated channels, which are what most cells use to let calcium in, and these are primarily controlled by hormones or neurotransmitters. The second type are voltage-gated channels, which are mostly found in muscle and nerve cells, and these are primarily controlled by changes in the electrical membrane potential. So, calcium flows in through these channels, and to prevent calcium levels from getting too high, cells kick excess calcium right back out with ATP-dependent calcium pumps as well as sodium calcium exchangers. In addition, most of the intracellular calcium is stored within organelles like the mitochondria and smooth endoplasmic reticulum, and it's released only when it's needed **(Figure 14.4)**.

Now, the majority of the extracellular calcium, the calcium in the blood and interstitium, is split almost equally between two groups: calcium that is diffusible and calcium that is not diffusible. Diffusible calcium is separated into two subcategories. First, there's free-ionized calcium, which is involved in all sorts of cellular processes, like neuronal action potentials, contraction of skeletal, smooth, and cardiac muscle, hormone secretion, and blood coagulation, all of which are tightly regulated by enzymes and hormones. The other category is complexed calcium, which is where the positively charged calcium is ionically linked to tiny negatively charged molecules like oxalate, a small anion that normally found in our blood in small amounts. The complexed calcium forms a molecule that's electrically neutral but, unlike free-ionized calcium, is not useful for cellular processes. Both of these are called diffusible because they're small enough to diffuse across cell membranes. Finally, there's the non-diffusible calcium, which is bound to negatively charged proteins like albumin. The resulting protein-calcium complex is too large and charged to cross membranes, leaving this calcium also uninvolved in cellular processes **(Figure 14.5)**.

Changes in the body's levels of extracellular calcium are detected by a surface receptor in parathyroid cells that's called the calcium-sensing receptor. These changes affect the amount of parathyroid hormone that's released by the parathyroid gland. The parathyroid hormone gets the bones to release calcium, it gets the kidneys to reabsorb more calcium so it's not lost in the urine, and it synthesizes calcitriol, which is also known as 1,25-dihydroxycholecalciferol, or active Vitamin D. Active Vitamin D then goes on to cause the gastrointestinal tract to increase calcium absorption. Altogether, these effects help to keep the extracellular levels of calcium within a narrow range that's between 8.5 to 10 mg/dl **(Figure 14.6)**.

**Figure 14.6**

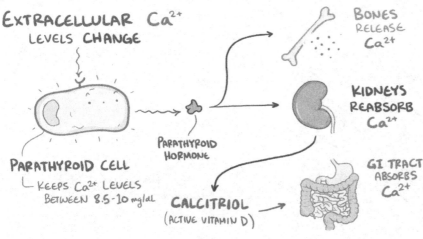

**Figure 14.7**

(THE BLOOD)

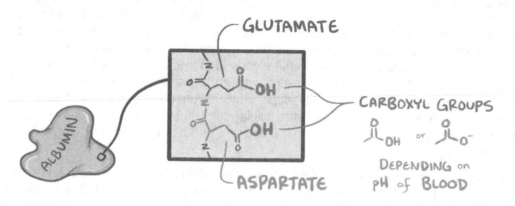

**Figure 14.8**

(THE BLOOD)

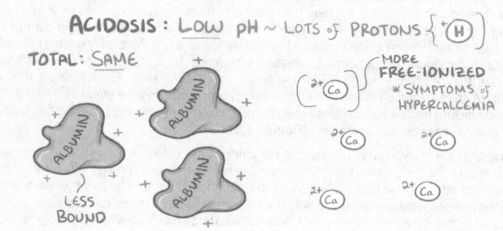

**Figure 14.9**

(THE BLOOD)

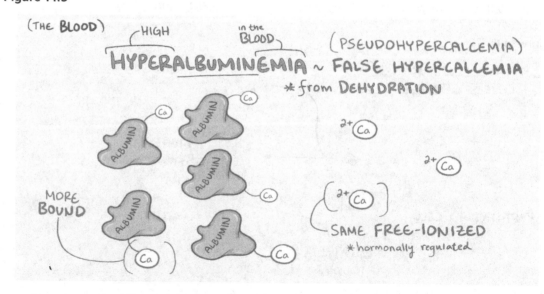

Sometimes, though, total calcium levels in the blood, a measurement that includes both diffusible and non-diffusible calcium, can vary a bit thanks to the blood's pH and protein levels. This happens because albumin has acidic amino acids, like glutamate and aspartate, which have some carboxyl groups that are in the form of COO- or COOH. Overall, the balance of COO- and COOH changes based on the pH of the blood **(Figure 14.7)**.

Now, when there's a low pH, or acidosis, there are plenty of protons or H+ ions floating around, and a lot of those COO- groups pick up a proton and become COOH. More COOH groups make albumin more positively charged, and since calcium is positively charged, these two repel each other, decreasing bound calcium and increases the proportion of free ionized calcium in blood. As more protons bind albumin, more free ionized calcium builds up in the blood, and so even though total levels calcium are the same, there's less bound calcium and *more* ionized calcium. Remember, free ionized calcium is important for cellular processes, but too much of it can lead to symptoms of hypercalcemia **(Figure 1.8)**.

Any condition that results in hyperalbuminemia, or high albumin levels, causes a higher concentration of protein-bound calcium, but here, free ionized calcium concentrations stay essentially the same due to hormonal regulation. This is therefore called *false hypercalcemia* or *pseudohypercalcemia*, since the concentration of bound calcium increases but the concentration of free ionized calcium stays the same. Even though this is rare, it can happen in people with dehydration because their albumin gets very concentrated **(Figure 14.9)**.

## CAUSES

Now, *true hypercalcemia* is most commonly caused by increased osteoclastic bone resorption, which is where osteoclasts, which are little bone eating cells, frantically break down the bones and release calcium into the blood. This might happen when the parathyroid gland becomes overgrown and releases more parathyroid hormone **(Figure 14.10)**. Another well-known cause of hypercalcemia is malignant tumors, some of which secrete parathyroid hormone-related protein, or PTHrP, a hormone that mimics the effect of parathyroid hormone and therefore stimulates the osteoclasts. Alongside these osteoclast cells, there're also osteo*blast* cells, the bone-building cells, and some tumors cause osteoblasts to die off. Overstimulated osteoclasts without enough osteoblasts can result in lytic bone lesions, which are commonly seen in some malignancies **(Figure 14.11)**.

**Figure 14.10**

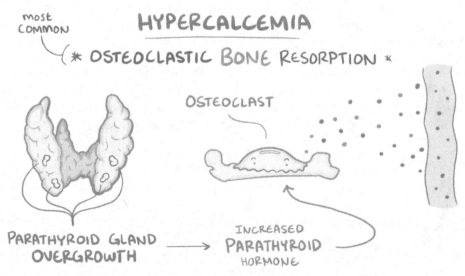

**Figure 14.11**

# HYPERCALCEMIA

most COMMON

\* OSTEOCLASTIC BONE RESORPTION \*

LYTIC BONE LESION

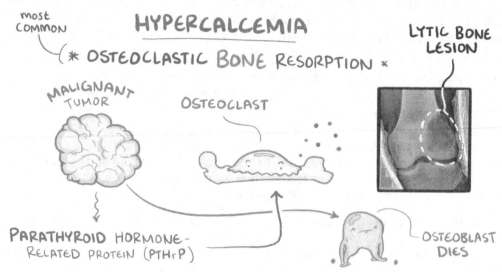

MALIGNANT TUMOR

OSTEOCLAST

PARATHYROID HORMONE-RELATED PROTEIN (PTHrP)

OSTEOBLAST DIES

**Figure 14.12**

# HYPERCALCEMIA

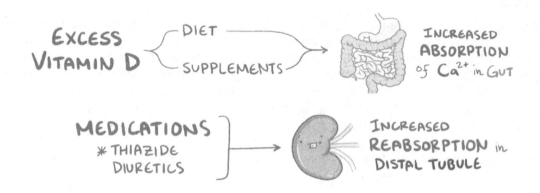

EXCESS VITAMIN D
- DIET
- SUPPLEMENTS

INCREASED ABSORPTION of $Ca^{2+}$ in GUT

MEDICATIONS
\* THIAZIDE DIURETICS

INCREASED REABSORPTION in DISTAL TUBULE

**Figure 14.13**

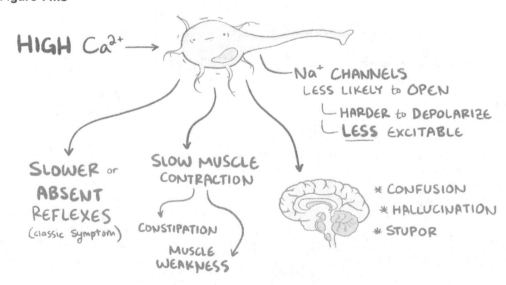

HIGH $Ca^{2+}$ →

$Na^+$ CHANNELS LESS LIKELY to OPEN
- HARDER to DEPOLARIZE
- LESS EXCITABLE

SLOWER or ABSENT REFLEXES (classic symptom)

SLOW MUSCLE CONTRACTION
- CONSTIPATION
- MUSCLE WEAKNESS

\* CONFUSION
\* HALLUCINATION
\* STUPOR

Another cause of hypercalcemia is excess Vitamin D, and this is caused either through diet or through supplements, and it can lead to too much calcium being absorbed in the gut. Finally, there are some medications that contribute to hypercalcemia; for example, thiazide diuretics increase calcium reabsorption in the distal tubule of the kidney **(Figure 14.12)**.

High levels of ionized calcium affect a variety of cellular processes, particularly those involving electrically active neurons. Normally, calcium ions stabilize the resting state of sodium channels, preventing them from spontaneously opening and letting sodium ions enter the cell.

With high levels of extracellular calcium, voltage-gated sodium channels are less likely to open up, making the neuron less excitable and therefore making it harder to reach depolarization. This is causes slower or absent reflexes, classic symptoms of hypercalcemia. This sluggish firing of neurons also leads to slower muscle contraction, which causes constipation and generalized muscle weakness. In the central nervous system, hypercalcemia causes confusion, hallucinations, and stupor **(Figure 14.13)**.

In most cases, when there's too much calcium in the blood, the kidneys try to dump it into the urine, causing hypercalciuria, which is excess calcium in the urine. Hypercalciuria leads to a loss of excess fluid in the kidneys, which causes dehydration, and the combination of hypercalciuria and dehydration can lead to calcium oxalate kidney stones **(Figure 14.14)**.

**Figure 14.14**

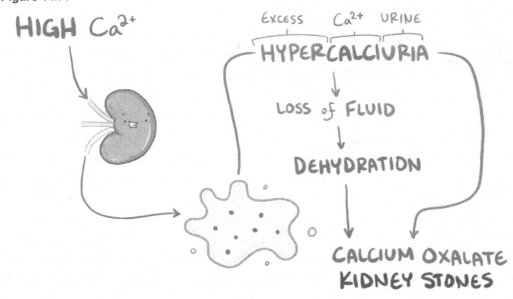

## DIAGNOSIS

Hypercalcemia is diagnosed based on high level of calcium in the blood, so generally above 10.5 mg/dL. An electrocardiogram might have changes like bradycardia, AV block, shortening of the QT interval, and sometimes in the precordial leads, we'll see the appearance of an Osborn wave. To identify the cause of hypercalcemia, healthcare professionals conduct lab tests that look at parathyroid hormone, vitamin D, albumin, phosphorus, and magnesium levels.

## TREATMENT

The main goal of treatment is to lower calcium levels by using medications that reduce calcium in blood. One approach is to increase urinary excretion of calcium, which can be done by rehydrating an individual, which causes more calcium to get filtered out of the body. In addition, loop diuretics can be helpful because they inhibit calcium reabsorption in the loop of Henle, leaving calcium in the lumen of the nephron so that it will be excreted. Another approach is to increase gastrointestinal excretion by using glucocorticoids to decrease intestinal calcium absorption, allowing calcium to instead simply pass through the gut without being absorbed. Finally, bone resorption can be prevented by using bisphosphonates or calcitonin to inhibit osteoclasts.

## SUMMARY

All right, as a quick recap: hypercalcemia describes a *high* concentration of free ionized calcium in the blood, which most commonly results from excess parathyroid hormone as well as malignancies. High calcium levels causes excitable cells to be less...well, excitable, resulting in slow reflexes, muscle weakness, and constipation **(Figure 14.15)**.

**Figure 14.15**

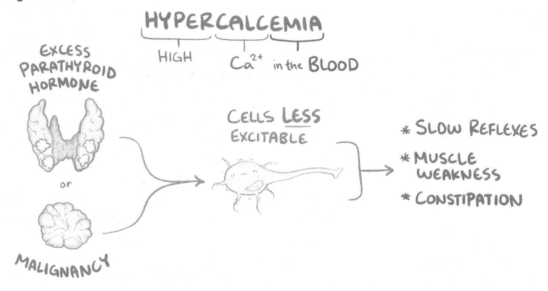

# Hyperkalemia

osmosis.org/learn/hyperkalemia

**W**ith hyperkalemia, *hyper-* means over, *kal-* refers to potassium, and *-emia* refers to the blood, so hyperkalemia means higher than normal potassium levels in the blood, so generally over 5.5 mEq/L **(Figure 15.1)**.

## PHYSIOLOGY

Now, total body potassium can essentially be split into two components, intracellular and extracellular potassium, or potassium inside and outside the cells, respectively. The extracellular component includes both the intravascular space, which is the space within the blood and lymphatic vessels, and the interstitial space, the space between cells where you typically find fibrous proteins and long chains of carbohydrates that are called glycosaminoglycans **(Figure 15.2)**.

**Figure 15.1**

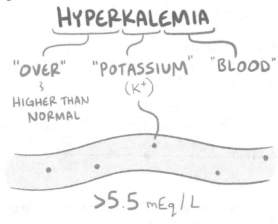

**Figure 15.2**

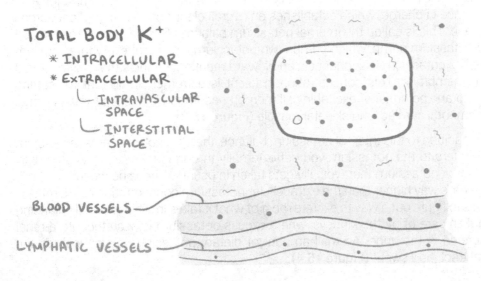

**Figure 15.3**

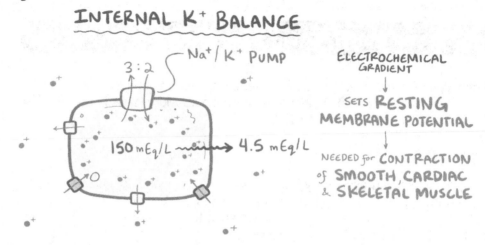

INTERNAL K⁺ BALANCE

Na⁺/K⁺ PUMP

3:2

150 mEq/L → 4.5 mEq/L

ELECTROCHEMICAL GRADIENT
↓
SETS RESTING MEMBRANE POTENTIAL
↓
NEEDED for CONTRACTION of SMOOTH, CARDIAC & SKELETAL MUSCLE

**Figure 15.4**

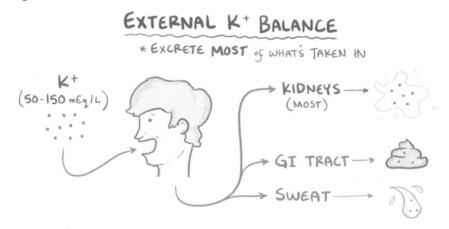

EXTERNAL K⁺ BALANCE

*EXCRETE MOST of WHAT'S TAKEN IN

K⁺
(50-150 mEq/L)

KIDNEYS (MOST) →

GI TRACT →

SWEAT →

Now, the vast majority, around 98%, of all of the body's potassium is intracellular, or inside of the cells. In fact, the concentration of potassium inside the cells is about 150 mEq/L, whereas outside the cells it's only about 4.5 mEq/L.

Keep in mind that these potassium ions carry a charge, so the difference in concentration also leads to a difference in charge, which establishes an overall electrochemical gradient across the cell membrane. This is called the internal potassium balance. This balance is maintained by the sodium-potassium pump, which pumps two potassium ions in for every three sodium ions out, as well as potassium leak channels and inward rectifier channels that are scattered throughout the membrane. This concentration gradient is extremely important for setting the resting membrane potential of excitable cell membranes, which is needed for the normal contraction of smooth, cardiac, and skeletal muscle **(Figure 15.3)**.

Also, though, in addition to this internal potassium balance, there's also an external potassium balance, which refers to the potassium you get externally through diet every day. On a daily basis, the amount of potassium that typically gets taken in usually ranges between 50 mEq/L to 150 mEq/L. That's way higher than the extracellular potassium concentration of 4.5 mEq/L, so your body has to figure out a way to excrete most of what it takes in. This external balancing act is largely taken care of by the kidneys, where excess potassium is secreted into a renal tubule and excreted in the urine. A small amount of dietary potassium is also lost via the gastrointestinal tract and sweat **(Figure 15.4)**.

# INTERNAL CAUSES

So, in order for there to be too much potassium in the blood, which is called hyperkalemia, there are two possibilities. The first is an external balance shift, which is most often caused by an decrease in sodium excretion in the kidneys, which raises the level of potassium in the blood. The second is an internal balance shift where potassium moves out of cells, and into the interstitium and blood **(Figure 15.5)**.

One potential cause of an internal potassium balance shift is insulin deficiency. This is because, after a meal, glucose increases in the blood, and at the same time, insulin is released and binds to cells, stimulating uptake of that glucose. Insulin also increases the activity of the sodium/potassium pump, which pulls potassium into cells **(Figure 15.6)**.

People with Type I diabetes don't make enough insulin, so when they eat a meal, especially a meal with a lot of potassium, that potassium sits in the blood instead of being taken into cells, and this causes hyperkalemia.

**Figure 15.5**

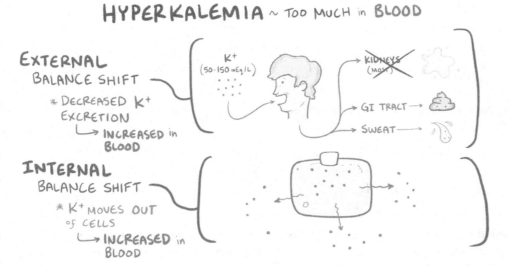

**Figure 15.6**

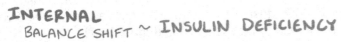

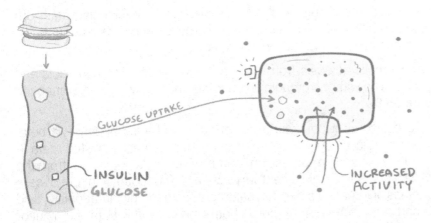

**Figure 15.7**

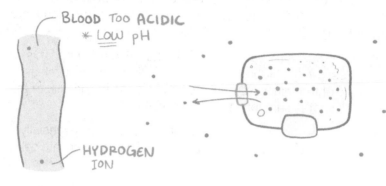

INTERNAL
BALANCE SHIFT ~ ACIDOSIS

- BLOOD TOO ACIDIC
  * LOW pH

- HYDROGEN ION

**Figure 15.8**

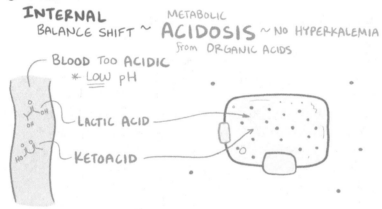

INTERNAL
BALANCE SHIFT ~ METABOLIC
ACIDOSIS ~ NO HYPERKALEMIA
from ORGANIC ACIDS

- BLOOD TOO ACIDIC
  * LOW pH

- LACTIC ACID

- KETOACID

Another cause of an internal potassium balance shift could be acidosis, which is when the blood becomes too acidic. In other words, a higher concentration of hydrogen ions lowers blood pH. One way the body can increase the blood pH is by moving hydrogen ions out of the blood and into cells. To accomplish this, cells use a special ion transporter that exchanges the hydrogen ion for a potassium ion across the cell membrane. So, to help compensate for an acidosis, hydrogen ions enter cells and potassium ions leave the cells and enter the blood. This might help with the acidosis, but it results in hyperkalemia **(Figure 15.7)**.

This isn't always the case for acidosis, though. For example, in respiratory acidosis, potassium levels aren't affected because $CO_2$ is lipid soluble and freely moves into cells without being exchanged for potassium; therefore, no hyperkalemia occurs.

Similarly, when there's a metabolic acidosis from excess organic acids, like lactic acid and ketoacids, protons can enter cells with the organic anion rather than having to be exchanged for potassium ions **(Figure 15.8)**.

Certain catecholamines can also shift potassium out of cells, and this happens via beta-2-adrenergic and alpha-adrenergic receptors on cell membranes. When activated, beta-2-adrenergic receptors stimulate the sodium-potassium pump, which pulls potassium from the blood into cells. Meanwhile alpha-adrenergic receptors cause a shift of potassium out of cells via calcium-dependent potassium channels. So, that said, beta-2-adrenergic antagonists, also known as beta blockers, and alpha-adrenergic agonists both cause a shift in potassium out of the cells and into the blood **(Figure 15.9)**.

**Figure 15.9**

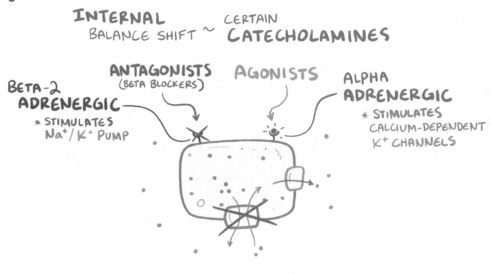

**Figure 15.10**

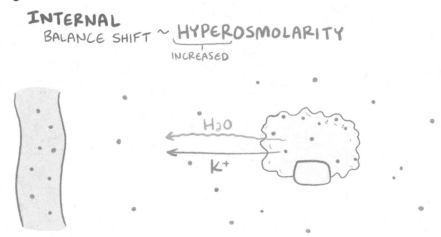

Another important mechanism is hyperosmolarity, which is where there is an increased extracellular osmolarity in relation to the intracellular space. This osmotic gradient pulls water out of cells and into the extracellular space. Less water in the cells increases the intracellular potassium concentration, which increases the potassium's concentration gradient and pushes more of it out of the cell and into the interstitium and blood **(Figure 15.10)**.

Cell lysis is yet another cause of hyperkalemia. Since so much potassium is kept within the cell, when a large number of cells die, or lyse, potassium is released into the blood, which causes hyperkalemia. Examples of large-scale cell lysis are severe burns, rhabdomyolysis, or breakdown of skeletal muscle, and tumor lysis as a result of chemotherapy **(Figure 15.11)**.

A final example of internal potassium balance leading to hyperkalemia is exercise. During exercise while the body and the body's cells are working harder, more cellular ATP, which is the molecular unit of currency, gets consumed. The depletion of ATP triggers potassium channels on the membrane of muscle cells to open up, which allows potassium to moves down its electrochemical gradient and out of the cell. Usually this shift is small, but if combined with beta-blockers or kidney issues, strenuous exercise can lead to hyperkalemia **(Figure 15.12)**.

**Figure 15.11**

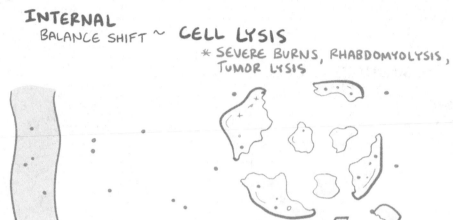

INTERNAL BALANCE SHIFT ~ CELL LYSIS
* SEVERE BURNS, RHABDOMYOLYSIS, TUMOR LYSIS

**Figure 15.12**

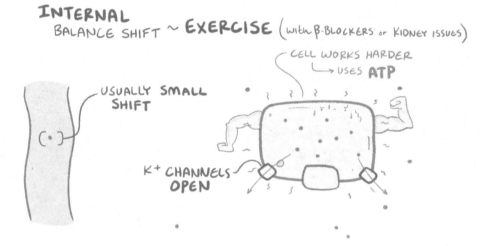

INTERNAL BALANCE SHIFT ~ EXERCISE (with β-BLOCKERS or KIDNEY ISSUES)

CELL WORKS HARDER → USES **ATP**

USUALLY SMALL SHIFT

K+ CHANNELS OPEN

**Figure 15.13**

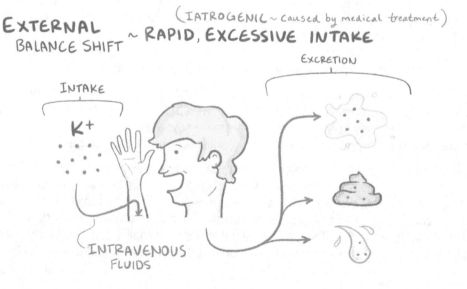

EXTERNAL BALANCE SHIFT ~ RAPID, EXCESSIVE INTAKE (IATROGENIC ~ caused by medical treatment)

INTAKE

EXCRETION

K+

INTRAVENOUS FLUIDS

**Figure 15.14**

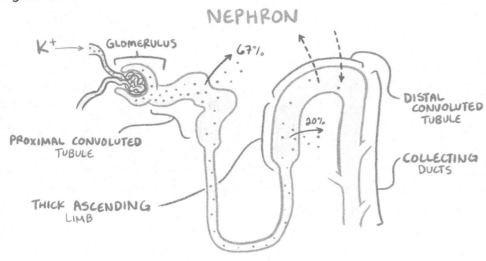

**Figure 15.15**

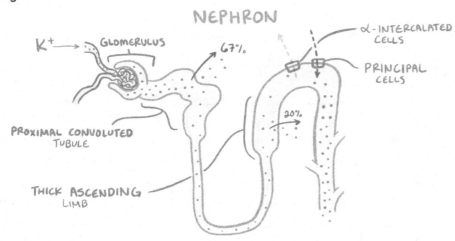

# EXTERNAL CAUSES

External potassium balance shifts resulting in hyperkalemia have to do with potassium intake and excretion. Taking in too much potassium can lead to hyperkalemia, but this would typically from rapid, excessive infusion of potassium into the bloodstream, as in patients receiving intravenous fluids. This would be considered an iatrogenic cause, meaning it results from a medical treatment or procedure **(Figure 15.13)**. Most other cases, though have to do with the kidneys and their ability to regulate what stays in the blood and gets excreted into the urine.

The kidney does this by the processes of filtration, reabsorption, and secretion in the nephron. First off, potassium is freely filtered from the blood into the urine at the glomerulus. After that, about 67% is reabsorbed in the proximal convoluted tubule, and an additional 20% is reabsorbed in the thick ascending limb, and that leaves about 13% of the initial amount. At this point, the distal tubule and collecting ducts of the nephron can either reabsorb or secrete potassium, depending on what the body needs **(Figure 15.14)**.

Now, reabsorption in this area is taken care of by the alpha-intercalated cells, while secretion is controlled by the principal cells. Typically for people on a normal diet, more potassium is secreted than reabsorbed at this stage, and it could be that all of the remaining potassium is secreted out if it's simply not needed **(Figure 15.15)**.

**Figure 15.16**

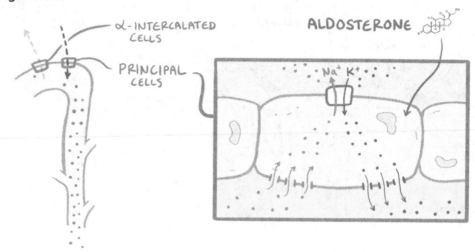

- α-INTERCALATED CELLS
- PRINCIPAL CELLS
- ALDOSTERONE
- Na⁺ K⁺

**Figure 15.17**

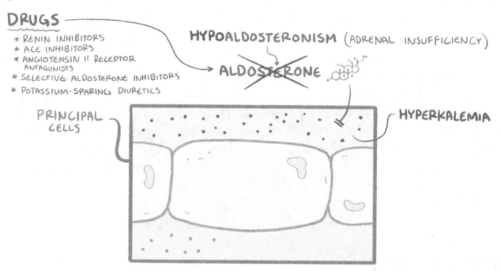

DRUGS
* RENIN INHIBITORS
* ACE INHIBITORS
* ANGIOTENSIN II RECEPTOR ANTAGONISTS
* SELECTIVE ALDOSTERONE INHIBITORS
* POTASSIUM-SPARING DIURETICS

HYPOALDOSTERONISM (ADRENAL INSUFFICIENCY)

~~ALDOSTERONE~~

PRINCIPAL CELLS

HYPERKALEMIA

**Figure 15.18**

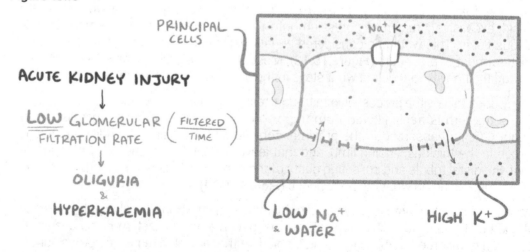

PRINCIPAL CELLS

ACUTE KIDNEY INJURY
↓
LOW GLOMERULAR FILTRATION RATE ( FILTERED / TIME )
↓
OLIGURIA & HYPERKALEMIA

Na⁺ K⁺

LOW Na⁺ & WATER

HIGH K⁺

Now, an important hormone that helps regulate potassium reabsorption or secretion in the kidneys is aldosterone. Aldosterone increases the number of sodium channels and the number of potassium channels on the lumen side of the principal cell as well as the number of sodium-potassium pumps on the basolateral side of the principal cells. This allows sodium to move from the tubule into the cell, and then to be pumped into the blood by the sodium-potassium pumps. As the pumps collectively move more sodium into the blood under the influence of aldosterone, more potassium is pumped into the cell, which raises the intracellular potassium concentration. Having more intracellular potassium and also having more potassium channels promotes potassium secretion **(Figure 15.16)**.

All that being said, in situations where somebody's unable to produce enough aldosterone, which is called hypoaldosteronism or adrenal insufficiency, there's less potassium secretion by the principal cells, and therefore more potassium is retained, leading to hyperkalemia. Along the same lines, drugs that reduce the effect of aldosterone can also cause hyperkalemia, and these are drugs like renin inhibitors, ACE inhibitors, angiotensin II receptor antagonists, selective aldosterone blockers, and potassium-sparing diuretics **(Figure 15.17)**.

Now, acute kidney injury can cause a low glomerular filtration rate, which is the volume of blood filtered through the kidney over a period of time, and this can lead to oliguria and hyperkalemia. In these situations, the nephron tries to hold on to salt and water, so by the time filtrate has moved into the distal tubule, there's very little of both sodium and water remaining in the lumen. Having little water in the lumen, creates a relatively high potassium concentration in the lumen. In addition to this, because less sodium is in the distal tubule, less of it moves through the luminal sodium channel into the principal cell and gets pumped over to the other side by the basolateral sodium-potassium pump. This means less potassium gets into the principal cell, creating a relatively low potassium concentration in the principal cell, leading to more potassium in the blood and hyperkalemia **(Figure 15.18)**.

## SYMPTOMS

All right, so there are all these ways to develop hyperkalemia, but what happens when somebody has hyperkalemia? Well, remember that the concentrations of potassium inside and outside of cells is really important for maintaining the resting cell membrane potential, and ultimately for allowing a cell to depolarize and a muscle to contract, and that includes the skeletal, smooth, and cardiac muscles. So, with too much potassium outside the cell, the membrane potential can become more positive, even to the point of causing contraction. Initially, this might cause mild intestinal cramping **(Figure 15.19)**.

But eventually, the resting membrane potential gets so high that it's above the threshold potential, meaning that once the muscle depolarizes and contracts, it can't repolarize to allow another contraction. In skeletal muscles, this can cause weakness and flaccid paralysis that starts in the lower extremities and ascends upward. Hyperkalemia also affects cardiac muscle contractions, which can lead to cardiac arrhythmias and cardiac arrest **(Figure 15.20)**.

## DIAGNOSIS

Hyperkalemia is diagnosed based on the presence of an elevated potassium levels in the blood, generally over 5.5 mEq/L. It's also important to get an electrocardiogram, which typically shows tall, peaked T waves with a narrow base best seen in the precordial leads $V_1$ through $V_6$, as well as a shortened QT interval, and ST-segment depression. In severe cases, hyperkalemia can also cause a prolonged PR interval, a diminished or absent P wave, and a widened QRS complex **(Figure 15.21)**.

**Figure 15.19**

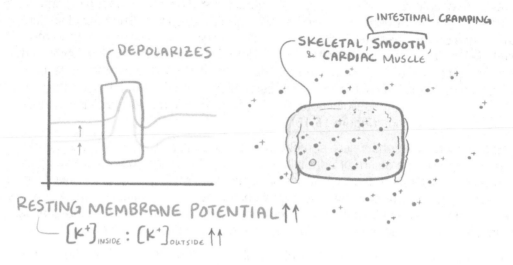

DEPOLARIZES

SKELETAL, SMOOTH, & CARDIAC MUSCLE

INTESTINAL CRAMPING

RESTING MEMBRANE POTENTIAL ↑↑
└ $[K^+]_{INSIDE} : [K^+]_{OUTSIDE}$ ↑↑

**Figure 15.20**

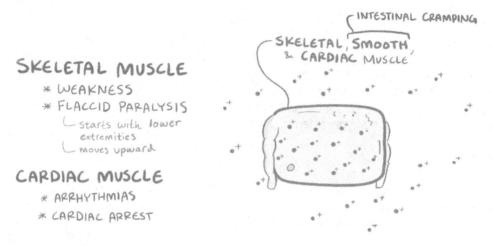

SKELETAL MUSCLE
* WEAKNESS
* FLACCID PARALYSIS
  └ starts with lower extremities
  └ moves upward

CARDIAC MUSCLE
* ARRHYTHMIAS
* CARDIAC ARREST

SKELETAL, SMOOTH, & CARDIAC MUSCLE

INTESTINAL CRAMPING

**Figure 15.21**

# DIAGNOSIS

* ↑ $[K^+]$ in BLOOD ~ > 5.5 mEq/L

* ELECTROCARDIOGRAM

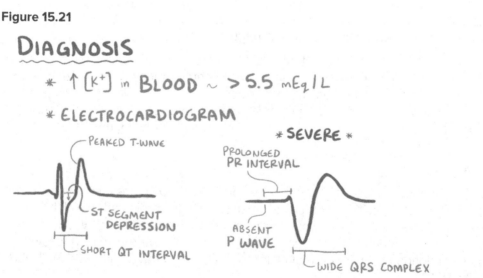

PEAKED T-WAVE

ST SEGMENT DEPRESSION

SHORT QT INTERVAL

* SEVERE *

PROLONGED PR INTERVAL

ABSENT P WAVE

WIDE QRS COMPLEX

## TREATMENT

With severe hyperkalemia, treatment might include using calcium to stabilize the myocardial cell membrane, using insulin, glucose, beta-adrenergic agonists, and sodium bicarbonate to shift potassium into the intracellular space, using resins that bind potassium to promote potassium elimination in the gastrointestinal tract, using potassium-wasting diuretics to promote potassium elimination in the kidneys, and in severe cases, dialysis.

## SUMMARY

All right, a quick recap: hyperkalemia describes a high concentration of potassium in the blood, which can be the result of shifts in internal potassium balance where potassium moves out of the body's cells, as well as external potassium balance problems having to do with the intake of potassium and typically the kidney's ability to regulate its excretion. Either way, the high potassium leads to muscle problems that could involve the smooth, skeletal, or cardiac muscles **(Figure 15.22)**.

**Figure 15.22**

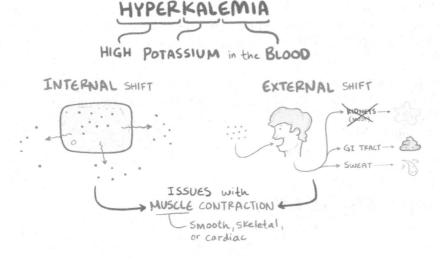

# Hypermagnesemia

osmosis.org/learn/hypermagnesemia

With hypermagnesemia, *hyper-* means "higher," *magnes-* refers to magnesium, and *-emia* refers to the blood, so hypermagnesemia means higher than normal magnesium levels in the blood. Symptoms typically develop at a level over 4 mEq/L **(Figure 16.1)**.

## PHYSIOLOGY

An average adult has about 25 grams of magnesium in their body. About half is stored in the bones, and most of the other half is found within the cells. In fact, magnesium is a really common positively charged ion found within the cell; it's second only to potassium. A very tiny fraction, roughly 1%, of the total magnesium in the body is in the extracellular space, which includes both the intravascular space, or the blood vessels and lymphatic vessels, and the interstitial space, or the space between cells **(Figure 16.2)**.

About 20% of the magnesium in the extracellular space, which would be about 0.2% of the total magnesium, is bound to negatively charged proteins like albumin. The other 80% of magnesium in the extracellular space, or 0.8% of the total magnesium, can be filtered into the kidneys **(Figure 16.3)**.

So inside the kidney, that magnesium gets filtered into the nephron, and about 30% is reabsorbed at the proximal convoluted tubule, 60% is reabsorbed in the ascending loop of Henle, and 5% is reabsorbed at the distal convoluted tubule. There's only 5% left, and that's excreted by the kidneys **(Figure 16.4)**.

**Figure 16.1**

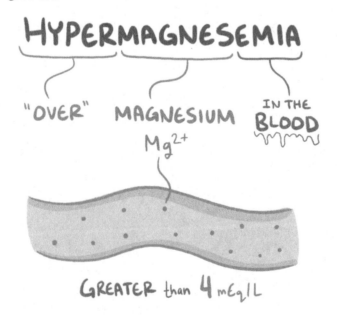

**Figure 16.2**

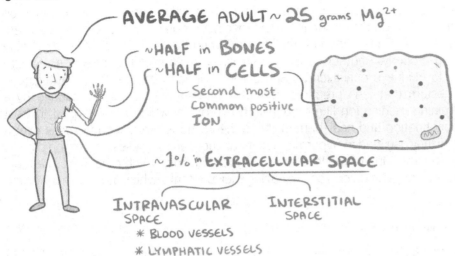

AVERAGE ADULT ~ 25 grams Mg²⁺

~HALF in BONES
~HALF in CELLS
    └ Second most common positive ION

~1% in EXTRACELLULAR SPACE

INTRAVASCULAR SPACE
    * BLOOD VESSELS
    * LYMPHATIC VESSELS

INTERSTITIAL SPACE

**Figure 16.3**

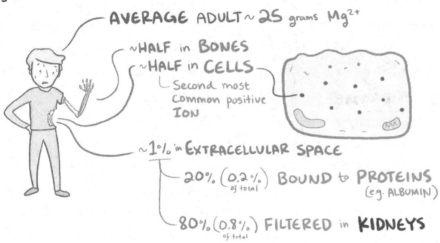

AVERAGE ADULT ~ 25 grams Mg²⁺

~HALF in BONES
~HALF in CELLS
    └ Second most common positive ION

~1% in EXTRACELLULAR SPACE

20% (0.2% of total) BOUND to PROTEINS (e.g. ALBUMIN)

80% (0.8% of total) FILTERED in **KIDNEYS**

**Figure 16.4**

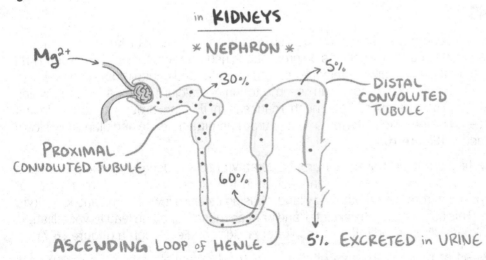

in **KIDNEYS**

* NEPHRON *

Mg²⁺

30%

5%
DISTAL CONVOLUTED TUBULE

PROXIMAL CONVOLUTED TUBULE

60%

ASCENDING LOOP of HENLE

5% EXCRETED in URINE

## CAUSES

So, in order for there to be too much magnesium in the blood, this normal balance has to be disturbed. The most common disruption is when those nephrons in the kidneys can't excrete magnesium properly. This can happen in renal failure, when the kidneys typically aren't able to excrete anything properly. Another cause of hypermagnesemia is the ingestion of more magnesium then the kidneys can excrete. Sometimes, this can be due to an intravenous infusion of magnesium that isn't prepared correctly. Other times, it can be caused by a magnesium containing medication like magnesium hydroxide, which can be used to treat symptoms like constipation and heartburn. If these medications are taken in excess over a long period of time, they can lead to hypermagnesemia. There are some less common causes of hypermagnesemia, too. One of these is tumor lysis syndrome, which results from a rapid number of cancer cells dying in unison and releasing their contents, which include magnesium **(Figure 16.5)**.

Figure 16.5

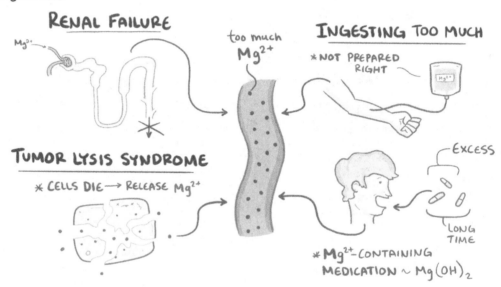

## SYMPTOMS

Hypermagnesemia can cause some serious complications. At the neuromuscular junction there are voltage-gated calcium channels on presynaptic neurons, and these need to open and let calcium in so that the neuron can release neurotransmitter and cause muscle contraction. Under normal circumstances, magnesium seems to inhibit calcium influx a little bit, which actually helps stabilize the axon. Too much magnesium floating around tends to inhibit calcium influx even more, which interferes with neurotransmitter release and ultimately slows muscle contraction **(Figure 16.6)**.

Also, normally the parathyroid hormone from the parathyroid gland usually stimulates calcium release into the blood. High levels of magnesium in the blood seem to inhibit release of parathyroid hormone from the parathyroid gland, causing calcium levels to fall and leading to hypocalcemia. This affects smooth, skeletal, and cardiac muscle and can lead to vasodilation, muscular weakness, diminished reflexes, respiratory failure, and even coma **(Figure 16.7)**.

Really high levels of magnesium also alter the electrical potential across the cardiac cell membrane, which can lead to cardiac arrhythmias like heart block and asystole **(Figure 16.8)**.

**Figure 16.6**

NEUROMUSCULAR JUNCTION

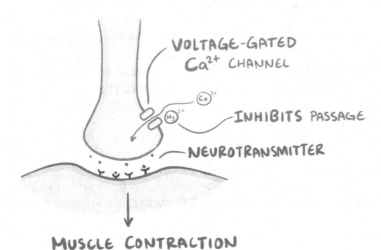

- VOLTAGE-GATED Ca²⁺ CHANNEL
- INHIBITS PASSAGE
- NEUROTRANSMITTER

MUSCLE CONTRACTION

**Figure 16.7**

PARATHYROID GLAND

HYPOCALCEMIA
- * VASODILATION
- * MUSCLE WEAKNESS
- * DIMINISHED REFLEXES
- * RESPIRATORY FAILURE
- * COMA

PARATHYROID HORMONE

~~CALCIUM RELEASE~~

HIGH MAGNESIUM

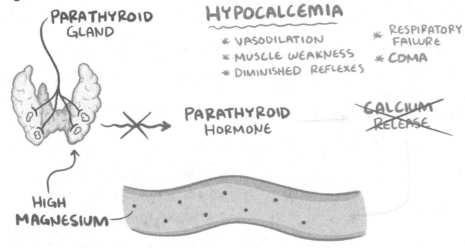

**Figure 16.8**

REALLY HIGH Mg²⁺ LEVELS

↓

ALTERS ELECTRICAL POTENTIAL ACROSS CARDIAC CELL MEMBRANE

↓

CARDIAC ARRHYTHMIAS
- * HEART BLOCK
- * ASYSTOLE

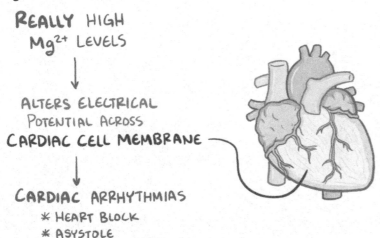

## TREATMENT

Anytime hypermagnesemia is causing symptoms, the level of free magnesium ions in the blood is usually over 4 meq/L. Treatment depends on the cause of hypermagnesemia. If it's due to excessive intake, then interrupting the source cures the condition. Because calcium and magnesium compete for binding, some of the symptoms of hypermagnesemia can be countered by injecting calcium, usually in the form of calcium gluconate, which acts as a physiological antagonist. Sometimes, furosemide can be used to promote kidney excretion of magnesium, and hemodialysis can also be used in severe cases **(Figure 16.9)**.

## SUMMARY

All right, as a quick recap: hypermagnesemia refers to an elevated free magnesium ion level that usually causes symptoms once it's over 4 meq/L. This can be caused by impaired excretion by the kidneys or an increased intake of magnesium. The excess magnesium antagonizes calcium and can lead to a neuromuscular blockade, causing symptoms like vasodilation, muscle weakness, and even cardiac arrhythmias.

**Figure 16.9**

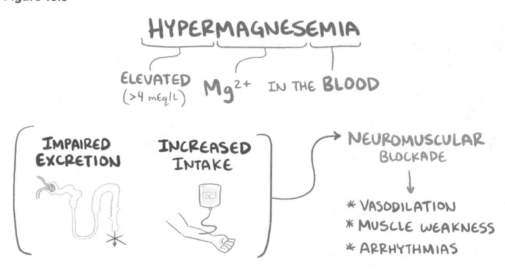

# Hypernatremia

**W**ith hypernatremia, *hyper-* means "above," *-natrium* is Latin for sodium, and *-emia* refers to the blood, so hypernatremia means a higher than normal concentration of sodium in the blood, generally above 145 mEq/L **(Figure 17.1)**.

## PHYSIOLOGY

The concentration of sodium in the blood depends on both sodium and water levels in the body. About 60% of our body weight comes from just water, and it basically sits in two places or fluid compartments: either outside the cells in the extracellular fluid or inside the cells in the intracellular fluid. The extracellular fluid includes the fluid in blood vessels, lymphatic vessels, and the interstitial space, which is the space between cells that is filled with proteins and carbohydrates. One third of the water in the body is in the extracellular compartment, whereas two thirds of it is in the intracellular compartment **(Figure 17.2)**.

Normally, the two compartments have the same osmolarity, or total solute concentration, and that allows water to move freely between the two spaces. But the exact composition of solutes differs quite a bit. The most common cation in the extracellular compartment is sodium, whereas in the intracellular compartment, it's potassium and magnesium. The most common anion in the extracellular compartment is chloride, whereas in the intracellular compartment, it's phosphate and negatively charged proteins. Of all of these, sodium is the ion the flits back and forth across cell membranes, and subtle changes in sodium concentration tilts the osmolarity balance in one direction or another and that moves water. This is why we say "wherever salt goes, water flows" **(Figure 17.3)**.

## PATHOLOGY

So, the concentration of sodium in the extracellular fluid, and therefore in the blood, can be increased either by losing more water than sodium or by gaining more sodium than water. An increased sodium concentration in the extracellular fluid draws water out of the cells. When hypernatremia develops over a long period of time, the cells get time to adapt and they start generating osmotically active particles to prevent the loss of free water via osmosis. However, when hypernatremia develops acutely, the cells get no time to adapt, and the loss of water leaves them shriveled up and can cause them to die **(Figure 17.4; Figure 17.5)**.

**Figure 17.1**

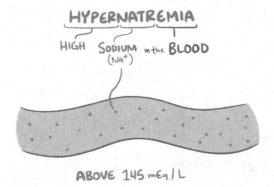

**Figure 17.2**

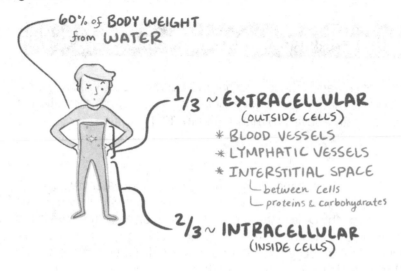

60% OF BODY WEIGHT from WATER

1/3 ~ **EXTRACELLULAR**
(OUTSIDE CELLS)
* BLOOD VESSELS
* LYMPHATIC VESSELS
* INTERSTITIAL SPACE
  └ between cells
  └ proteins & carbohydrates

2/3 ~ **INTRACELLULAR**
(INSIDE CELLS)

**Figure 17.3**

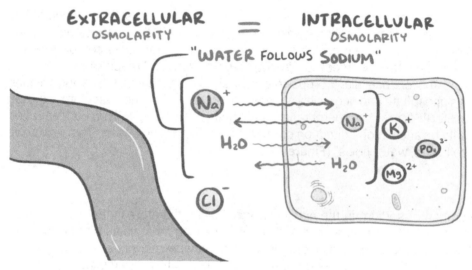

EXTRACELLULAR OSMOLARITY = INTRACELLULAR OSMOLARITY

"WATER FOLLOWS SODIUM"

**Figure 17.4**

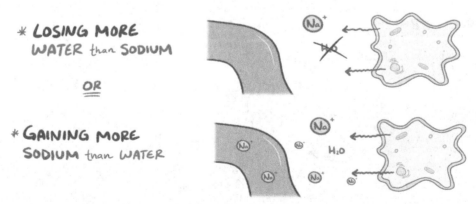

# HYPERNATREMIA
* HIGH CONCENTRATION *

* **LOSING MORE** WATER than SODIUM

OR

* **GAINING MORE** SODIUM than WATER

**Figure 17.5**

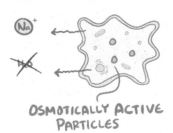

**HYPERNATREMIA**
* HIGH CONCENTRATION *

DEVELOPS OVER TIME
↳ CELLS ADAPT

Na⁺

H₂O

OSMOTICALLY ACTIVE
PARTICLES

**Figure 17.6**

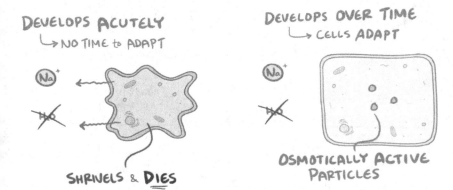

**HYPERNATREMIA**
* HIGH CONCENTRATION *

DEVELOPS ACUTELY
↳ NO TIME to ADAPT

Na⁺

H₂O

SHRIVELS & **DIES**

DEVELOPS OVER TIME
↳ CELLS ADAPT

Na⁺

H₂O

OSMOTICALLY ACTIVE
PARTICLES

## CAUSES

Now, all of us lose some free water everyday without even realizing it, like through sweat and normal breathing, since we breathe out humidified air. Under normal conditions, this loss is replaced by the water we drink, but this balance can be tipped when you have a high fever or exercise a lot on a hot summer day. In those situations, you can have temporary hypernatremia, which is easily fixed by drinking lots of water (**Figure 17.7**).

Another way that the body can lose free water is through the kidneys. When the nephrons filter blood and form urine, some of the water in the filtrate is reabsorbed in the distal convoluted tubule and the collecting duct. When you're dehydrated, antidiuretic hormone, also called ADH or vasopressin, gets released from the hypothalamus, and it boosts the nephron's ability to reabsorb water (**Figure 17.8**). So, if there's brain damage affecting the part of the hypothalamus that controls the release of ADH, then ADH levels could fall and the nephron wouldn't reabsorb as much water, making the urine dilute. This is called *central* diabetes insipidus because the fault lies *centrally*, in the hypothalamus (**Figure 17.9**). Another possibility is that the hypothalamus makes ADH normally, but the receptors in the kidney stop responding to it. This time the fault is in the kidneys, so it's known as *nephrogenic* diabetes insipidus. In both cases, the body loses free water and the sodium concentration goes up, causing hypernatremia.

**Figure 17.7**

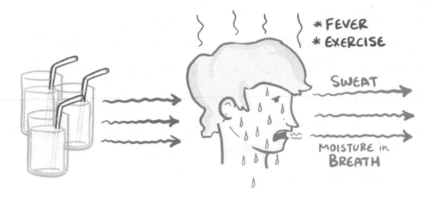

CAUSES ~ WATER LOSS

* FEVER
* EXERCISE

SWEAT

MOISTURE in BREATH

**Figure 17.8**

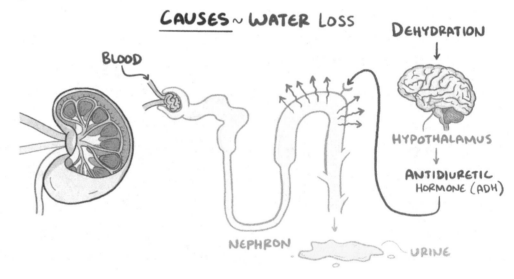

CAUSES ~ WATER LOSS

BLOOD

DEHYDRATION

HYPOTHALAMUS

ANTIDIURETIC HORMONE (ADH)

NEPHRON

URINE

**Figure 17.9**

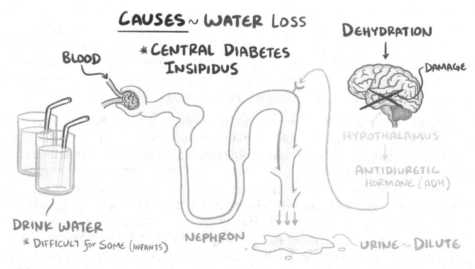

CAUSES ~ WATER LOSS

* CENTRAL DIABETES INSIPIDUS

BLOOD

DEHYDRATION

DAMAGE

HYPOTHALAMUS

ANTIDIURETIC HORMONE (ADH)

DRINK WATER
* DIFFICULT for SOME (INFANTS)

NEPHRON

URINE ~ DILUTE

**Figure 17.10**

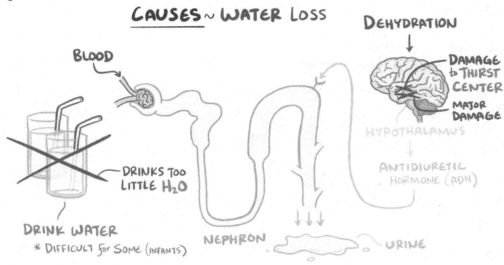

**Figure 17.11**

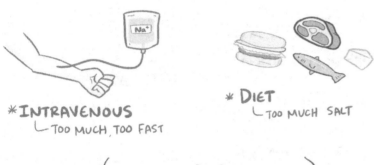

People with central and nephrogenic diabetes insipidus make up for losing too much water in their urine by just drinking more water. But any individual that doesn't compensate enough, like infants who can't drink water on their own, can develop severe hypernatremia.

Alternatively, there might be brain damage that only affects the thirst center in the hypothalamus rather than the ADH secreting part of the hypothalamus. Here, the kidneys aren't losing water, but the person is drinks too little water while still losing some through sweat, urination, and breathing, again resulting in hypernatremia. In rare cases, when there's major damage to the hypothalamus, ADH may not get released *and* the thirst center may be destroyed, which means that the person will lose a lot of water in the urine and still won't feel thirsty, which is a dangerous combination **(Figure 17.10)**.

Instead of a decrease in water, hypernatremia can also be caused by an increase in sodium. This happens most commonly when a patient in the hospital is given sodium intravenously to help increase their sodium level, and too much is given too quickly. This can also happen simply because there's too much salt in a person's diet. But in either situation, the kidneys usually do a good job of getting rid of too much sodium, so hypernatremia only usually happens under these conditions if there's a problem with how the kidneys are functioning **(Figure 17.11)**.

**Figure 17.12**

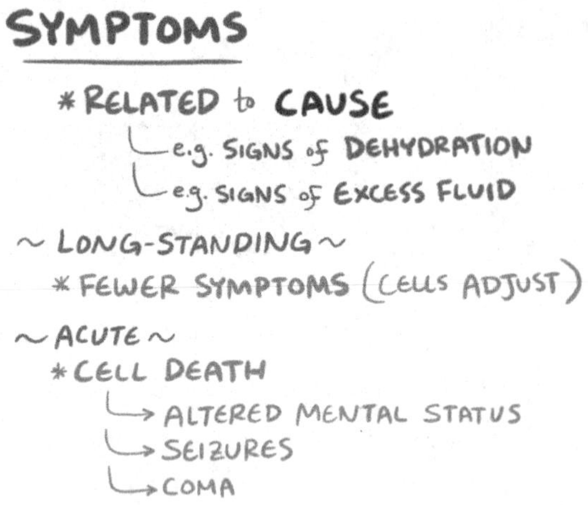

## SYMPTOMS

* RELATED to **CAUSE**
  - e.g. SIGNS of DEHYDRATION
  - e.g. SIGNS of EXCESS FLUID

~ LONG-STANDING ~
* FEWER SYMPTOMS (CELLS ADJUST)

~ ACUTE ~
* CELL DEATH
  - → ALTERED MENTAL STATUS
  - → SEIZURES
  - → COMA

**Figure 17.13**

## DIAGNOSIS

**BLOOD VOLUME**

HYPOVOLEMIC
~ LOW ~
* TOO LITTLE $H_2O$
* SWEATING TOO MUCH

* KIDNEYS LOSING $Na^+$
  - LOOP DIURETICS
  - DISEASE

EUVOLEMIC
~ NORMAL ~
* KIDNEYS DUMPING $H_2O$

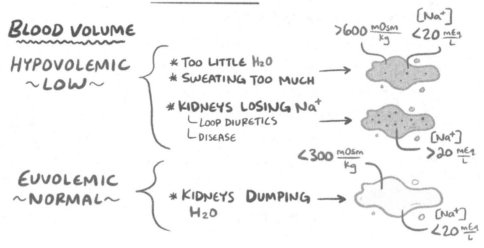

$>600 \frac{mOsm}{kg}$   $[Na^+] <20 \frac{mEq}{L}$

$[Na^+] >20 \frac{mEq}{L}$

$<300 \frac{mOsm}{kg}$

$[Na^+] <20 \frac{mEq}{L}$

**Figure 17.14**

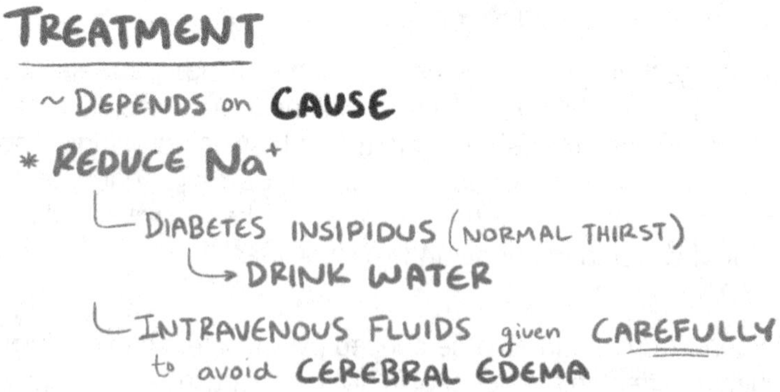

## TREATMENT

~ DEPENDS on **CAUSE**

* REDUCE $Na^+$
  - DIABETES INSIPIDUS (NORMAL THIRST)
    - → DRINK WATER
  - INTRAVENOUS FLUIDS given CAREFULLY to avoid **CEREBRAL EDEMA**

## SYMPTOMS

Symptoms of hypernatremia are related to the underlying cause. Patients may show signs of dehydration, or signs of excess fluid in their tissues. Long-standing hypernatremia typically causes fewer symptoms because the cells have a chance to adjust, whereas acute hypernatremia can cause cell death, particularly in the central nervous system, resulting in serious problems like altered mental status, seizures, or even a coma **(Figure 17.12)**.

## DIAGNOSIS

The first step in diagnosing hypernatremia is to figure out if a patient's intravascular volume is low, or "hypovolemic," or normal, or "euvolemic." If a person is hypovolemic, they're usually drinking too little water or sweating a lot. In this situation, the kidneys are trying to hold on to water by peeing out thick, concentrated urine with osmolarity of over 600 mOsm/kg. At the same time, the kidneys are also trying to preserve sodium so they have a urine sodium concentration less than 20 mEq/L. If the urine sodium concentration is higher than 20 mEq/L in a hypovolemic patient, it could be because the kidneys are doing a poor job at holding on to sodium ions. This could be the result of medications like osmotic and loop diuretics or even due to kidney disease. If a person is euvolemic, then it's usually because their kidneys are dumping water, like in diabetes insipidus. Their urine osmolality is usually below 300 mOsm/kg, and they have a urine sodium concentration less than 20 mEq/L **(Figure 17.13)**.

## TREATMENT

Treatment of hypernatremia depends on the underlying cause, but ultimately the goal is to reduce the sodium concentration in the blood. Individuals with diabetes insipidus with a normal thirst mechanism can do this by drinking water. If intravenous fluids have to be given, this has to be done carefully to avoid complications like cerebral edema **(Figure 17.14)**.

## SUMMARY

All right, as a quick recap: hypernatremia is an electrolyte disorder that describes a *high* concentration of sodium in the blood, which can be caused either by increased water loss or decreased water intake. Hypernatremia can cause water to shift out of the cells, and, in severe cases, it can cause brain cells to shrink and die. Diagnosing hypernatremia involves checking the volume status and measuring the urine osmolarity and urine sodium concentration. Treatment generally involves slowly and carefully giving back free water to normalize the sodium concentration over time **(Figure 17.15)**.

**Figure 17.15**

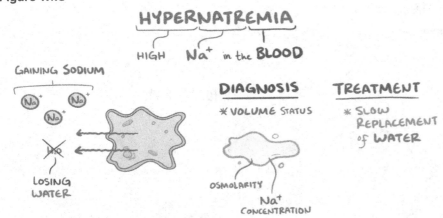

# Hyperphosphatemia

osmosis.org/learn/hyperphosphatemia

*H*yper- means over, *phosphat-* refers to phosphate, and *-emia* refers to the blood, so hyperphosphatemia means having a high phosphate level in the blood. Typically, that's above 4.5 mg/dL.

## PHYSIOLOGY

Now, phosphate is made up of one central phosphorus atom surrounded by four oxygen atoms in a tetrahedral arrangement, like a mini pyramid. It has a charge of minus 3, and it's written $PO_4^{3-}$ (**Figure 18.1**).

In the body, about 85% of the phosphate is stored in the bones, where it combines with calcium to make a tough compound called hydroxyapatite, which is the stuff that makes bones hard. Of the remaining phosphate, a tiny amount is extracellular, or outside cells, like in the blood, and this is the bit that gets measured. The majority of the phosphate is intracellular, or inside cells, where it does all sorts of things. It's responsible for phosphorylation, where it binds to fats and proteins. It forms the high energy bonds of adenosine triphosphate, or ATP, which is the most common energy currency in the cell. It's part of the DNA and RNA backbone that links individual nucleotides together, and it's also part of cellular signaling molecules like cyclic-adenosine monophosphate, or cAMP for short. The bottom line is that phosphate is super important (**Figure 18.2**).

Because most phosphate is locked up with calcium in the bones, the levels of phosphate are heavily tied to the levels of ionized calcium in the body. If calcium levels fall, the four parathyroid glands buried within the thyroid gland will release parathyroid hormone, which frees up both calcium and phosphate ions from the bones. Parathyroid hormone does this by stimulating osteoclasts, the cells that break bone down, to release hydrogen ions, which dissolve the hard, mineralized hydroxyapatite. As soon as the positively-charged calcium and negatively-charged phosphate are released from the bones, they grab onto each other again like a pair of star-crossed lovers, meaning that the ionized calcium level doesn't really go up very much at all (**Figure 18.3**).

Figure 18.1

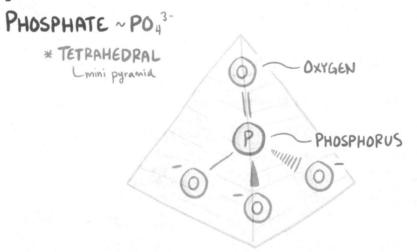

PHOSPHATE ~ $PO_4^{3-}$

\* TETRAHEDRAL
 └ mini pyramid

OXYGEN

PHOSPHORUS

Figure 18.2

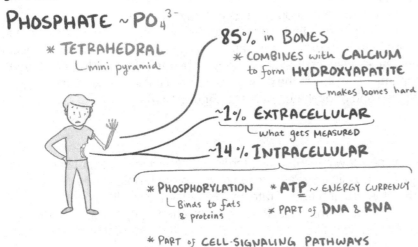

Figure 18.3

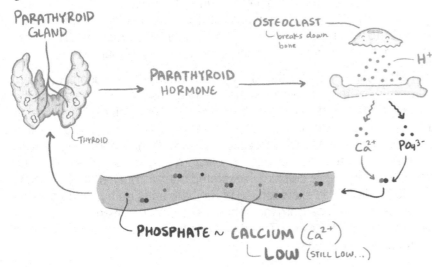

Figure 18.4

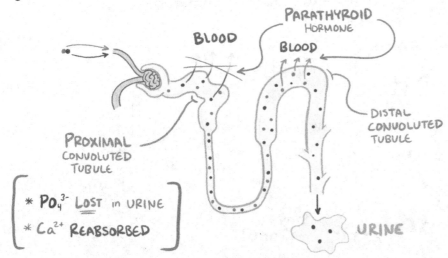

Now, these two make their way to the nephron of the kidney, and at this point in the proximal convoluted tubule, phosphate usually gets reabsorbed back into the blood via sodium-phosphate cotransporters. It turns out, though, that parathyroid hormone also shuts this process down. That means that phosphate is left in the lumen and then eventually sent out in the urine. Now, that calcium's still in the lumen, but parathyroid hormone also affects the distal convoluted tubule and increases calcium reabsorption. So, when the dust settles, parathyroid hormone results in phosphate being lost in the urine while ionized calcium is kept in the blood, so ionized calcium levels rise and phosphate levels fall **(Figure 18.4)**.

## CAUSES

With all that in mind, we can see how hyperphosphatemia might develop, and that can happen a few different ways. The first possibility is as a result of acute or chronic kidney disease. So, let's say that normally the glomerular filtration rate, or GFR, which is the fluid filtered into the kidney per unit time, is 180 L / day. If the phosphate concentration of that blood is 0.04 g / L, that means that 7.2 g of phosphate is filtered per day. Let's say that 90% of that is reabsorbed, so that's 6.48 g, leaving 10%, or 0.72 grams, to be excreted per day.

Now, with kidney disease, the GFR falls to 28.8 L/day, which means only 1.2 g of phosphate is filtered per day and that only 0.12 g is excreted in a day. So, where there were 0.72 grams being excreted per day, now there's only 0.12 g. That means that the difference stays in the blood every day, and this contributes to hyperphosphatemia. This number, 28.8 L/day, or 20 mL/min, is the point at which it's thought that excretion can't keep up with intake **(Figure 18.5)**.

Hyperphosphatemia can also happen when the kidneys are unable to reabsorb calcium, which means that more is excreted. Remember that in response to low calcium, the parathyroid glands release parathyroid hormone. However, since calcium keeps being wasted, the parathyroid gland keeps releasing parathyroid hormone. This condition is called secondary hyperparathyroidism because the primary problem is with the kidneys. Secondary hyperparathyroidism causes a continuous release of calcium and phosphate from the bones, sort of like an open tap. Here, while calcium is excreted due to impaired reabsorption, phosphate is reabsorbed due to impaired excretion, so phosphate ends up building up in the blood. To make matters worse, all this loss from the bones makes them thin and weak, which is part of a process called renal osteodystrophy. This describes the overall bone changes that happen in people with chronic kidney disease.

**Figure 18.5**

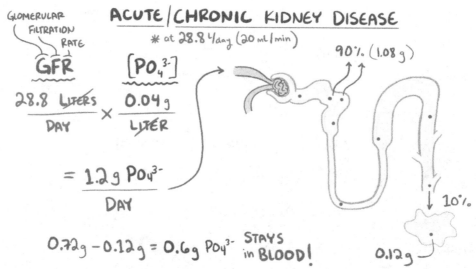

**Figure 18.6**

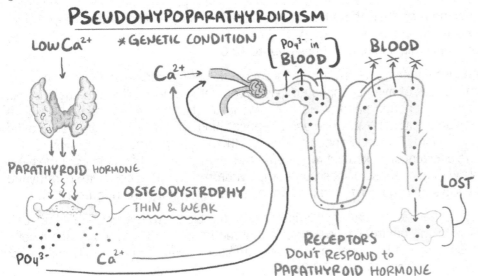

## PSEUDOHYPOPARATHYROIDISM

*GENETIC CONDITION

Low Ca²⁺

$PO_4^{3-}$ in BLOOD

BLOOD

Ca²⁺

PARATHYROID HORMONE

OSTEODYSTROPHY
THIN & WEAK

$PO_4^{3-}$    Ca²⁺

LOST

RECEPTORS
DON'T RESPOND to
PARATHYROID HORMONE

**Figure 18.7**

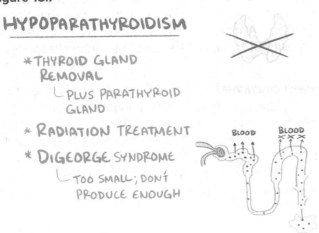

## HYPOPARATHYROIDISM

* THYROID GLAND
  REMOVAL
  └ PLUS PARATHYROID
    GLAND

* RADIATION TREATMENT

* DIGEORGE SYNDROME
  └ TOO SMALL; DON'T
    PRODUCE ENOUGH

BLOOD    BLOOD

**Figure 18.8**

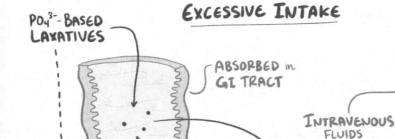

## EXCESSIVE INTAKE

$PO_4^{3-}$-BASED
LAXATIVES

ABSORBED in
GI TRACT

INTRAVENOUS
FLUIDS

$PO_4^+$

Related to this is pseudohypoparathyroidism, which is where the kidneys simply don't respond to parathyroid hormone because of a genetic defect in the parathyroid hormone receptor. Since parathyroid hormone tells the kidneys to save calcium and get rid of phosphate, calcium is again lost while phosphate builds up in the blood, following the same pattern as kidney disease, including the thinning of the bones **(Figure 18.6)**.

All right, so because parathyroid hormone causes excretion of phosphate and reabsorption of calcium, another cause of hyperphosphatemia is hypoparathyroidism, where the parathyroid glands don't produce enough parathyroid hormone in the first place. Hypoparathyroidism results in the same situation of increased reabsorption of phosphate and decreased reabsorption of calcium. This can happen following a thyroid gland removal surgery when the parathyroids are accidentally taken out too or after radiation treatment for cancer of the head or neck. People with the genetic disease DiGeorge syndrome are often born with parathyroid glands that are too small and can't produce enough parathyroid hormone **(Figure 18.7)**.

Alternatively, phosphate levels can rapidly increase in the blood from excessive intake and absorption through the gastrointestinal tract or through the bloodstream via intravenous fluids. One cause is taking too much of a phosphate-based laxative either orally, as pills or liquid, or rectally, as an enema **(Figure 18.8)**.

A final cause of hyperphosphatemia relates to the fact that most phosphate in the body is within the cells. Any time a lot of cells die, that phosphate is spilled into the bloodstream, causing hyperphosphatemia. This cause includes things like crush injuries, like when a piano falls on someone's legs, or tumor lysis syndrome, which is cancer treatment that causes lots of tumor cells to die all at once, or rhabdomyolysis, which is the rapid destruction of skeletal muscle cells **(Figure 18.9)**.

Another situation is when living cells are affected by respiratory acidosis, which is when the carbon dioxide levels rise because a person isn't breathing or ventilating it out of the lungs quickly enough. That carbon dioxide can diffuse into a cell and react with water to form carbonic acid which quickly breaks into a proton and bicarbonate. The bicarbonate goes back into the blood in exchange for a chloride ion, leaving behind a proton. All this ends up lowering the cellular pH. Now, normally glycolysis in the cell uses up a lot of phosphate, but this lower pH tends to inhibit glycolysis. As a result, the cells don't pull as much phosphate out of the blood, and this allows levels in the blood to rise.

**Figure 18.9**

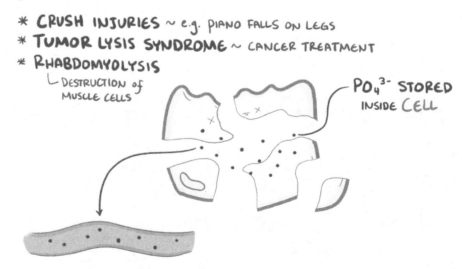

**Figure 18.10**

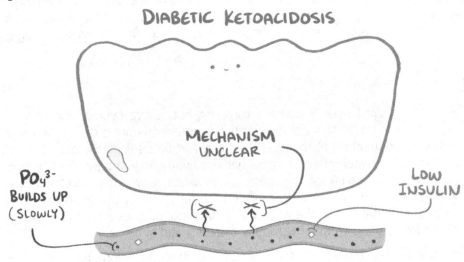

DIABETIC KETOACIDOSIS

MECHANISM UNCLEAR

$PO_4^{3-}$ BUILDS UP (SLOWLY)

LOW INSULIN

**Figure 18.11**

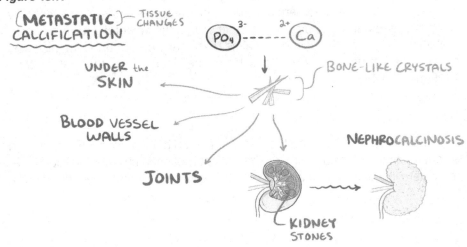

(METASTATIC) CALCIFICATION — TISSUE CHANGES

$PO_4^{3-}$ ----- $Ca^{2+}$

BONE-LIKE CRYSTALS

UNDER the SKIN

BLOOD VESSEL WALLS

JOINTS

KIDNEY STONES

NEPHROCALCINOSIS

**Figure 18.12**

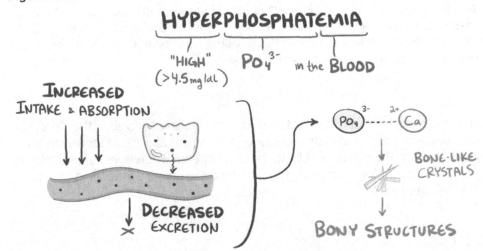

HYPERPHOSPHATEMIA

"HIGH" (>4.5 mg/dL) $PO_4^{3-}$ in the BLOOD

INCREASED INTAKE & ABSORPTION

DECREASED EXCRETION

$PO_4^{3-}$ ----- $Ca^{2+}$

BONE-LIKE CRYSTALS

BONY STRUCTURES

Somewhat similarly, in diabetic ketoacidosis, there are low levels of insulin. Although the exact mechanism is unclear, this reduces the amount of phosphate that cells extract from the blood, causing it to build up in the blood. In this case, though, it's a slower process, since there's also an osmotic diuresis, or increased urination, from the hyperglycemia, or high blood sugar (**Figure 18.10**).

## SYMPTOMS

Mild hyperphosphatemia doesn't usually cause symptoms, but severe hyperphosphatemia can make neurons more excitable. This can trigger the spontaneous firing of neurons and tetany, or the involuntary contraction of muscles. This can end up causing Chvostek's sign, which is when facial muscles twitch after the facial nerve is lightly finger tapped 1 cm below the zygomatic process. It can also cause Trousseau's sign, which is where a blood pressure cuff occludes the brachial artery, and that pressure on the nerve is enough to make it fire, resulting in a muscle spasm that makes the wrist and metacarpophalangeal joints flex. It can also cause symptoms like tingling around the mouth, seizures, and bone pain.

High levels of phosphate also cause phosphate to find and stick to calcium, forming bone-like crystals containing calcium and phosphate in places that they shouldn't be, like just beneath the skin, in the walls of blood vessels, in the joints, or in the kidneys, where they can form kidney stones. With long-term hyperphosphatemia, the whole kidney can eventually turn into bone, which is called nephrocalcinosis. In other words, flesh literally turns to bone. This widespread calcification of healthy tissues is called metastatic calcification. In this case, *metastatic* means that the tissue rapidly changes from one thing to another, rather than referring to cancer (**Figure 18.11**).

## DIAGNOSIS

Diagnosis of hyperphosphatemia is based on the phosphate level being above 4.5 mg/dL, and treatment involves decreasing phosphate intake. This is accomplished by avoiding foods that contain a lot of phosphate like dairy, meat, and soda; in other words, no more pepperoni pizza with cola.

## TREATMENT

To decrease the amount of phosphate that's absorbed from the gastrointestinal tract, people can given medications called phosphate binders. Now, you can also try to increase excretion of phosphate, and in people with healthy kidneys, a combination of intravenous saline and a loop diuretic like furosemide can increase excretion. This is called forced diuresis, and it essentially overwhelms the proximal convoluted tubule of the nephron with so much fluid that it's unable to effectively reabsorb solutes, including phosphate.

## SUMMARY

All right, as a quick recap: hyperphosphatemia describes high phosphate levels in the blood, so above 4.5 mg/dL. This can result from increased absorption and intake, decreased excretion, or a shift of phosphate from the inside of cells to the bloodstream. High levels of phosphate ions in the blood also like to bind with calcium, forming bone-like crystals that can slowly turn into bony structures (**Figure 18.12**).

# Hypocalcemia

**W**ith hypocalcemia, *hypo-* means below, *calc-* refers to calcium, and *-emia* refers to the blood, so hypocalcemia means *lower* than normal calcium levels in the blood, so generally less than 8.5 mg/dL **(Figure 19.1)**.

## PHYSIOLOGY

Now, calcium, or $Ca^{2+}$, exists as an ion with a double positive charge, and it's the most abundant metal in the human body. So, I know what you're thinking; yeah, we're all pretty much cyborgs. Anyway, about 99% of that calcium is in our bones in the form of calcium phosphate, also called hydroxyapatite. The last 1% is split so that the majority, about 0.99%, is extracellular, which means in the blood and in the interstitial space between cells, and 0.01% is intracellular **(Figure 19.2)**.

**Figure 19.1**

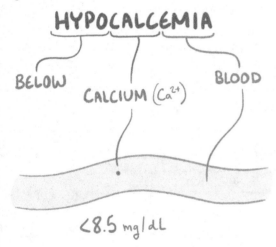

**Figure 19.2**

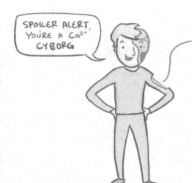

**Figure 19.3**

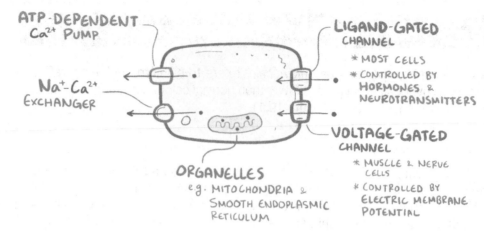

**Figure 19.4**

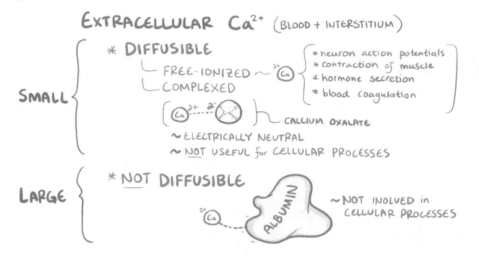

**Figure 19.5**

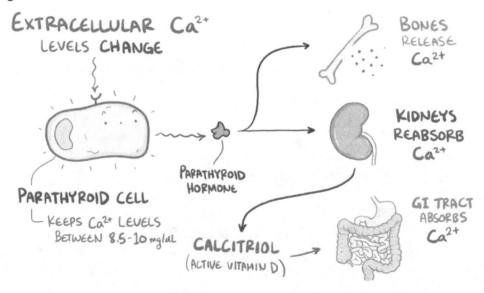

High levels of intracellular calcium cause cells to die. In fact, that's exactly what happens during apoptosis, which is also known as programmed cell death. For that reason, cells end up using a ton of energy just by keeping their intracellular calcium levels low. Now, calcium gets into the cell through two types of channels, or cell doors, within the cell membrane. The first type are ligand-gated channels, which are what most cells use to let calcium in, and these are primarily controlled by hormones or neurotransmitters. The second type are voltage-gated channels, which are mostly found in muscle and nerve cells, and these are primarily controlled by changes in the electrical membrane potential. So, calcium flows in through these channels, and to prevent calcium levels from getting too high, cells kick excess calcium right back out with ATP-dependent calcium pumps as well as sodium calcium exchangers. In addition, most of the intracellular calcium is stored within organelles like the mitochondria and smooth endoplasmic reticulum, and it's released only when it's needed **(Figure 19.3)**.

Now, the majority of the extracellular calcium, the calcium in the blood and interstitium, is split almost equally between two groups: calcium that is diffusible and calcium that is not diffusible. Diffusible calcium is separated into two subcategories. First, there's free-ionized calcium, which is involved in all sorts of cellular processes, like neuronal action potentials, contraction of skeletal, smooth, and cardiac muscle, hormone secretion, and blood coagulation, all of which are tightly regulated by enzymes and hormones. The other category is complexed calcium, which is where the positively charged calcium is ionically linked to tiny negatively charged molecules like oxalate, a small anion that normally found in our blood in small amounts. The complexed calcium forms a molecule that's electrically neutral but, unlike free-ionized calcium, is not useful for cellular processes. Both of these are called diffusible because they're small enough to diffuse across cell membranes. Finally, there's the non-diffusible calcium, which is bound to negatively charged proteins like albumin. The resulting protein-calcium complex is too large and charged to cross membranes, leaving this calcium also uninvolved in cellular processes **(Figure 19.4)**.

Changes in the body's levels of extracellular calcium are detected by a surface receptor in parathyroid cells that's called the calcium-sensing receptor. These changes affect the amount of parathyroid hormone that's released by the parathyroid gland. The parathyroid hormone gets the bones to release calcium, it gets the kidneys to reabsorb more calcium so it's not lost in the urine, and it synthesizes calcitriol, which is also known as 1,25-dihydroxycholecalciferol, or active Vitamin D. Active Vitamin D then goes on to cause the gastrointestinal tract to increase calcium absorption. Altogether, these effects help to keep the extracellular levels of calcium within a narrow range that's between 8.5 to 10 mg/dl **(Figure 19.5)**.

**Figure 19.6**

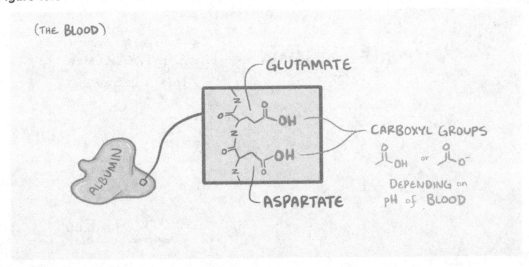

**Figure 19.7**

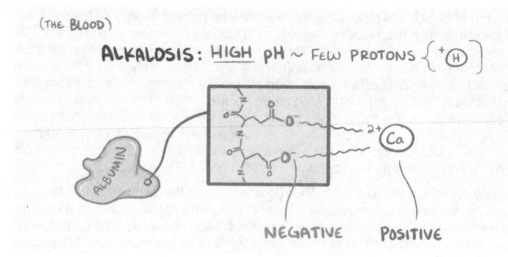

(THE BLOOD)

ALKALOSIS: HIGH pH ~ FEW PROTONS { $^+$(H) }

NEGATIVE      POSITIVE

**Figure 19.8**

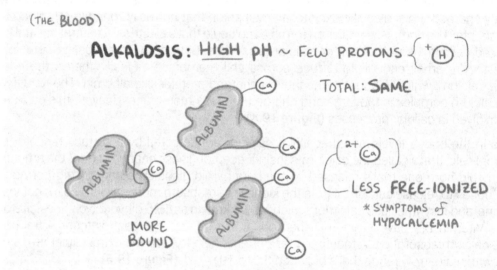

(THE BLOOD)

ALKALOSIS: HIGH pH ~ FEW PROTONS { $^+$(H) }

TOTAL: SAME

LESS FREE-IONIZED
*SYMPTOMS of HYPOCALCEMIA

MORE BOUND

**Figure 19.9**

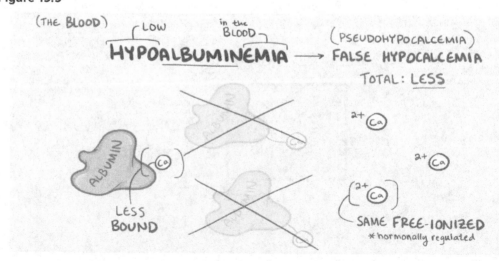

(THE BLOOD)      LOW      in the BLOOD      (PSEUDOHYPOCALCEMIA)

HYPOALBUMINEMIA → FALSE HYPOCALCEMIA

TOTAL: LESS

LESS BOUND

SAME FREE-IONIZED
*hormonally regulated

Sometimes, though, total calcium levels in the blood, a measurement that includes both diffusible and non-diffusible calcium, can vary a bit thanks to the blood's pH and protein levels. This happens because albumin has acidic amino acids, like glutamate and aspartate, which have some carboxyl groups that are in the form of COO- or COOH. Overall, the balance of COO- and COOH changes based on the pH of the blood **(Figure 19.6)**.

When there's a high pH, or alkalosis, there are very few protons floating around, and so those carboxyl groups tend to be in the COO- form. More COO- groups tend to make albumin negatively charged, and since calcium is positively charged, opposites attract, and the negatively charged albumin latches onto calcium, which means there's more bound calcium and less free-ionized calcium in the blood **(Figure 19.7)**.

So that means that even though the total levels of calcium are the same, there's *less* ionized calcium, and that's the one that's important for cellular processes. This can lead to symptoms of hypocalcemia **(Figure 19.8)**.

Also, any condition that results in hypoalbuminemia or low albumin levels, would lead to a loss of bound calcium, while at the same time free ionized calcium concentrations stay essentially the same due to hormonal regulation. This is therefore called *false hypocalcemia* or *pseudohypocalcemia*, since there's less overall calcium due to less bound calcium but the free ionized calcium levels are still the same **(Figure 19.9)**.

## CAUSES

All right, so too little calcium in the blood, which is true hypocalcemia, can be caused either by less calcium entering the blood or by too much calcium leaving the blood. Less calcium entering the blood is the most common cause of hypocalcemia, and this can be due to hypoparathyroidism, which means lower levels or lower activity of parathyroid hormone. Hypoparathyroidism can be caused by surgical removal or autoimmune destruction of the parathyroid gland, by congenital problems involving the parathyroid gland, like DiGeorge syndrome, or by magnesium deficiency, since magnesium is needed for parathyroid hormone production. Low levels of vitamin D can also lead to hypocalcemia, and these can be caused by a deficient diet, malabsorption, cirrhosis, lack of sunlight, or chronic renal failure, among other causes **(Figure 19.10)**.

**Figure 19.10**

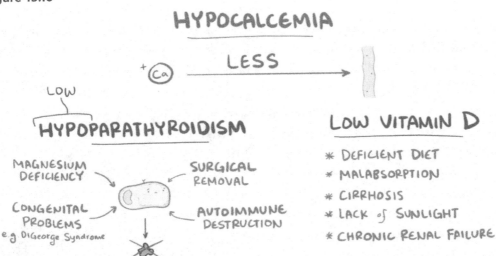

**Figure 19.11**

# HYPOCALCEMIA

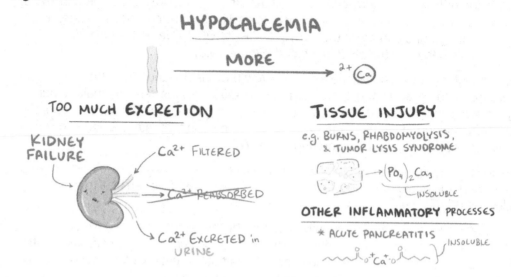

MORE ⟶ $Ca^{2+}$

## TOO MUCH EXCRETION

KIDNEY FAILURE

$Ca^{2+}$ FILTERED

$Ca^{2+}$ REABSORBED

$Ca^{2+}$ EXCRETED in URINE

## TISSUE INJURY

e.g. BURNS, RHABDOMYOLYSIS, & TUMOR LYSIS SYNDROME

⟶ $(PO_4)_2Ca_3$ — INSOLUBLE

### OTHER INFLAMMATORY PROCESSES

* ACUTE PANCREATITIS

$Ca^+$ — INSOLUBLE

**Figure 19.12**

# HYPOCALCEMIA

## * TOO MANY BLOOD TRANSFUSIONS *

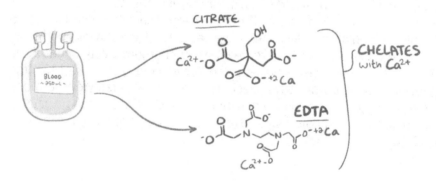

CITRATE

$Ca^{2+}$ $+2Ca$

CHELATES with $Ca^{2+}$

EDTA

$+2Ca$

$Ca^{2+}$

BLOOD ~250mL~

**Figure 19.13**

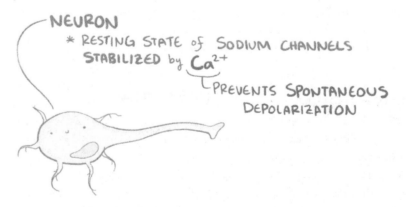

NEURON
* RESTING STATE of SODIUM CHANNELS STABILIZED by $Ca^{2+}$
— PREVENTS SPONTANEOUS DEPOLARIZATION

**Figure 19.14**

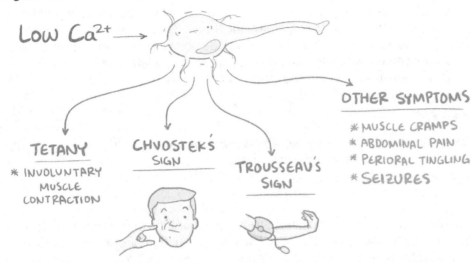

Then, there's the second cause of hypocalcemia, which is too much calcium leaving the blood. This might happen when too much ionized calcium is excreted. Normally, calcium filters from the blood into the glomerulus of the kidney, but then it's reabsorbed back into the blood by the nephron so that it isn't lost. In kidney failure, the nephron doesn't effectively re-absorb calcium, which means that calcium is excreted into the urine. Another cause of calcium leaving the blood is tissue injury, like burns, rhabdomyolysis, and tumor lysis syndrome, where large numbers of cells die and release intracellular phosphate into the blood. This phosphate binds to the ionized calcium and forms calcium phosphate, making the calcium insoluble and effectively decreasing the total amount of calcium in the blood. Other inflammatory processes can also cause too much calcium to leave the blood; for example, in acute pancreatitis, free fatty acids end up binding to ionized calcium, making it insoluble and precipitating out as a soap-like substance **(Figure 19.11)**.

Finally, ionized calcium levels can fall as a result of having too many blood transfusions. This is because additives to the blood, like citrate and ethylenediaminetetraacetic acid, or EDTA, can chelate or bind to calcium, forming complexed calcium, which is an inactive molecule **(Figure 19.12)**. Low levels of ionized calcium affect a variety of cellular processes, particularly those involving electrically active neurons. Normally, the resting state of sodium channels is stabilized by calcium ions, which prevent them from spontaneously opening and potentially causing depolarization **(Figure 19.13)**.

When levels of extracellular calcium are low, voltage-gated sodium channels are less stable and more likely to open up, allowing the cell to depolarize more easily and making the neuron more excitable. This can trigger tetany, or the involuntary contraction of muscles, a classic symptom of hypocalcemia. The spontaneous firing of neurons also causes Chvostek's sign, which is when facial muscles twitch after the facial nerve is lightly finger tapped 1 cm below the zygomatic process. It also can cause Trousseau's sign, which is where the pressure from a blood pressure cuff occluding the brachial artery is enough to make it fire, resulting in a muscle spasm that makes the wrist and metacarpophalangeal joints flex. Other symptoms of low extracellular calcium include muscle cramps, abdominal pain, perioral tingling which is tingling around the mouth, and in extreme cases, seizures **(Figure 19.14)**.

## DIAGNOSIS

Hypocalcemia is diagnosed based on a low level of calcium in the blood, meaning that it's generally below 8.5 mg/dL. An electrocardiogram might show changes, such as a prolonged QT, prolonged ST segment, and arrhythmias, like torsade de pointes and atrial fibrillation. To identify the cause of hypocalcemia, healthcare professionals conduct lab tests for parathyroid hormone, Vitamin D, albumin, phosphorus, and magnesium.

## TREATMENT

The main goal of treatment is to normalize calcium levels using formulations like calcium gluconate, and if appropriate, Vitamin D supplementation.

## SUMMARY

All right, as a quick recap: hypocalcemia describes a low concentration of free ionized calcium in the blood, which most commonly results from defective production of calcium controlling hormones, like parathyroid hormone and active Vitamin D. Low calcium levels, can cause certain excitable cells to be even more excitable, resulting in tetany, muscle spasms, and cardiac dysfunction (**Figure 19.15**).

**Figure 19.15**

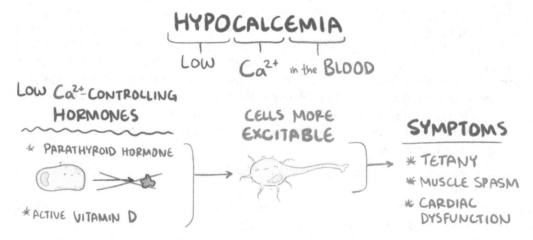

# Hypokalemia

osmosis.org/learn/hypokalemia

With hypokalemia, *hypo-* means under, *kal-* refers to potassium, and *-emia* refers to the blood, so hypokalemia means lower than normal potassium levels in the blood, which generally means under 3.5 mEq/L.

## PHYSIOLOGY

Total body potassium can essentially be split into two components, intracellular and extracellular potassium, or potassium inside and outside the cells. The extracellular component includes both the intravascular space, the space within the blood and lymphatic vessels and the interstitial space, the space between cells where you typically find fibrous proteins and long chains of carbohydrates that are called glycosaminoglycans. The vast majority, around 98%, of all of the body's potassium is intracellular, or inside the cells **(Figure 20.1)**.

In fact, the concentration of potassium inside the cells is about 150 mEq/L, whereas outside the cells, it's only about 4.5 mEq/L. Keep in mind that these potassium ions carry a charge, so the difference in concentration also leads to a difference in charge, which establishes an overall electrochemical gradient across the cell membrane **(Figure 20.2)**.

This is called the internal potassium balance. This balance is maintained by the sodium-potassium pump, which pumps two potassium ions in for every three sodium ions out, as well as potassium leak channels and inward rectifier channels that are scattered throughout the membrane. This concentration gradient is extremely important for setting the resting membrane potential of excitable cell membranes, which is needed for normal contraction of smooth, cardiac, and skeletal muscle **(Figure 20.3)**.

In addition to this internal potassium balance, there's also an external potassium balance, which refers to the potassium you get externally through the diet every day. On a daily basis, the amount of potassium that typically gets taken in usually ranges between 50 mEq/L to 150 mEq/L, which is way higher than the extracellular potassium concentration of 4.5 mEq/L, so your body has to figure out a way to excrete most of what it takes in. This external balancing act is largely taken care of by the kidneys, where excess potassium is secreted into a renal tubule and excreted in the urine. A small amount of dietary potassium is also lost via the gastrointestinal tract and the sweat **(Figure 20.4)**.

**Figure 20.1**

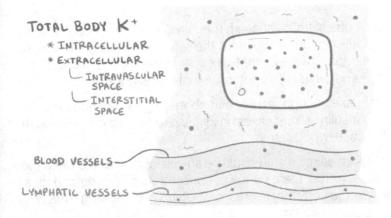

TOTAL BODY K⁺
* INTRACELLULAR
* EXTRACELLULAR
  └ INTRAVASCULAR SPACE
  └ INTERSTITIAL SPACE

BLOOD VESSELS
LYMPHATIC VESSELS

**Figure 20.2**

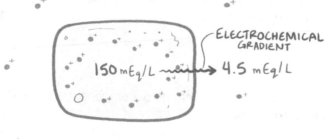

TOTAL BODY K⁺
* INTRACELLULAR (~98%)
* EXTRACELLULAR (~2%)

ELECTROCHEMICAL
GRADIENT
150 mEq/L → 4.5 mEq/L

**Figure 20.3**

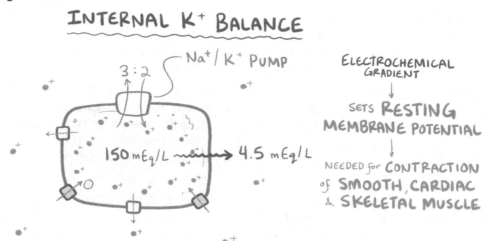

INTERNAL K⁺ BALANCE

Na⁺/K⁺ PUMP
3:2

ELECTROCHEMICAL
GRADIENT
↓
SETS RESTING
MEMBRANE POTENTIAL
↓
NEEDED for CONTRACTION
of SMOOTH, CARDIAC
& SKELETAL MUSCLE

150 mEq/L → 4.5 mEq/L

## INTERNAL CAUSES

So, in order for there to be too little potassium in the blood, or hypokalemia, there are two possibilities, the first is an external balance shift most often caused by an increase in potassium excretion in the kidneys, which lowers the level of potassium in the blood, and the second is an internal balance shift where potassium moves into the cells from the interstitium and blood **(Figure 20.5)**.

One potential cause of an internal potassium balance shift is having excess insulin. This is because, after a meal, glucose increases in the blood, and at the same time insulin is released, which binds to cells and stimulates the uptake of that glucose. Insulin also increases the activity of the sodium/potassium pump, which pulls potassium into cells **(Figure 20.6)**.

People with Type I diabetes don't make enough insulin, and so they use exogenous insulin, meaning an injection or infusion of insulin. In rare cases, insulin overdose can cause enough potassium uptake into cells as to cause hypokalemia.

Another cause of an internal potassium balance shift could be an alkalosis, which is when the blood becomes too alkaline. In other words, there's a lower concentration of hydrogen ions, meaning a higher blood pH. One way the body can decrease blood pH is by moving hydrogen

**Figure 20.4**

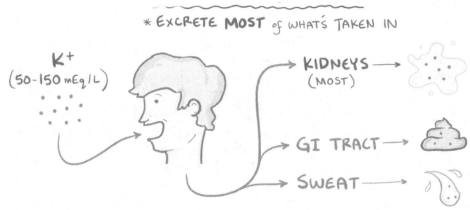

**Figure 20.5**

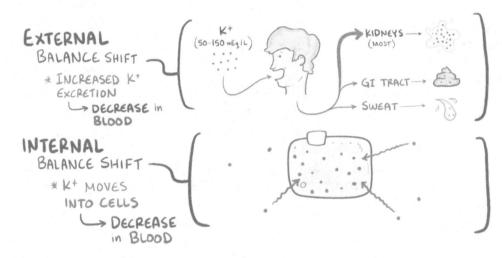

ions out of cells and into the blood. To accomplish this, cells use a special ion transporter that exchanges the hydrogen ion for a potassium ion across the cell membrane. So, in order to help compensate for an alkalosis, hydrogen ions leave cells and potassium ions enter the cells and leave the blood, resulting in hypokalemia.

That being said, not all acid-base disturbances affect potassium levels. For example, in respiratory alkalosis due to low carbon dioxide levels in the blood, potassium levels aren't typically affected because CO2 is lipid soluble and freely moves into or out of cells without being exchanged for potassium; therefore, it doesn't lead to hypokalemia **(Figure 20.7)**.

Certain catecholamines can shift potassium movement into cells via the beta-2-adrenergic and alpha-adrenergic receptors on cell membranes. When activated, beta-2-adrenergic receptors stimulate the sodium-potassium pump, pulling potassium from the blood into cells. Meanwhile, alpha-adrenergic receptors cause a shift of potassium out of cells via calcium-dependent potassium channels. So, beta-2-adrenergic agonists and alpha-adrenergic antagonists both cause a shift in potassium into cells and out of the blood **(Figure 20.8)**.

**Figure 20.6**

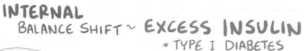

INTERNAL BALANCE SHIFT ~ **EXCESS INSULIN**
* TYPE I DIABETES

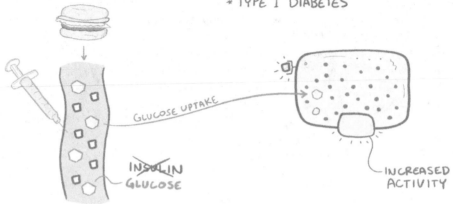

GLUCOSE UPTAKE

INSULIN
GLUCOSE

INCREASED ACTIVITY

**Figure 20.7**

INTERNAL BALANCE SHIFT ~ RESPIRATORY **ALKALOSIS** ~ <u>NO</u> HYPOKALEMIA

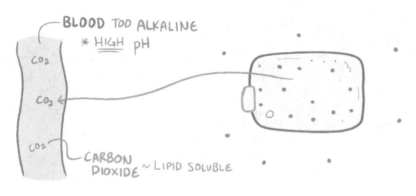

BLOOD TOO ALKALINE
* <u>HIGH</u> pH

$CO_2$

$CO_2$

$CO_2$

CARBON DIOXIDE ~ LIPID SOLUBLE

**Figure 20.8**

INTERNAL BALANCE SHIFT ~ CERTAIN **CATECHOLAMINES**

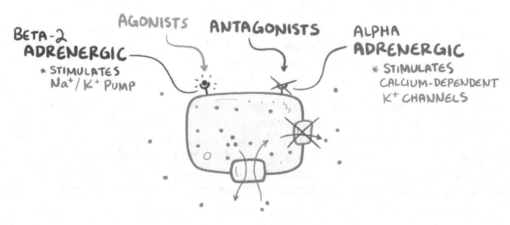

AGONISTS    ANTAGONISTS

BETA-2 **ADRENERGIC**
* STIMULATES $Na^+/K^+$ PUMP

ALPHA **ADRENERGIC**
* STIMULATES CALCIUM-DEPENDENT $K^+$ CHANNELS

# EXTERNAL CAUSES

All right, on to external potassium balance shifts resulting in hypokalemia, which has to do with potassium intake or excretion. With regards to intake, not taking enough potassium in can lead to hypokalemia, like in cases of anorexia, prolonged fasting, or specific types of diets. Most other cases, though, have to do with the kidney's ability to regulate what stays in the blood and gets excreted into the urine. The kidney does this by the processes of filtration, reabsorption, and secretion in the nephron **(Figure 20.9)**.

First off, potassium is freely filtered from the blood into the urine at the glomerulus. After that, about 67% is reabsorbed in the proximal convoluted tubule, and an additional 20% is reabsorbed in the thick ascending limb. And that leaves 13% of the initial amount, right? At this point, the distal tubule and collecting ducts of the nephron can either reabsorb or secrete potassium depending on what the body needs **(Figure 20.10)**.

Now, reabsorption in this area is taken care of by the alpha-intercalated cells, while secretion is controlled by the principal cells. Typically for people on a normal diet, more potassium is secreted than reabsorbed at this stage, and it could even be that all of the remaining potassium is secreted out if it's simply not needed.

Now, an important hormone that helps regulate potassium reabsorption or secretion in the kidneys is aldosterone. Aldosterone increases the number of sodium channels on the lumen side of the principal cell and and sodium-potassium pumps on the basolateral side of the principal cells. This allows sodium to move from the tubule into the cell, and then get pumped into the blood by the sodium-potassium pumps. As the pumps collectively move more sodium into the blood under the influence of aldosterone, more potassium gets pumped into the cell, which raises the intracellular potassium concentration. Having more intracellular potassium and also having more potassium channels promotes potassium secretion **(Figure 20.11)**.

Having said all that, in situations where somebody produces too much aldosterone, like primary hyperaldosteronism, there's more potassium secretion by the principal cells, meaning more gets excreted, and that means less potassium is retained, causing hypokalemia. Other pathological conditions that cause increased aldosterone levels include compensated heart failure and cirrhosis **(Figure 20.12)**.

Commonly used diuretics, like loop diuretics and thiazide diuretics, also increase potassium excretion and can lead to hypokalemia. These diuretics inhibit sodium reabsorption upstream of the principal cells, which means more sodium is delivered downstream to the principal cells. As a result, more sodium enters the principal cells and is available for the sodium-potassium pump, which pumps sodium out into the blood and pumps potassium into the cell, creating a relatively high potassium concentration in the principal cell. These diuretics also allow more water to remain in the lumen, creating a relatively low potassium concentration in the lumen. Together, a relatively high potassium concentration in the principal cell and a relatively low potassium concentration in the lumen increase the potassium gradient and cause a lot of potassium to get secreted and excreted in the urine, leading to hypokalemia **(Figure 20.13)**.

Another external balance shift causing hypokalemia is increased losses of gastrointestinal secretions, typically due to vomiting and diarrhea. Now, the upper GI tract actually only secretes a small amount of potassium, so direct losses via vomiting are usually minimal. But the loss of stomach acid leads to metabolic alkalosis, which as we already saw, can lead to hypokalemia. Relative to the upper GI tract, the lower GI tract secretes more potassium, so more gets directly lost in the feces in cases of chronic diarrhea, like those from infections, inflammatory bowel diseases, and laxative abuse **(Figure 20.14)**.

Finally, a very small amount of potassium is also lost in sweat, which could be relevant for individuals who exercise a lot in a hot climate.

**Figure 20.9**

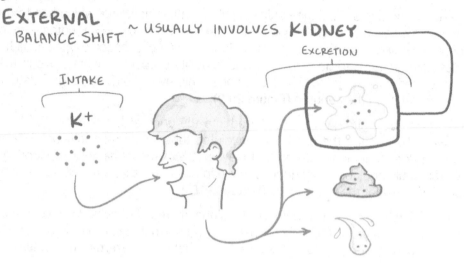

**Figure 20.10**

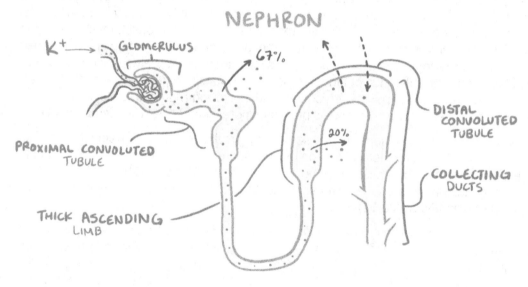

**Figure 20.11**

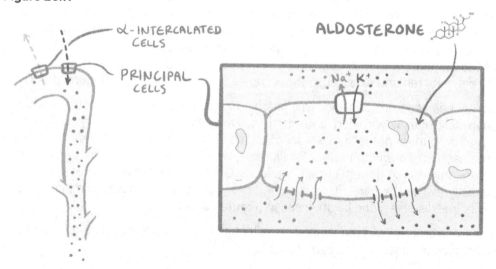

**Figure 20.12**

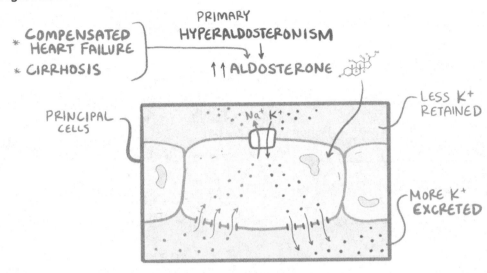

**Figure 20.13**

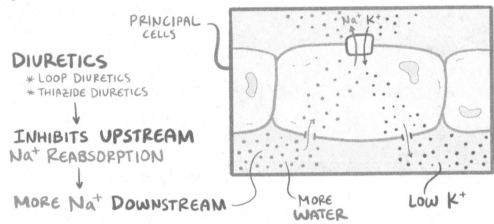

**Figure 20.14**

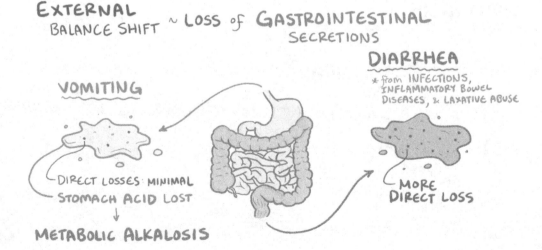

**Figure 20.15**

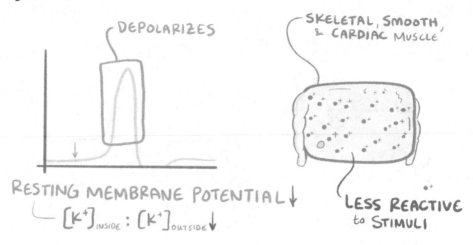

DEPOLARIZES

SKELETAL, SMOOTH, & CARDIAC MUSCLE

RESTING MEMBRANE POTENTIAL↓
└ $[K^+]_{INSIDE} : [K^+]_{OUTSIDE}$ ↓

LESS REACTIVE to STIMULI

**Figure 20.16**

DIMINISHED CONTRACTIONS of...

* SMOOTH MUSCLE
  └→ CONSTIPATION

* SKELETAL MUSCLE
  └→ WEAKNESS
  └→ CRAMPS
  └→ FLACCID PARALYSIS

* RESPIRATORY MUSCLES
  └→ RESPIRATORY DEPRESSION

* CARDIAC MUSCLES
  └→ ARRHYTHMIAS & CARDIAC ARREST

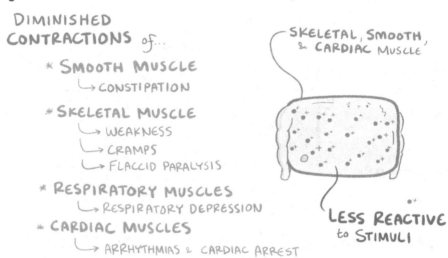

SKELETAL, SMOOTH, & CARDIAC MUSCLE

LESS REACTIVE to STIMULI

**Figure 20.17**

DIAGNOSIS

* LOW POTASSIUM ($< 3.5$ mEq/L)

* ELECTROCARDIOGRAM

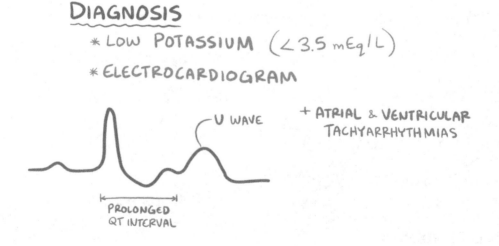

U WAVE

+ ATRIAL & VENTRICULAR TACHYARRHYTHMIAS

PROLONGED QT INTERVAL

## SYMPTOMS

All right, so there are all these ways to develop hypokalemia, but what happens when somebody has hypokalemia? Well, remember that the concentrations of potassium inside and outside of cells is really important for maintaining the resting cell membrane potential, and ultimately for allowing a cell to depolarize and a muscle to contract, and that includes all of the skeletal, smooth, and cardiac muscles. So, with low potassium in the blood, the membrane potential can hyperpolarize, or become more negative. This means that these muscle cells become less reactive to stimuli **(Figure 20.15)**.

Diminished contractions of smooth muscles can lead to constipation. Diminished skeletal muscle contractions can lead to muscle weakness, cramps, and flaccid paralysis, which tends to begins in the lower extremities and ascends upward. Respiratory muscles may also be affected, which leads to respiratory depression. Finally, hypokalemia can affect cardiac muscle contractions, which can lead to cardiac arrhythmias as well as cardiac arrest **(Figure 20.16)**.

## DIAGNOSIS & TREATMENT

Hypokalemia is diagnosed based on the presence of low levels of potassium in the blood, generally below 3.5 mEq/L. It's also important to get an electrocardiogram, which typically shows a prolonged QT interval, appearance of a U wave, and atrial or ventricular tachyarrhythmias **(Figure 20.17)**.

In patients with severe hypokalemia, the main goal of treatment is to normalize potassium levels. This is done by reducing ongoing potassium losses by treating underlying causes like vomiting and diarrhea, using potassium-sparing diuretics if diuretic therapy is required, and replenishing potassium stores with supplementation.

## SUMMARY

All right, as a quick recap: hypokalemia describes a low concentration of potassium in the blood, which can be the result of internal potassium balance shift where potassium moves into the body's cells, as well as an external potassium balance shift having to do with either low intake or high excretion of potassium. Either way, the low potassium levels leads to issues with muscle contractions of smooth, skeletal, or cardiac muscles **(Figure 20.18)**.

**Figure 20.18**

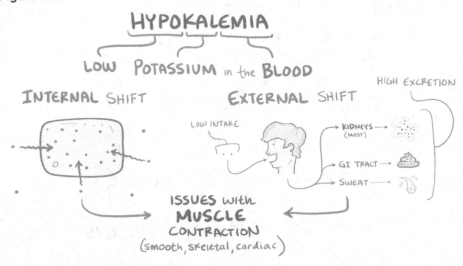

# Hypomagnesemia

osmosis.org/learn/hypomagnesemia

**W**ith hypomagnesemia, *hypo-* means "lower," *magnes-* refers to magnesium, and *-emia* refers to the blood, so hypomagnesemia means lower than normal magnesium levels in the blood. Symptoms typically develop at a level below 1 mEq/L **(Figure 21.1)**.

An average adult has about 25 grams of magnesium in their body. About half is stored in the bones, and most of the other half is found within the cells. In fact, magnesium is a really common positively charged ion found within the cell; it's second only to potassium. A very tiny fraction, roughly 1%, of the total magnesium in the body is in the extracellular space, which includes both the intravascular space, or the blood vessels and lymphatic vessels, and the interstitial space, or the space between cells. About 20% of the magnesium in the extracellular space, which would be about 0.2% of the total magnesium, is bound to negatively charged proteins like albumin. The other 80% of magnesium in the extracellular space, or 0.8% of the total magnesium, can be filtered into the kidneys **(Figure 21.2)**.

**Figure 21.1**

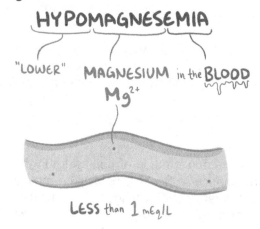

**Figure 21.2**

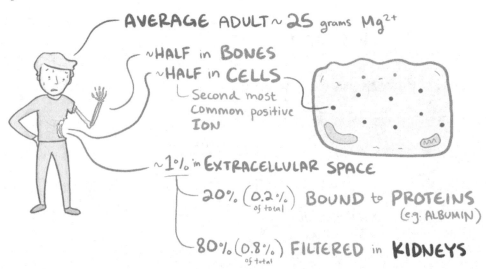

**Figure 21.3**

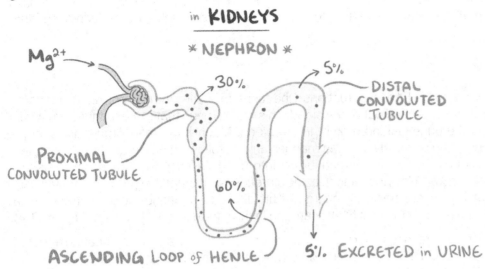

**Figure 21.4**

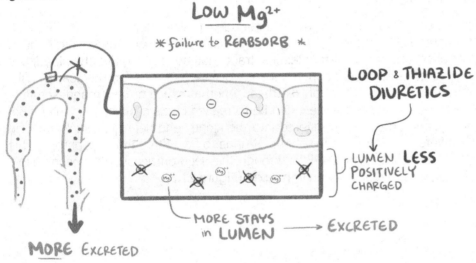

**Figure 21.5**

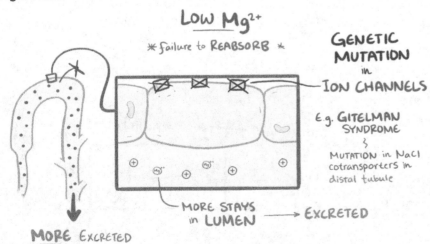

Inside the kidney, that magnesium gets filtered into the nephron. About 30% is reabsorbed at the proximal convoluted tubule, 60% is reabsorbed in the ascending loop of Henle, and 5% is reabsorbed at the distal convoluted tubule. The last 5% is excreted by the kidneys (**Figure 21.3**).

## CAUSES

Magnesium levels can fall in a few situations. One scenario is when the nephron fails to reabsorb the magnesium that's filtered out of the blood. This would mean that more magnesium would be excreted in the urine instead of kept in the blood. Magnesium reabsorption is mostly a passive process. The positively charged magnesium ion follows the electrochemical gradient and moves from the positively charged lumen into the cells lining the lumen, which usually have a negative charge. Now, loop and thiazide diuretics can disrupt that process because they both make the lumen less positively charged. This diminishes magnesium's electrochemical gradient, causing more of the ions to stick around in the filtrate and get peed out (**Figure 21.4**).

Another scenario where magnesium levels can fall is when there's a genetic mutation affecting channels regulating ion flow. Again, this could change the electrochemical gradient and cause more magnesium to stick around in the lumen and then be peed out. An example of this is Gitelman syndrome, where there's a mutation in the gene coding for the Na-Cl cotransporters in the distal tubule (**Figure 21.5**).

Another mechanism for hypomagnesemia is prolonged malnutrition, where not enough magnesium is consumed. Alternatively, enough magnesium may be consumed, but enough of it might not be absorbed in the gastrointestinal tract. Instead of going into the blood, this magnesium is excreted—this could happen because of interference from medications like proton pump inhibitors or from a bout of diarrhea. Another cause of hypomagnesemia is uncontrolled diabetes mellitus, where there can be increased levels of glucose in the blood. This means that there's more glucose filtered into the kidney and nephron, which ends up attracting a lot of water, causing a large volume of urine to flow through the nephrons. This high flow carries ions like magnesium right through the nephron because it doesn't allow enough time for magnesium reabsorption to happen (**Figure 21.6**).

**Figure 21.6**

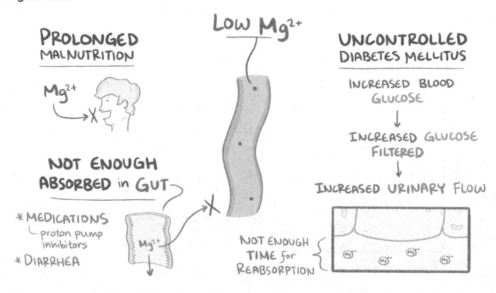

**Figure 21.7**

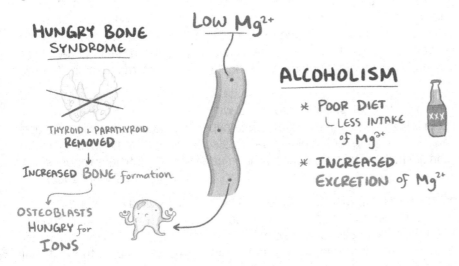

**Figure 21.8**

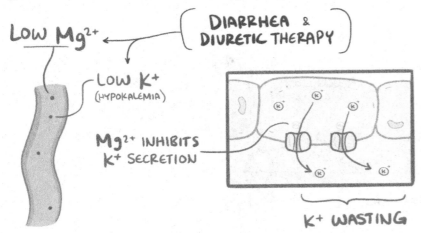

**Figure 21.9**

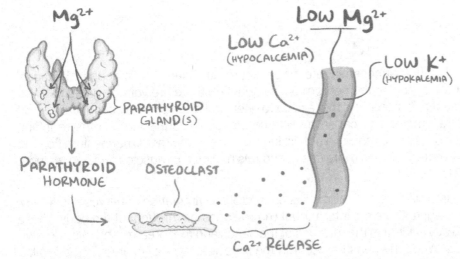

Yet another cause of hypomagnesemia is hungry bone syndrome, which is when the thyroid or the parathyroid glands are surgically removed, leading to increased bone formation. In this case, the osteoblasts, or bone-forming cells, are literally hungry for ions to make more mineralised matrix, and they consume the blood's magnesium. Alcoholism can contribute to hypomagnesemia in two ways: often these individuals have a poor diet, meaning they might have low magnesium intake; also, alcohol increases renal excretion of magnesium **(Figure 21.7)**.

Low magnesium in the blood is commonly associated with low potassium in the blood, or hypokalemia, because a lot of the conditions that cause hypomagnesemia, like diarrhea and diuretic therapy, are also responsible for hypokalemia. It's also thought that magnesium in the cells of the nephron can get in the way of potassium channels a little bit. With less magnesium, more potassium is secreted, excreted, and wasted, leading to hypokalemia **(Figure 21.8)**.

Now, severe hypomagnesemia can also lead to low calcium in the blood, or hypocalcemia, since the parathyroid gland needs magnesium in order to release parathyroid hormone, which normally causes osteoclast cells to release calcium from the bones into the blood. So, without magnesium, there's impaired release of parathyroid hormone. It's also thought that magnesium is needed in order to respond to parathyroid hormone as well, so less magnesium means less calcium in the blood here, too **(Figure 21.9; Figure 21.10)**.

**Figure 21.10**

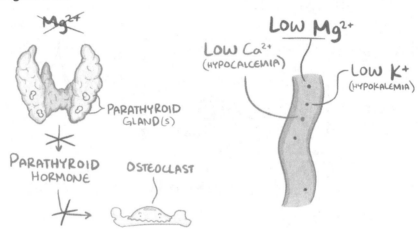

## SYMPTOMS

Early symptoms of hypomagnesemia are often neuromuscular. This happens because, under normal circumstances, at the neuromuscular junction there are voltage-gated calcium channels on presynaptic neurons, and these need to open and let calcium in so that the neuron can release neurotransmitter and cause muscle contraction. Magnesium seems to inhibit calcium influx a little bit, and this ends up stabilizing the axon. So, without magnesium floating around, calcium can enter neurons more easily, and this makes the muscles and nerves more excitable **(Figure 21.11)**.

This can lead to neuromuscular symptoms like uncontrolled stimulation of nerves and tetany, which is a condition where there are intermittent muscle spasms throughout the body. These spasms are particularly evident in the muscles of the hands and the forearm, and this is known as Trousseau's sign. When the spasms occur in the muscles of facial expression, it's called Chvostek's sign. Severe hypomagnesemia can even lead to convulsions or seizures, as well as abnormal heart rhythms **(Figure 21.12)**.

**Figure 21.11**

NEUROMUSCULAR JUNCTION

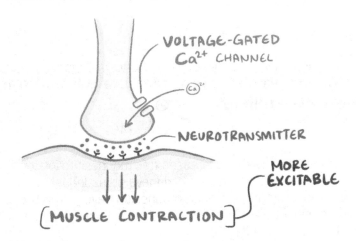

VOLTAGE-GATED Ca²⁺ CHANNEL

Ca²⁺

NEUROTRANSMITTER

MORE EXCITABLE

[MUSCLE CONTRACTION]

**Figure 21.12**

NEUROMUSCULAR SYMPTOMS

* UNCONTROLLED NERVE STIMULATION

* TETANY ~ INTERMITTENT MUSCLE SPASMS

* SEIZURES
* CONVULSIONS
* ABNORMAL HEART RHYTHMS

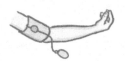

TROUSSEAU SIGN

CHOVSTEK SIGN

**Figure 21.13**

HYPOMAGNESEMIA

LOW    Mg²⁺    in the BLOOD

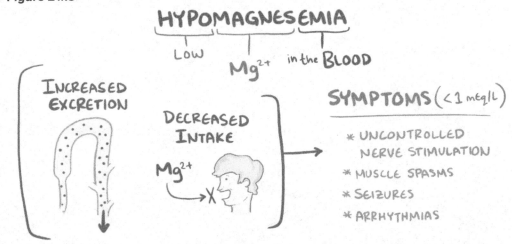

INCREASED EXCRETION

DECREASED INTAKE

Mg²⁺ → X

SYMPTOMS (< 1 meq/L)

* UNCONTROLLED NERVE STIMULATION
* MUSCLE SPASMS
* SEIZURES
* ARRHYTHMIAS

## DIAGNOSIS

Hypomagnesemia is usually diagnosed by measuring the level of free unbound magnesium in the serum or by doing a 24-hour urine collection.

## TREATMENT

Treatment here depends on the cause, and if hypomagnesemia is due to inadequate intake, then it can be supplemented orally. In more severe cases, magnesium can be given in the form of magnesium sulphate either intravenously or intramuscularly.

## SUMMARY

All right, as a quick recap: hypomagnesemia refers to a decreased free magnesium ion levels in the blood. This can be caused by excessive excretion by the kidneys or inadequate intake of magnesium. These situations can lead to symptoms once magnesium levels drop below 1 meq/L, and these symptoms include uncontrolled firing of the neurons, leading to muscle spasms, seizures, and cardiac arrhythmias **(Figure 21.13)**.

# Hyponatremia

With hyponatremia, *hypo-* means "under" or "low," *-natrium* is Latin for sodium, and *-emia* refers to the blood, so hyponatremia means a lower than normal concentration of sodium in the blood, generally below 135 mEq/L **(Figure 22.1)**.

## PHYSIOLOGY

The concentration of sodium in the blood depends on both sodium and water levels in the body. About 60% of our body weight comes from just water, and it basically sits in two places or fluid compartments: either outside the cells in the extracellular fluid or inside the cells in the intracellular fluid. The extracellular fluid includes the fluid in blood vessels, lymphatic vessels, and the interstitial space, which is the space between cells that is filled with proteins and carbohydrates. One third of the water in the body is in the extracellular compartment, whereas two thirds of it is in the intracellular compartment **(Figure 22.2)**.

Normally, the two compartments have the same osmolarity, or total solute concentration, and that allows water to move freely between the two spaces. But the exact composition of solutes differs quite a bit. The most common cation in the extracellular compartment is sodium, whereas in the intracellular compartment, it's potassium and magnesium. The most common anion in the extracellular compartment is chloride, whereas in the intracellular compartment, it's phosphate and negatively charged proteins. Of all of these, sodium is the ion the flits back and forth across cell membranes, and subtle changes in sodium concentration tilts the osmolarity balance in one direction or another and that moves water. This is why we say "wherever salt goes, water flows" **(Figure 22.3)**.

**Figure 22.1**

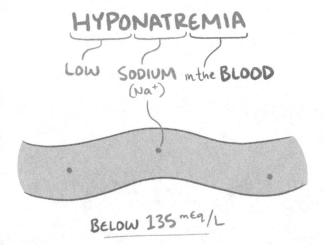

## PATHOLOGY

That being said, hyponatremia, or low concentration of sodium in the extracellular fluid and therefore the blood, can be caused by either *losing* more sodium than water, or *gaining* more water than sodium. Broadly speaking, hyponatremia can be divided into three categories based on water volume status **(Figure 22.4)**.

**Figure 22.2**

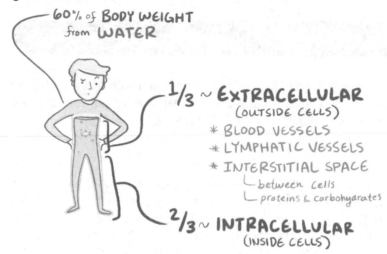

60% of BODY WEIGHT from WATER

1/3 ~ **EXTRACELLULAR**
(OUTSIDE CELLS)
* BLOOD VESSELS
* LYMPHATIC VESSELS
* INTERSTITIAL SPACE
    └ between cells
    └ proteins & carbohydrates

2/3 ~ **INTRACELLULAR**
(INSIDE CELLS)

**Figure 22.3**

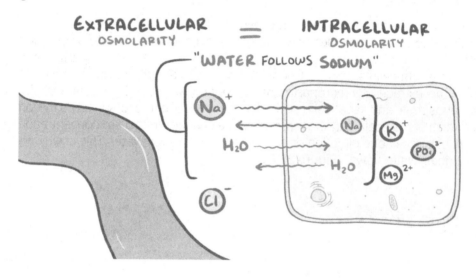

**EXTRACELLULAR** OSMOLARITY = **INTRACELLULAR** OSMOLARITY

"WATER FOLLOWS SODIUM"

**Figure 22.4**

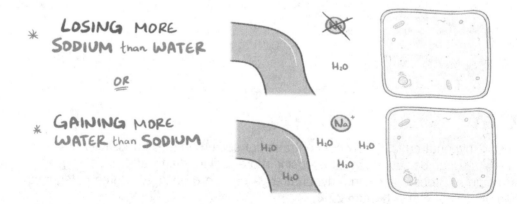

**HYPONATREMIA**
* LOW CONCENTRATION *

* LOSING MORE SODIUM than WATER

OR

* GAINING MORE WATER than SODIUM

**Figure 22.5**

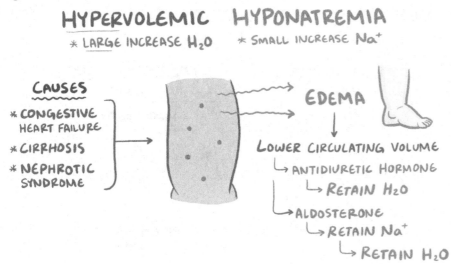

HYPERVOLEMIC HYPONATREMIA

* LARGE INCREASE $H_2O$    * SMALL INCREASE $Na^+$

CAUSES

* CONGESTIVE HEART FAILURE
* CIRRHOSIS
* NEPHROTIC SYNDROME

EDEMA

LOWER CIRCULATING VOLUME
↳ ANTIDIURETIC HORMONE
  ↳ RETAIN $H_2O$
↳ ALDOSTERONE
  ↳ RETAIN $Na^+$
    ↳ RETAIN $H_2O$

The first category is *hypervolemic* hyponatremia, where there's an enormous increase in total body water with a less significant increase in total body sodium. Typically, this is seen in conditions like congestive heart failure, cirrhosis, or nephrotic syndrome where a lot of fluid leaks out of the blood vessels and into the interstitial space. This causes edema, especially in the ankles. Even though there's more water in the body overall, there's a decrease in the effective circulating volume, which is the amount of blood flowing in the body. That, though, stimulates the release of antidiuretic hormone, which retains pure water, leading to an increase in water, as well as aldosterone, which retains sodium. Remember, though, since water follows sodium, the body retains even more water, so ultimately there's a *large* increase in water but a small increase in sodium, leading to hyponatremia **(Figure 22.5)**.

The second category is *hypovolemic* hyponatremia, where there's a small decrease in total body water with a large decrease in total body sodium. This can occur in conditions like diarrhea or vomiting, where the cells lining the gastrointestinal tract actually pump sodium ions into the digestive juices, but then those ions don't get reabsorbed because the undigested food and the digestive juices are tossed out of the body. It can also develop in response to using certain medications like diuretics, where sodium ions are pumped into the renal tubule and lost in the urine. Another, more nuanced condition is cerebral salt wasting, which is when an intracranial injury like meningitis disrupts the normal sympathetic nervous system stimulation of the kidneys, leading to disproportionate loss of sodium **(Figure 22.6)**.

A third category is *euvolemic* hyponatremia, or normal volume hypovolemia, which is where there's a normal body sodium with an increase in total body water, even though that's contrary to the name. The reason that it's given that name is that you don't have fluid pouring into the interstitial space, and therefore there's no edema. So no clinical signs of hypervolemia. Euvolemic hyponatremia can be split into cases with dilute urine and concentrated urine. Cases that cause dilute urine include adrenal insufficiency, hypothyroidism, and drinking too much water called polydipsia or beer which is called potomania. Basically the body has a lot of water and the kidneys are trying to get rid of it as best they can. The main condition that causes concentrated urine is syndrome of inappropriate antidiuretic hormone secretion, which can be shortened to SIADH. This is where inappropriate presence of antidiuretic hormone causes water retention, which means the urine gets more concentrated **(Figure 22.7)**.

There is one final type of hyponatremia, and it's sometimes called a *false hyponatremia* or *pseudohyponatremia*. This is where the body water and sodium levels are normal, but there's an excessive amount of lipids, like in hypertriglyceridemia, or proteins, like in multiple myeloma.

**Figure 22.6**

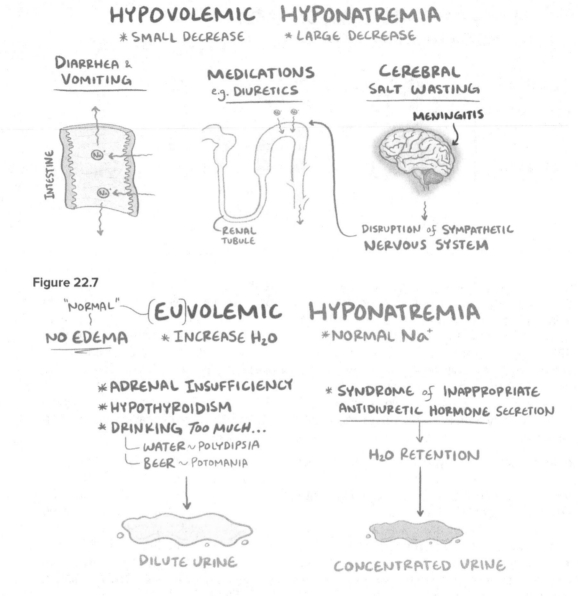

# HYPOVOLEMIC HYPONATREMIA
* SMALL DECREASE    * LARGE DECREASE

DIARRHEA & VOMITING

MEDICATIONS
e.g. DIURETICS

CEREBRAL SALT WASTING

MENINGITIS

INTESTINE

RENAL TUBULE

DISRUPTION of SYMPATHETIC NERVOUS SYSTEM

**Figure 22.7**

"NORMAL" — (EU)VOLEMIC HYPONATREMIA
NO EDEMA    * INCREASE H₂O    * NORMAL Na⁺

* ADRENAL INSUFFICIENCY
* HYPOTHYROIDISM
* DRINKING TOO MUCH...
  └ WATER ~ POLYDIPSIA
  └ BEER ~ POTOMANIA

DILUTE URINE

* SYNDROME of INAPPROPRIATE ANTIDIURETIC HORMONE SECRETION

H₂O RETENTION

CONCENTRATED URINE

High levels of lipids and proteins affects the laboratory instruments that measure the sodium concentration, making the instruments say the sodium concentration is too low, which is false **(Figure 22.8)**.

## SYMPTOMS

Hyponatremia can cause symptoms like nausea, vomiting, and muscle cramps. In severe hyponatremia, which is when the sodium concentration falls below 120 mEq/L, there can be cerebral edema, which can cause confusion, coma, and even death. This cerebral edema results from water shifting from the extracellular compartment to the intracellular compartment, causing the cells in the central nervous system to swell up and get damaged or die. It can also cause increased intracranial pressure, which can squash the blood vessels heading in and out of the brain causing ischemia and possibly brain herniation, which can damage respiratory centers in the brain and cause respiratory failure **(Figure 22.9)**.

**Figure 22.8**

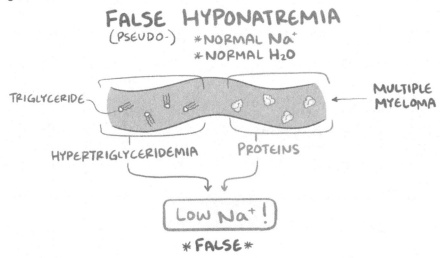

FALSE HYPONATREMIA
(PSEUDO-) *NORMAL Na⁺
*NORMAL H₂O

TRIGLYCERIDE

MULTIPLE MYELOMA

HYPERTRIGLYCERIDEMIA     PROTEINS

Low Na⁺!

*FALSE*

**Figure 22.9**

## SYMPTOMS

* NAUSEA, VOMITING, MUSCLE CRAMPS

~ SEVERE (<120 mEq/L) ~

* CEREBRAL EDEMA
   ↳ CONFUSION, COMA, DEATH
   ↳ INCREASED INTRACRANIAL PRESSURE → ISCHEMIA
   ↳ HERNIATION → RESPIRATORY FAILURE

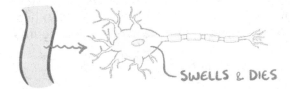

SWELLS & DIES

## DIAGNOSIS

Hyponatremia is usually diagnosed by looking at physical exam findings and labs from the urine and blood. For example, a normal serum osmolality suggests true hyponatremia versus a pseudohyponatremia. In addition, signs of edema suggest hypervolemic hyponatremia, whereas signs of dehydration suggest hypovolemic hyponatremia. Finally, urine osmolality can help differentiate between the two main types of euvolemic hyponatremia. If the urine osmolality is really concentrated, or greater than 100 mOsm/kg, then the problem may be SIADH. On the other hand, if the urine osmolality is dilute, or less than 100 mOsm/kg, then the problem may be due to taking in too much fluid. The urinary sodium concentration can also be helpful, with greater than 20-40 mEq/L suggesting SIADH and cerebral salt wasting, and less than 20 mEq/L suggesting hypovolemia.

**Figure 22.10**

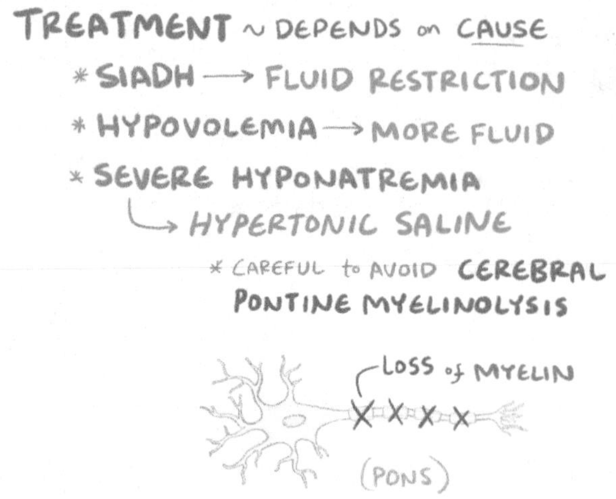

TREATMENT ~ DEPENDS on CAUSE
* SIADH → FLUID RESTRICTION
* HYPOVOLEMIA → MORE FLUID
* SEVERE HYPONATREMIA
  ↳ HYPERTONIC SALINE
    * CAREFUL to AVOID CEREBRAL
    PONTINE MYELINOLYSIS

LOSS of MYELIN
X X X X
(PONS)

## TREATMENT

Treatment of hyponatremia depends on the underlying cause. In patients with SIADH, fluid restriction is generally first-line therapy, whereas in patients that are hypovolemic, giving more fluid is helpful. Generally speaking for severe hyponatremia, it's important to give hypertonic saline, but it has to be done carefully to avoid complications like cerebral pontine myelinolysis, which is where there's a loss of myelin in the pons, a structure in the brain, due to rapid shifts in sodium and water (**Figure 22.10**).

## SUMMARY

All right, as a quick recap: hyponatremia is an electrolyte disorder that describes a low concentration of sodium in the blood, which can be divided into hypervolemic, hypovolemic and euvolemic causes. Euvolemic causes can be split into those with concentrated urine and those with dilute urine. Hyponatremia can cause water to shift into cells, and, in severe cases, it can lead to cerebral edema and death. Sodium levels can be increased with hypertonic saline, but this needs to be done slowly to avoid cerebral pontine myelinolysis (**Figure 22.11**).

**Figure 22.11**

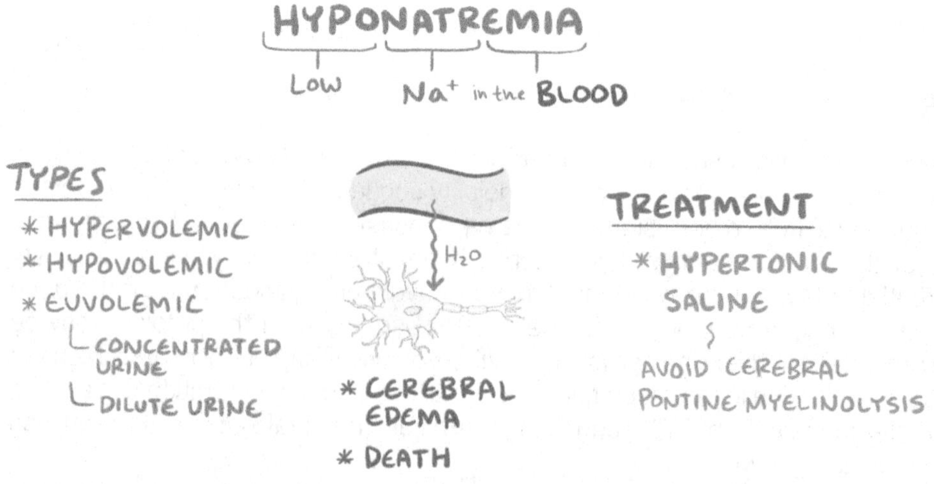

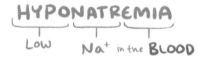

HYPONATREMIA
LOW   Na$^+$ in the BLOOD

TYPES
* HYPERVOLEMIC
* HYPOVOLEMIC
* EUVOLEMIC
  ↳ CONCENTRATED URINE
  ↳ DILUTE URINE

H$_2$O

* CEREBRAL EDEMA
* DEATH

TREATMENT
* HYPERTONIC SALINE
  ⟩
  AVOID CEREBRAL PONTINE MYELINOLYSIS

# Hypophosphatemia

**H**ypo- means "under," *phosphat-* refers to phosphate, and *-emia* refers to the blood, so hypophosphatemia means having a low level of phosphate in the blood. Typically, that's below 2.5 mg/dL. Phosphate is made up of one central phosphorus atom surrounded by four oxygen atoms in a tetrahedral arrangement, like a mini pyramid. It has a charge of minus 3, and it's written $PO_4^{3-}$ **(Figure 23.1)**.

## PHYSIOLOGY

In the body, about 85% of the phosphate is stored in the bones, where it combines with calcium to make a tough compound called hydroxyapatite, which is the stuff that makes bones hard. Of the remaining phosphate, a tiny amount is extracellular, or outside cells, like in the blood, and this is the bit that gets measured. The majority of the phosphate is intracellular, or inside cells, where it does all sorts of things. It's responsible for phosphorylation, where it binds to fats and proteins. It forms the high energy bonds of adenosine triphosphate, or ATP, which is the most common energy currency in the cell. It's part of the DNA and RNA backbone that links individual nucleotides together, and it's also part of cellular signaling molecules like cyclic-adenosine monophosphate, or cAMP for short. The bottom line is that phosphate is super important **(Figure 23.2)**.

## PATHOLOGY

Because most phosphate is locked up with calcium in the bones, the levels of phosphate are heavily tied to the levels of ionized calcium in the body. If calcium levels fall, the four parathyroid glands buried within the thyroid gland will release parathyroid hormone, which frees up both calcium and phosphate ions from the bones. Parathyroid hormone does this by stimulating osteoclasts, the cells that break bone down, to release hydrogen ions, which dissolve the hard, mineralized hydroxyapatite. As soon as the positively-charged calcium and negatively-charged phosphate are released from the bones, they grab onto each other again like a pair of star-crossed lovers, meaning that the ionized calcium level doesn't really go up very much at all **(Figure 23.3)**.

**Figure 23.1**

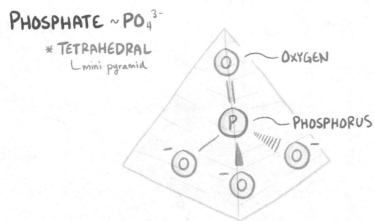

PHOSPHATE ~ $PO_4^{3-}$

\* TETRAHEDRAL
  └ mini pyramid

OXYGEN

PHOSPHORUS

**Figure 23.2**

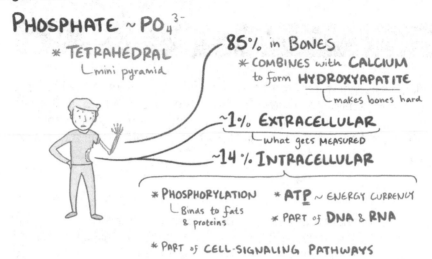

PHOSPHATE ~ $PO_4^{3-}$

* TETRAHEDRAL
  └ mini pyramid

85% in BONES
* COMBINES with CALCIUM to form HYDROXYAPATITE
  └ makes bones hard

~1% EXTRACELLULAR
  └ what gets MEASURED

~14% INTRACELLULAR

* PHOSPHORYLATION
  └ Binds to fats & proteins

* ATP ~ ENERGY CURRENCY
* PART of DNA & RNA

* PART of CELL-SIGNALING PATHWAYS

**Figure 23.3**

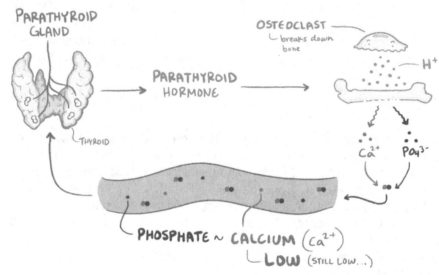

PARATHYROID GLAND

PARATHYROID HORMONE

THYROID

OSTEOCLAST
  └ breaks down bone

$H^+$

$Ca^{2+}$    $PO_4^{3-}$

PHOSPHATE ~ CALCIUM ($Ca^{2+}$)
  └ LOW (STILL LOW...)

**Figure 23.4**

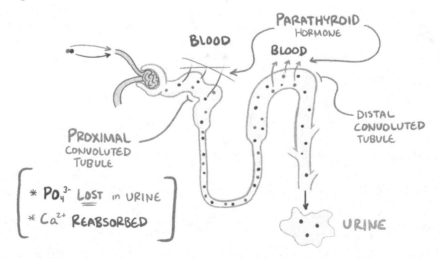

BLOOD

PARATHYROID HORMONE

BLOOD

DISTAL CONVOLUTED TUBULE

PROXIMAL CONVOLUTED TUBULE

[ * $PO_4^{3-}$ LOST in URINE
  * $Ca^{2+}$ REABSORBED ]

URINE

Now, these two make their way to the nephron of the kidney, and at this point in the proximal convoluted tubule, phosphate usually gets reabsorbed back into the blood via sodium-phosphate cotransporters. It turns out, though, that parathyroid hormone also shuts this process down. That means that phosphate is left in the lumen and then eventually sent out in the urine. Now, that calcium's still in the lumen, but parathyroid hormone also affects the distal convoluted tubule and increases calcium reabsorption. So, when the dust settles, parathyroid hormone results in phosphate being lost in the urine while ionized calcium is kept in the blood, so ionized calcium levels rise and phosphate levels fall **(Figure 23.4)**.

## CAUSES

With all of this in mind, we can see how hypophosphatemia might develop, and this can happen in a few ways. The first possibility is through the excessive loss of phosphate. This can result in conditions, like primary hyperparathyroidism, where the person produces too much parathyroid hormone, leading to excess phosphate being excreted in the urine. Another example of this kind of condition is Fanconi syndrome, which is where the proximal convoluted tubule essentially loses its capacity to reabsorb a variety of solutes, including phosphate, which once again means that it's excreted in the urine **(Figure 23.5)**.

Another thing that can lead to hypophosphatemia is not absorbing enough phosphate through the gastrointestinal tract. Some substances, like alcohol or medication, can impair phosphate absorption and lead to excretion. These medications include antacids containing aluminum, calcium, or magnesium, all of which are positive ions that can bind with the negatively charged phosphate to block absorption **(Figure 23.6)**.

Alternatively, a person may simply not be getting enough phosphate in their diet, although this is unusual because it's found in nearly all foods. The exception is someone who's starving and severely malnourished, or someone who is actively depriving themselves of food, like in anorexia nervosa. In both of these situations, blood glucose levels are low, and, as a result, cellular metabolism slows down considerably. When an individual in this state starts to suddenly eat healthy meals again, like in a hospital setting, they suddenly have a bunch of glucose in their blood, and insulin usually skyrockets in response to this in order to push that newfound glucose into the cells. This causes a demand for phosphate in cells because the first step in glucose metabolism is to have the enzyme hexokinase attach phosphate to the glucose. Also, the production of ATP molecules themselves requires a lot of phosphate **(Figure 23.7)**.

**Figure 23.5**

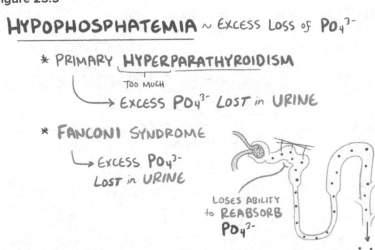

**Figure 23.6**

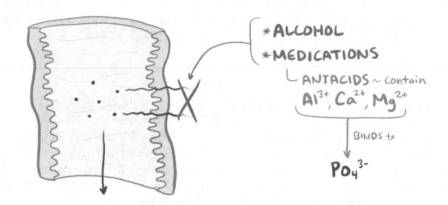

HYPOPHOSPHATEMIA ~ NOT ENOUGH ABSORBED in GASTROINTESTINAL TRACT

* ALCOHOL
* MEDICATIONS
  └ ANTACIDS ~ contain $Al^{3+}$, $Ca^{2+}$, $Mg^{2+}$

BINDS to $PO_4^{3-}$

**Figure 23.7**

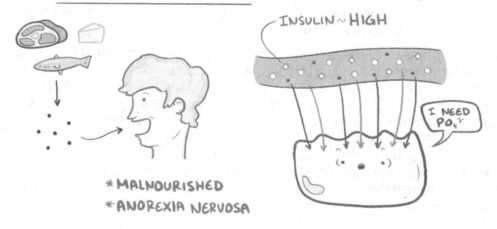

HYPOPHOSPHATEMIA ~ NOT ENOUGH in DIET

INSULIN ~ HIGH

I NEED $PO_4^{3-}$

* MALNOURISHED
* ANOREXIA NERVOSA

**Figure 23.8**

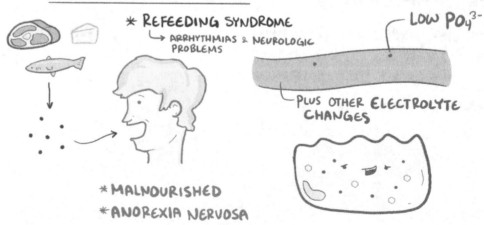

HYPOPHOSPHATEMIA ~ NOT ENOUGH in DIET

* REFEEDING SYNDROME
  └ ARRHYTHMIAS & NEUROLOGIC PROBLEMS

LOW $PO_4^{3-}$

└ PLUS OTHER ELECTROLYTE CHANGES

* MALNOURISHED
* ANOREXIA NERVOSA

**Figure 23.9**

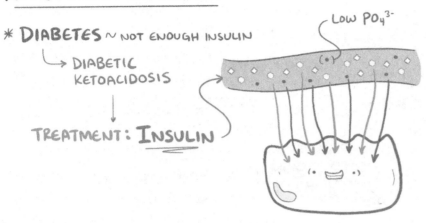

**Figure 23.10**

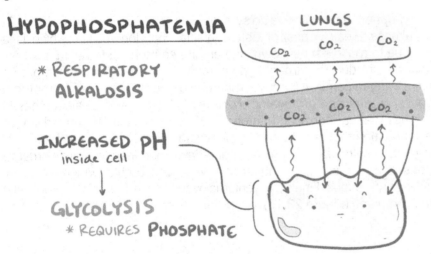

Now, because phosphate is needed but not readily available, this means that phosphate is extracted from the blood. Phosphate levels, which have remained relatively normal until this point, now plummet. This is called "refeeding syndrome," and it can cause levels of other electrolytes to rapidly change as well, putting these people at serious risk of developing cardiac arrhythmias and neurologic problems **(Figure 23.8)**.

Similarly, individuals with diabetes can't make enough insulin, so their cells are effectively "starving" even though they are surrounded by glucose in the blood. Sometimes these individuals can develop diabetic ketoacidosis, and to treat that complication, individuals are given insulin. Just like in refeeding syndrome, insulin causes the cells to extract glucose and phosphate from the blood, and so the blood phosphate levels can fall quickly **(Figure 23.9)**.

A final cause of hypophosphatemia is respiratory alkalosis, which causes extracellular carbon dioxide levels to decrease as it's ventilated out of the lungs. This causes intracellular carbon dioxide to freely diffuse out of the cell, raising the cellular pH. This stimulates glycolysis, a metabolic process that requires a lot of phosphate. As in refeeding syndrome, when cells need phosphate, they simply pull it out of the blood, causing hypophosphatemia **(Figure 23.10)**.

**Figure 23.11**

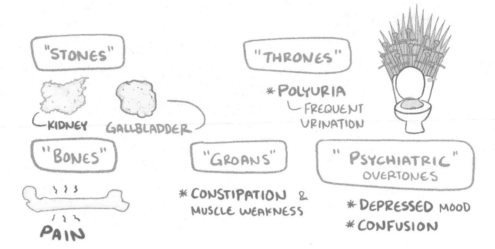

## SYMPTOMS

Most people with mild hypophosphatemia have no symptoms, but severe hypophosphatemia can cause muscle weakness, weak bones, or osteomalacia, rhabdomyolysis, which is a type of kidney damage due to muscle breakdown, and an altered mental status. In addition, hypophosphatemia that occurs due to primary hyperparathyroidism may show symptoms caused by the associated hypercalcemia. A common mnemonic to remember these symptoms is "stones, thrones, bones, groans, and psychiatric overtones." "Stones" is for calcium-based kidney stones or gallstones that can form, and "thrones" refers to the toilet to remind you of the polyuria or frequent urination that results from impaired sodium and water reabsorption. "Bones" is for bone pain that results after chronic hormone-driven demineralization in order to release calcium. "Groans" is for constipation and muscle weakness, both of which are partly due to decreased muscle contractions. Finally, "psychiatric overtones" refers to symptoms like a depressed mood and confusion **(Figure 23.11)**.

**Figure 23.12**

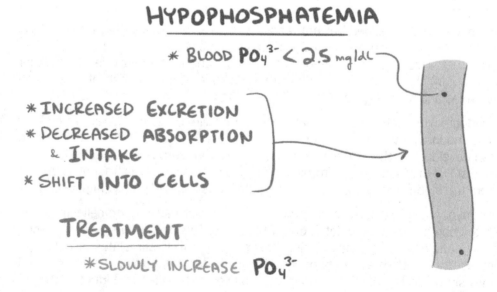

# HYPOPHOSPHATEMIA

* BLOOD $PO_4^{3-} < 2.5$ mg/dL

* INCREASED EXCRETION
* DECREASED ABSORPTION & INTAKE
* SHIFT INTO CELLS

## TREATMENT

* SLOWLY INCREASE $PO_4^{3-}$

# DIAGNOSIS & TREATMENT

Diagnosis of hypophosphatemia is based on the phosphate level being below 2.5 mg/dL, and treatment involves giving intravenous or oral phosphate and close monitoring of blood levels. In cases of malnutrition, it's important to gradually increase caloric intake and supplements over several days to avoid refeeding syndrome .

# SUMMARY

All right, as a quick recap: hypophosphatemia describes a blood phosphate level below 2.5 mg/dL. This can result from increased excretion, decreased absorption and intake, or a shift of phosphate from the bloodstream to the inside of cells. Regardless of the cause, the treatment is typically a slow increase in phosphate levels to bring them back to normal once again **(Figure 23.12)**.

# Hypospadias & epispadias

osmosis.org/learn/hypospadias_and_epispadias

With hypospadias and epispadias, *hypo-* means below, *epi-* means above, and *-spadias* refers to a slit or opening. So instead of having an opening at the tip of the urethra, hypospadias refers to an abnormal opening on the bottom of the urethra and epispadias refers to an abnormal opening on the top of the urethra **(Figure 24.1)**. Both of these can happen in boys and girls, but they're way, way more common in boys.

## PHYSIOLOGY

During genital development in the fetus, there's a point in the 8th week of gestation when both boys and girls have a similar bit of tissue called the genital tubercle that normally grows in the cranial direction, meaning that it grows towards the head. After that point, in boys, the genital tubercle responds to the hormone dihydrotestosterone and stretches out a bit into a primitive phallus **(Figure 24.2)**.

**Figure 24.1**

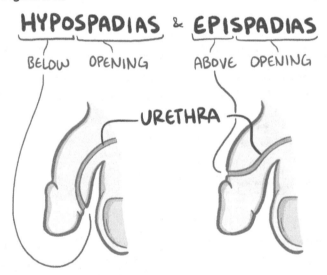

**Figure 24.2**

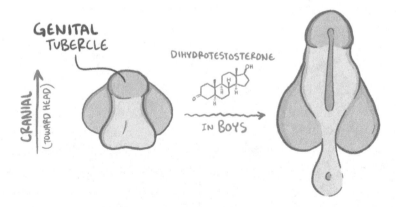

**Figure 24.3**

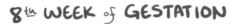

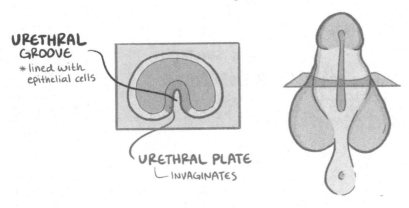

**Figure 24.4**

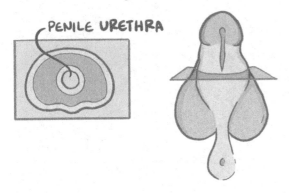

**Figure 24.5**

**Figure 24.6**

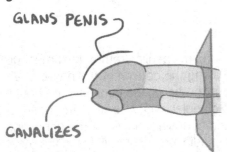
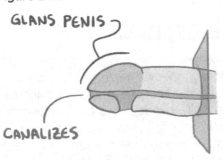

As it grows in length, an area of tissue on the underside called the urethral plate invaginates to form a urethral groove which is lined with epithelial cells **(Figure 24.3)**.

In the 14th week of gestation, the two urethral folds on the sides pinch off the groove to make it close, forming the penile urethra **(Figure 24.4)**.

In the 17th week of gestation, the ectodermal cells of the glans penis, which is the head of the penis, also undergo a process of canalization, and the urethral canal connects with the penile canal, and that means that the urethra eventually meets the outside world at the tip of the penis **(Figure 24.5; Figure 24.6)**.

**Figure 24.7**

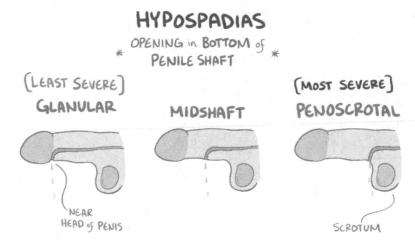

# HYPOSPADIAS
### OPENING in BOTTOM of PENILE SHAFT

* **(LEAST SEVERE)** GLANULAR
* MIDSHAFT
* **(MOST SEVERE)** PENOSCROTAL

NEAR HEAD of PENIS

SCROTUM

**Figure 24.8**

# EPISPADIAS

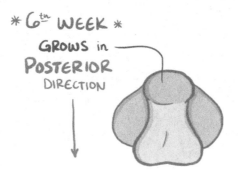

* 6ᵗʰ WEEK *
GROWS in POSTERIOR DIRECTION

## MALE GENITALIA

In a boy, hypospadias happens when the urethral folds along the penile urethra don't meet up and close properly. That leaves an opening somewhere along the bottom of the penile shaft and urine can leak out at that spot, instead of going out the tip of the penis like it should. Anatomically, hypospadias can happen in three areas: glanular, which is near the head of the penis; midshaft, which is the middle of the penis; and penoscrotal, where the penis and scrotum come together. Generally, the least severe hypospadiases are glanular, and the most severe are penoscrotal **(Figure 24.7)**.

Now, with regard to epispadias, the problem starts during the 6th week of gestation when the genital tubercle grows in a posterior direction, which means towards the rectal area, instead of the cranial direction **(Figure 24.8)**.

In a boy, this results in an opening along the upper surface of the penis. And anatomically, epispadias can happen in three areas: penopubic, where the base of the penis and the abdominal wall come together; penile, which is just somewhere along the penis; and, again, glanular, or near the head of the penis. Generally, the least severe epispadiases are glanular, and the most severe are penopubic **(Figure 20.9)**.

**Figure 24.9**

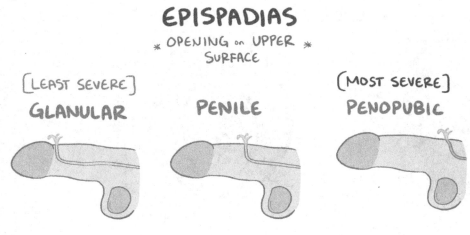

EPISPADIAS
* OPENING on UPPER *
SURFACE

[LEAST SEVERE]
GLANULAR

PENILE

(MOST SEVERE)
PENOPUBIC

**Figure 24.10**

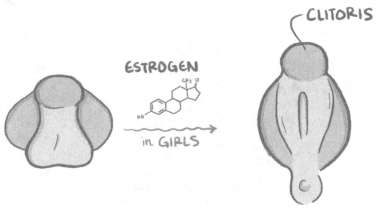

CLITORIS

ESTROGEN

in GIRLS

## FEMALE GENITALIA

All right so, switching gears to girls, during development, estrogens stimulate the development of the external genitalia. In this case, the genital tubercle elongates only gets a little bit longer and then forms the clitoris **(Figure 24.10)**. Here, the urethral folds and groove do not fuse but instead create the labia minora and the vestibule. In the 13th week of gestation, the urethra forms, and it's situated anterior to the vagina and is shorter than the one in boys **(Figure 24.11)**.

Hypospadias results in the urethra opening into the anterior vaginal wall, whereas epispadias results in the urethra developing too far anteriorly **(Figure 24.12)**.

## CAUSES

Now, the precise causes of hypospadias and epispadias are not fully understood, but they to be related to fetal exposure to abnormal levels of androgens and estrogens. Of the two, hypospadias is more common, and they're associated with other conditions like chordee, which is when the penis has a hook shape and curves inwardly, inguinal hernia, which is a protrusion of bowel through the inguinal canal, and cryptorchidism, which is the absence of testes from the scrotum. Epispadias, on the other hand, are usually associated with bladder exstrophy, where the bladder sticks out through the abdominal wall, and in females, they're often associated with a bifid clitoris, which is where the clitoris itself is divided into two parts.

**Figure 24.11**

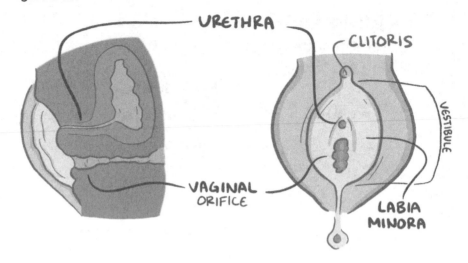

**Figure 24.12**

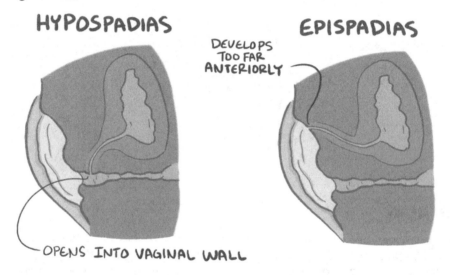

## SYMPTOMS

Symptoms of hypospadias and epispadias largely depends on the location of the abnormal urethral opening. In boys, the symptoms can range from making it slightly difficult to target the urine to incontinence. In girls, the diagnosis often happens later in life, and can cause frequent and painful urination, as well as recurrent urinary tract infections. As individuals mature, if the problem is left untreated, it can lead to sexual dysfunction, infertility, and psychosocial problems, especially in intimate relationships.

## DIAGNOSIS

The diagnosis of both hypospadias and epispadias is typically made when examining a newborn infant. Imaging studies, like an excretory urogram, can also be used to help with the diagnosis, and this is where a series of x-rays are used to visualize substances passing through the kidneys, the bladder, and the urethra.

# TREATMENT

To treat both hypospadias and epispadias, surgery can be done to reconstruct the urethra, close up the defect, and allow urine to come out the tip of the urethra. This is usually done within the first two years of life. Sometimes, hormone therapy can be useful as well, especially when there is an additional problem, like in a boy with a micropenis, which is an extremely small penis that results from low androgen levels during development. Finally, infants with hypospadias should not undergo circumcision, because the foreskin may be useful for future reconstruction **(Figure 24.13)**.

# SUMMARY

All right, as a quick recap: epispadias and hypospadias are generally seen in boys, although they can happen in both sexes. In boys with hypospadias, there is an abnormal opening on the underside of the penis, whereas with epispadias, there is an abnormal opening above, or on top of, the penis. Fortunately, both can be surgically corrected so that urine flows out of the tip of the urethra.

**Figure 24.13**

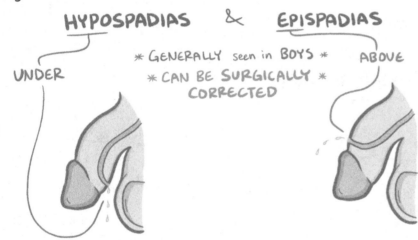

# IgA nephropathy (Berger disease)

## osmosis.org/learn/iga_nephropathy

gA is a class of immunoglobulin, or antibody, and *nephropathy* means kidney disease. IgA nephropathy, sometimes known as Berger disease, is the most common form of nephropathy worldwide, and it happens when an abnormal IgA forms and deposits in the kidneys, causing kidney damage **(Figure 25.1)**.

## PHYSIOLOGY

IgA is the main antibody found in breast milk, tears, saliva, and the mucosal secretions of the respiratory tract, the gastrointestinal tract, and the genitourinary tract **(Figure 25.2)**.

Unlike other antibodies, IgA can be secreted out in pairs in a *dimeric* form called *secretory* IgA, which is literally two IgA antibodies attached together. Being bound together helps both antibodies avoid degradation by proteolytic enzymes in harsh environments like the gut **(Figure 25.3)**.

**Figure 25.1**

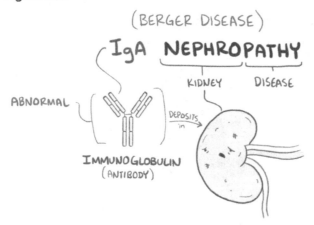

**Figure 25.2**

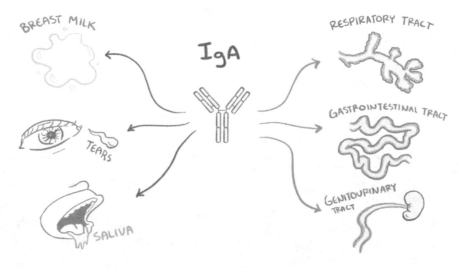

**Figure 25.3**

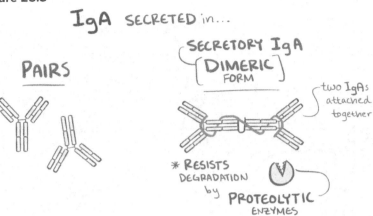

**Figure 25.4**

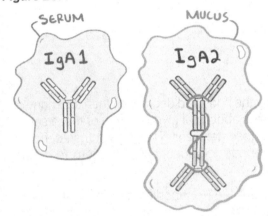

**Figure 25.5**

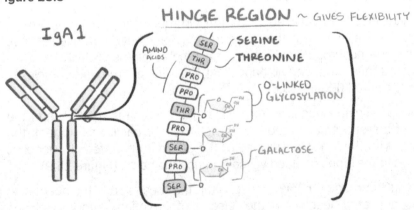

Now, IgA comes in subclasses: IgA1 and IgA2. IgA1 is found mainly in the serum, while IgA2 is more often found in the mucus secretions, typically in its dimeric form **(Figure 25.4)**.

Now, the hinge region of the IgA1 heavy chain—the part that gives the antibody a bit of flexibility to bind multiple antigens without being torn apart—is made up of a string of amino acids. Among these are serine and threonine residues which are O-linked glycosylated, meaning they have a sugar molecule, specifically galactose, attached to their oxygen **(Figure 25.5)**.

**Figure 25.6**

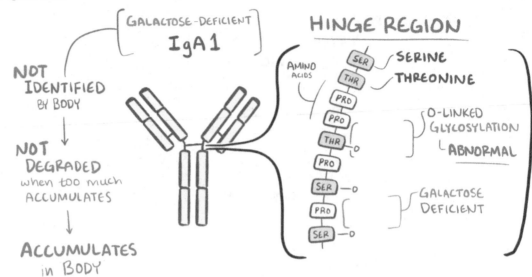

## CAUSES

These glycosylated IgA1 antibodies are identified by the body and degraded when too many of them accumulate. In IgA nephropathy, though, there is abnormal glycosylation of these serine and threonine residues, causing them to be galactose-deficient. These galactose-deficient IgA1s are *not* identified by the body, and therefore *not* degraded, allowing them to simply accumulate **(Figure 25.6)**.

In addition, it's thought that these galactose-deficient IgA1 antibodies are different enough from normal IgA1 antibodies that the body no longer recognizes them as self. In response, the body generates IgG antibodies that target the abnormally glycosylated residues. These are known as anti-glycan IgG antibodies **(Figure 25.7)**.

When these anti-glycan IgG antibodies bind to abnormal IgA1, immune complexes are formed. These immune complexes can travel through the bloodstream where they get trapped at sites of filtration, like the kidney. IgA nephropathy is therefore a Type III hypersensitivity disorder, meaning that pathology and inflammation will happen at the site the immune complexes deposit, not where they are formed **(Figure 25.8)**.

The immune complexes specifically deposit in the mesangium, which is the tissue in the Bowman's capsule that offers structural support to the glomerular capillaries. In fact, the mesangium is continuous with the smooth muscles of the afferent and efferent arterioles, and fills in the space between the loops of blood vessels, hence the name **(Figure 25.9)**.

When the abnormal IgA1-IgG immune complexes deposit in the mesangium, the alternative complement pathway is activated, leading to the release of proinflammatory cytokines and migration of macrophages into the kidney, all of which contribute to glomerular injury. Usually the glomerulus and mesangium help filter the blood to remove wastes while keeping larger proteins and cells, including red blood cells, from entering the urine. So, when there is glomerular injury, red blood cells sneak into the urine, causing hematuria, which contributes to this being a type of nephritic syndrome **(Figure 25.10)**.

**Figure 25.7**

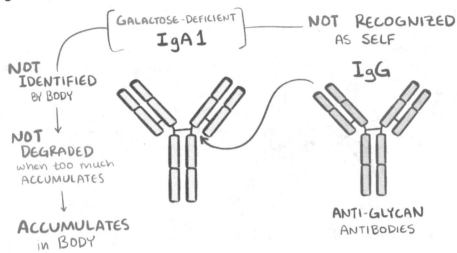

**Figure 25.8**

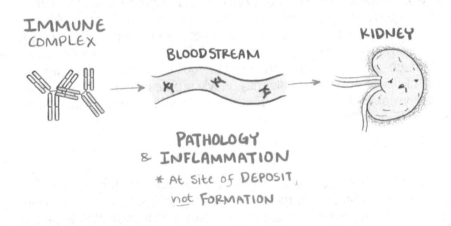

**Figure 25.9**

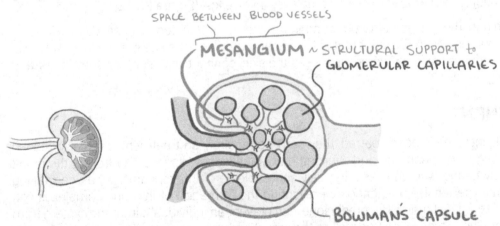

**Figure 25.10**

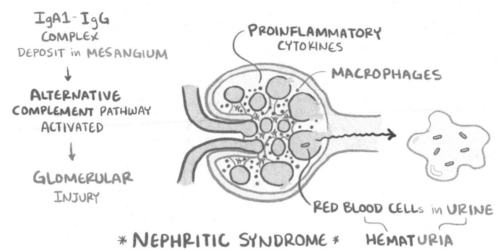

## SYMPTOMS

Typically, IgA nephropathy presents in childhood as either microscopic or gross hematuria, meaning seen under either a microscope or with the naked eye, and it typically develops during an infection involving the mucosal lining, like infections of the gastrointestinal or respiratory tract. In these sorts of infections, IgA1 antibody production gets ramped up, leading to IgG anti-glycan formation, and immune complex deposition in the glomerular mesangium, causing inflammation. With each mucosal infection, the glomeruli undergo inflammation and injury, so over time — on the scale of decades — individuals may slowly progress to renal failure. The exact reason why the abnormal IgA1 forms in the first place is unclear, but genetic factors likely play an important role (**Figure 25.11**).

## DIAGNOSIS

On light microscopy, there'll often be mesangial proliferation, or expansion of the mesangium, and upon a closer look with electron microscopy, there'll be immune complexes deposited within the mesangium. Those immune complexes can also be visualized on immunofluorescence, although one important finding that can help differentiate from other immune-complex mediated nephropathies is that these complexes involve IgA (**Figure 25.12**).

These findings, though, can also be found in another IgA-mediated disease, called Henoch-Schönlein purpura, or HSP, except that in IgA nephropathy only the kidney's involved, whereas in HSP the kidneys can be affected, as well as the skin, connective tissue, scrotum, joints, and GI tract (**Figure 25.13**).

## TREATMENT

Once the kidneys have been scarred, they can't be repaired, so treatment is mainly focused on preventing further damage and avoiding end stage kidney disease. Controlling the blood pressure, by eating well and reducing salt and cholesterol intake, can help, as can taking specific antihypertensive medications. Preventing the formation of immune complexes can help, and so corticosteroids, like prednisone, can prevent an individual's immune system from making both the defective IgA1 as well as the anti-glycan IgG, which bind together to form the immune complexes.

**Figure 25.11**

# IgA NEPHROPATHY

* PRESENTS in CHILDHOOD
  └ MICROSCOPIC or GROSS HEMATURIA
    └ naked eye

* DEVELOPS DURING INFECTION
  of MUCOSAL LINING

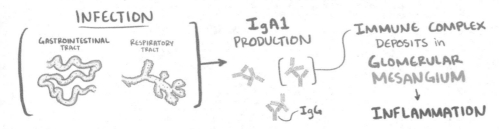

INFECTION — GASTROINTESTINAL TRACT, RESPIRATORY TRACT → IgA1 PRODUCTION, IgG → IMMUNE COMPLEX DEPOSITS in GLOMERULAR MESANGIUM → INFLAMMATION

**Figure 25.12**

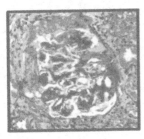
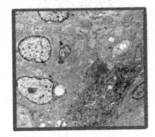
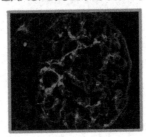

LIGHT MICROSCOPY — MESANGIAL PROLIFERATION (EXPANSION)

ELECTRON MICROSCOPY — IMMUNE DEPOSITS in MESANGIUM

IMMUNOFLUORESCENCE — IMMUNE COMPLEXES └ involve IgA

**Figure 25.13**

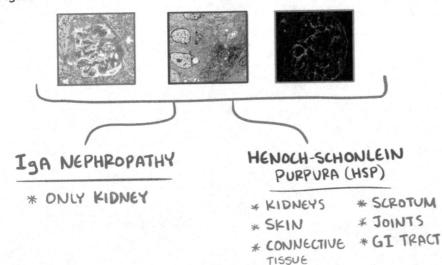

IgA NEPHROPATHY
* ONLY KIDNEY

HENOCH-SCHONLEIN PURPURA (HSP)
* KIDNEYS    * SCROTUM
* SKIN       * JOINTS
* CONNECTIVE * GI TRACT
  TISSUE

## SUMMARY

All right, as a quick recap: IgA nephropathy is the most common cause of nephropathy worldwide, and it's a type of nephritic syndrome in which abnormal IgA1 immunoglobulin is targeted by anti-glycan auto-antibodies, forming immune complexes that are then deposited in the glomerular mesangium, which starts up a Type III hypersensitivity reaction that causes glomerular injury and hematuria **(Figure 25.14)**.

**Figure 25.14**

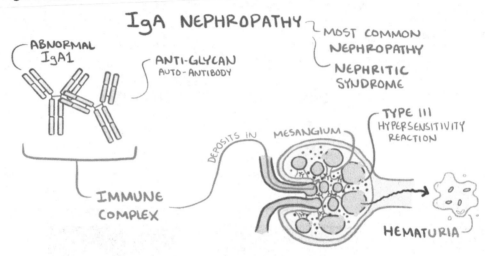

# Intrarenal acute kidney injury

osmosis.org/learn/intrarenal_acute_kidney_injury

Acute kidney injury, or AKI, is when the kidney isn't functioning at 100%, and this decrease in function develops relatively quickly, typically over a few days. Actually, AKI used to be known as acute renal failure, or ARF, but AKI is a broader term that also includes subtle decreases in kidney function. AKI can essentially be split into three types: prerenal AKI, meaning the cause of kidney injury comes from before the kidneys; postrenal AKI, meaning the injury is caused after the kidneys; or intrarenal AKI, meaning the injury happens within the kidneys **(Figure 26.1)**.

## PHYSIOLOGY

Now, the kidneys' job is to regulate what's in the blood, so they might remove waste, or make sure electrolyte levels are steady, or regulate the overall amount of water, and even make hormones; the kidneys do a lot of stuff! Blood gets into the kidney through the renal artery, into tiny clumps of arterioles called glomeruli, where it's initially filtered, with the filtrate, the stuff filtered out, moving into the renal tubule **(Figure 26.2)**.

**Figure 26.1**

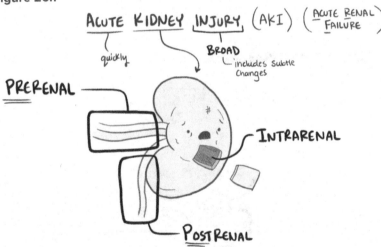

**Figure 26.2**

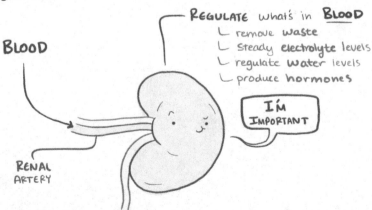

**Figure 26.3**

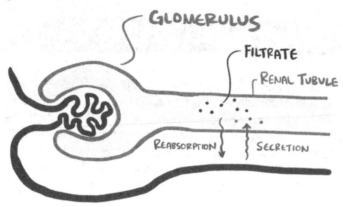

**Figure 26.4**

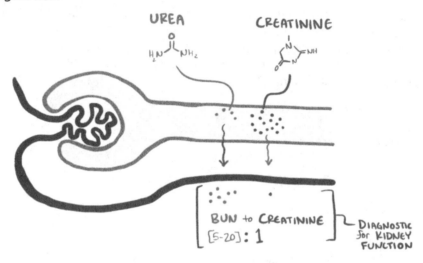

**Figure 26.5**

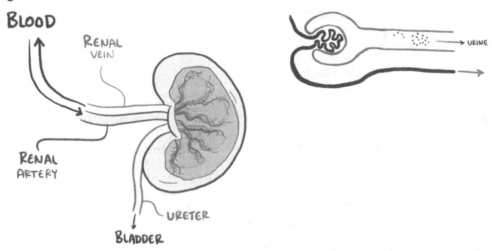

Sometimes, fluid or electrolytes can move back from the filtrate into the blood, which is called reabsorption, and sometimes more fluid or electrolytes can move from the blood to the filtrate, which is called secretion **(Figure 26.3)**.

Along with fluid and electrolytes, waste-containing compounds like urea and creatinine are also filtered, although some urea is actually *reabsorbed* back into the blood, whereas only a little bit of creatinine is reabsorbed. In fact, in the blood, the normal ratio of blood urea nitrogen, or BUN, to creatinine is between 5 and 20 to 1, meaning that the blood carries 5 to 20 molecules of urea for every one molecule of creatinine, and this is a pretty good diagnostic for looking at kidney function **(Figure 26.4)**! Ultimately, the filtrate is turned into urine and is excreted from the kidney through the ureter, into the bladder, and peed away. Meanwhile, the filtered blood drains into the renal vein **(Figure 26.5)**.

## CAUSES

Typically, intrarenal AKI's happen due to damage to the tubules, the glomerulus, or the interstitium, the space between tubules. The most common cause of intrarenal AKI is acute tubular necrosis, which is where the epithelial cells that line the tubules necrose, or die. One way this can happen is via ischemia, or a lack of blood supply to the cells **(Figure 26.6)**.

A lot of times, acute tubular necrosis due to ischemia is caused by a prerenal acute kidney injury, since prerenal AKI results in less blood sent to the kidneys, and those epithelial cells need oxygen from the blood just like any other cells. In fact, all that secretion and reabsorption in the tubules takes a *lot* of energy, and so these cells are particularly sensitive to a loss of blood supply, especially the cells in the proximal tubule and medullary segment of the thick ascending limb **(Figure 26.7; Figure 26.8)**.

**Figure 26.6**

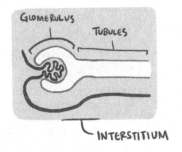

**Figure 26.7**

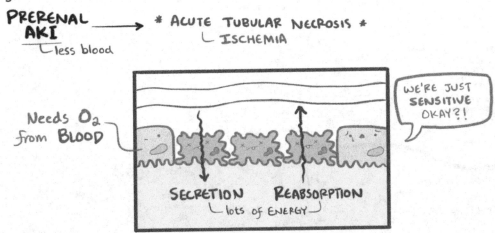

**Figure 26.8**

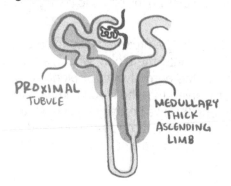

PROXIMAL TUBULE

MEDULLARY THICK ASCENDING LIMB

**Figure 26.9**

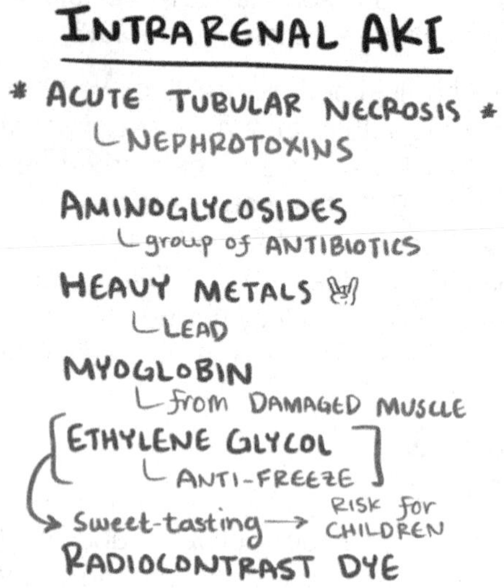

# INTRARENAL AKI

* **ACUTE TUBULAR NECROSIS** *
  └ NEPHROTOXINS

**AMINOGLYCOSIDES**
  └ group of ANTIBIOTICS

**HEAVY METALS**
  └ LEAD

**MYOGLOBIN**
  └ from DAMAGED MUSCLE

[**ETHYLENE GLYCOL**
  └ ANTI-FREEZE ]
  → Sweet-tasting → RISK for CHILDREN

**RADIOCONTRAST DYE**

**Figure 26.10**

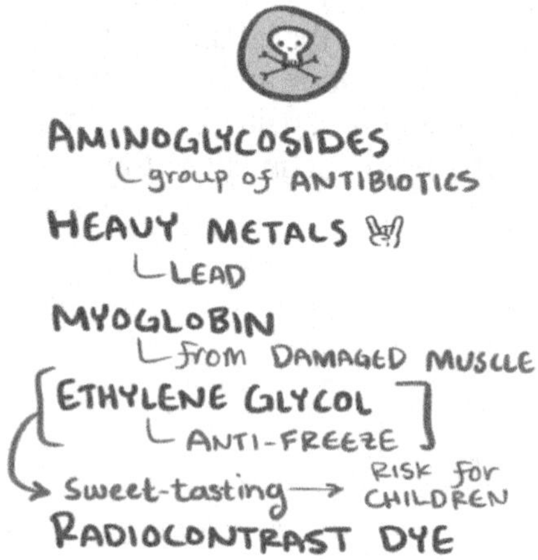

**AMINOGLYCOSIDES**
  └ group of ANTIBIOTICS

**HEAVY METALS**
  └ LEAD

**MYOGLOBIN**
  └ from DAMAGED MUSCLE

[**ETHYLENE GLYCOL**
  └ ANTI-FREEZE ]
  → Sweet-tasting → RISK for CHILDREN

**RADIOCONTRAST DYE**

**Figure 26.11**

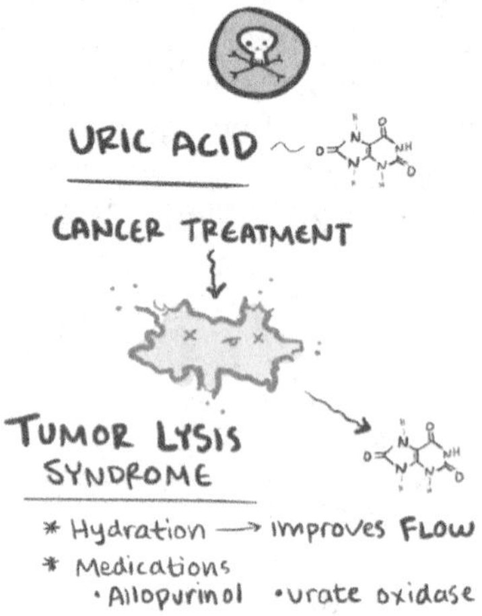

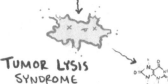

**URIC ACID** ~

**CANCER TREATMENT**

**TUMOR LYSIS** SYNDROME

* Hydration → improves FLOW
* Medications
  · Allopurinol  · urate oxidase

**Figure 26.12**

# INTRARENAL AKI

* **ACUTE TUBULAR NECROSIS** *

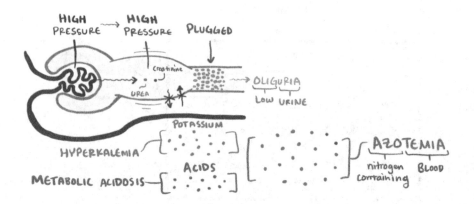

HIGH PRESSURE → HIGH PRESSURE   PLUGGED

creatinine

UREA

→ OLIGURIA
LOW URINE

HYPERKALEMIA — POTASSIUM

AZOTEMIA
nitrogen containing   BLOOD

METABOLIC ACIDOSIS — ACIDS

## NEPHROTOXINS

The other way epithelial cells can necrose is via nephrotoxins, which are substances that tend to damage the epithelial tubular cells **(Figure 26.9)**. A few of the common ones are aminoglycosides, a group of antibiotics; heavy metals like lead; myoglobin released from damaged muscles; ethylene glycol, essentially anti-freeze which is naturally sweet tasting and therefore a risk for poisoning children; radiocontrast dye; and uric acid **(Figure 26.10)**.

## TUMOR LYSIS SYNDROME

That last one, uric acid, is a waste product that can build up when cells die during cancer treatment. This is called tumor lysis syndrome, and it's the reason why staying well hydrated to improve flow through the tubules as well as using medications like allopurinol and urate oxidase to lower uric acid levels can be so important while on certain chemotherapies **(Figure 26.11)**.

## AZOTEMIA & HYPERKALEMIA

Whatever the cause of cell death is, when those cells die, they slough off into the tubule, and basically build up and plug the tubule. Just like in postrenal AKI, this generates higher pressures in the tubules, meaning that fluid's essentially trying to flow from high pressure arterioles to high pressure tubules, which doesn't really work very well. The fluid filtered across is lowered, which lowers the glomerular filtration rate, or GFR, which is how much blood the kidneys filter in mL through their glomeruli per minute. With less blood being filtered, less urine is produced, which is called oliguria, meaning abnormally low urine production. Then, less urea and creatinine get filtered out, so more stays in the blood, which is called azotemia, meaning there are high levels of nitrogen-containing compounds in the blood. Along with that, dead cells aren't very good at re-absorbing or secreting molecules anymore, right? So, other things start to build up in the blood as well, like potassium, which is called hyperkalemia, as well as acids, which is called metabolic acidosis **(Figure 26.12)**.

These dead, clumped-up cells in the tubule form a brown granular cast which is eventually excreted in the urine. It's called a cast because it stays in the same cylindrical shape as the tubule. If the underlying cause of the acute tubular necrosis is addressed, people can recover, because tubular cells can typically regenerate over the course of a few weeks **(Figure 26.13)**.

**Figure 26.13**

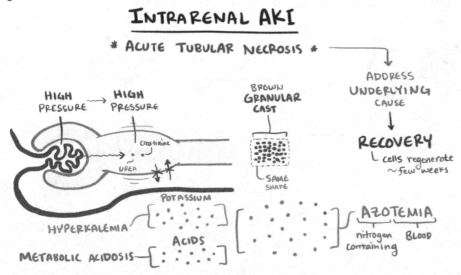

**Figure 26.14**

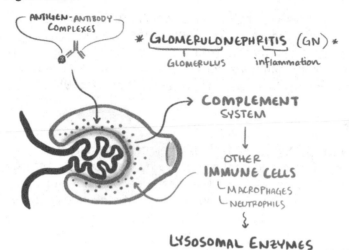

ANTIGEN-ANTIBODY COMPLEXES

*✳ GLOMERULONEPHRITIS (GN) ✳*
GLOMERULUS    inflammation

→ COMPLEMENT SYSTEM
↓
OTHER IMMUNE CELLS
└ MACROPHAGES
└ NEUTROPHILS
↓
LYSOSOMAL ENZYMES

**Figure 26.15**

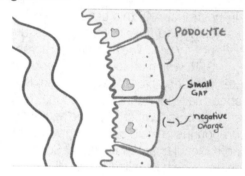

PODOCYTE
Small GAP
(−) negative charge

**Figure 26.16**

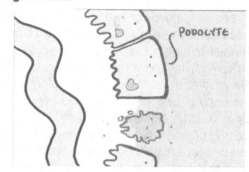

PODOCYTE

**Figure 26.17**

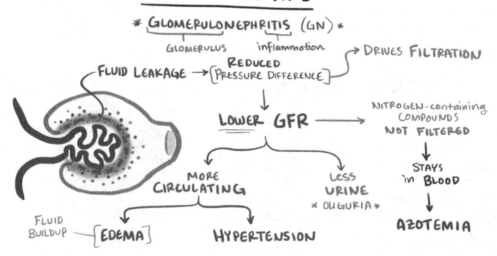

# INTRARENAL AKI

✳ GLOMERULONEPHRITIS (GN) ✳
GLOMERULUS    inflammation

FLUID LEAKAGE → REDUCED [PRESSURE DIFFERENCE] → DRIVES FILTRATION
↓
LOWER GFR → NITROGEN-containing COMPOUNDS NOT FILTERED
↓
STAYS in BLOOD
↓
AZOTEMIA

MORE CIRCULATING          LESS URINE ✳ OLIGURIA ✳

FLUID BUILDUP → [EDEMA]    HYPERTENSION

# GLOMERULONEPHRITIS

All right, another type of intrarenal AKI is glomerulonephritis, or GN, which means inflammation of the glomerulus. GN is often caused by antigen-antibody complexes depositing in the glomerular tissue. This deposition activates the complement system, which is a cascade of enzymes that attracts other immune cells like macrophages and neutrophils to the site, which release lysosomal enzymes, causing inflammation and damaging the podocytes, which are the cells that line the glomerulus **(Figure 26.14)**.

These normally have small gaps between them and have a negative electrical charge, both of which prevent large molecules from filtering through **(Figure 26.15)**. When the podocytes are damaged, therefore, membrane permeability increases and large molecules are allowed to be filtered into the urine proteins, which is called proteinuria, and even red blood cells can be filtered in, which is called hematuria **(Figure 26.16)**.

Also, this fluid leakage reduces the pressure difference that drives filtration of small molecules and electrolytes like sodium, and so the GFR actually goes down because of the leakage. Lower GFR means less blood gets filtered and so less urine is produced, causing oliguria. That means more fluid is circulating in the blood, which leads to edema, or fluid buildup, in the tissues, as well as hypertension from excess fluid volume. Finally, if those nitrogen-containing compounds aren't being filtered out, more stays *in* the blood, causing azotemia **(Figure 26.17)**.

# ACUTE INTERSTITIAL NEPHRITIS

All right, finally, we have damage to the kidney interstitium as a cause of *intra*renal AKI, one key example being acute interstitial nephritis, which is inflammation of the interstitium over the course of days to weeks. This inflammation is caused by the infiltration of immune cells, like neutrophils and eosinophils, which then causes inflammation. This is thought to be a type I or type IV hypersensitivity reaction, and is typically a response to a medication like NSAIDs, penicillin, and diuretics. Early symptoms include oliguria and eosinophiluria, which is eosinophils in the urine, but also general symptoms, like a fever and a rash. These symptoms usually subside if the medication is stopped. If the medication *isn't* removed, and the immune cells continue to damage the connective tissue in the interstitium, those kidney cells can start to die off, which is called renal papillary necrosis, where the renal papillae are destroyed. This can again cause hematuria, blood in the urine, as well as flank pain. Other potential causes of renal papillary necrosis are chronic use of analgesics, like aspirin, as well as diabetes mellitus, sickle cell disease, and pyelonephritis **(Figure 26.18)**.

**Figure 26.18**

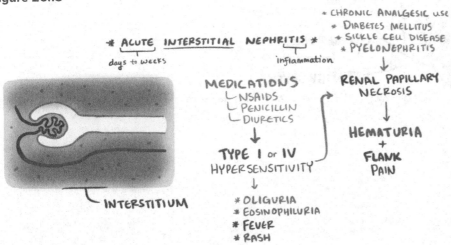

## SUMMARY

In general, with intrarenal AKI, the kidneys lose the ability to filter the blood properly, and the cells are often damaged such that reabsorption and secretion are impaired. If the urea isn't reabsorbed, less urea stays in the blood relative to creatinine, and the BUN:Cr ratio falls to less than 15 to 1. Also, those cells can't reabsorb sodium, meaning the urine's Na+ goes above 40 mEq/L, and the $FE_{Na}$, which is the fraction of sodium excreted in the urine, of total sodium filtered, expressed as a percentage, goes above 2%. Finally, since water's not being reabsorbed as much, urine osmolality falls below 350 mOsm/kg **(Figure 26.19)**.

So, as a quick recap, intrarenal AKI is kidney injury caused by something within the kidneys themselves, which could be the tubules as in acute tubular necrosis, the glomerulus as in glomerulonephritis, or the interstitium as in acute interstitial nephritis **(Figure 26.20)**.

**Figure 26.19**

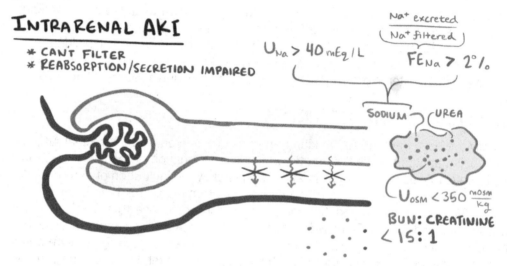

**Figure 26.20**

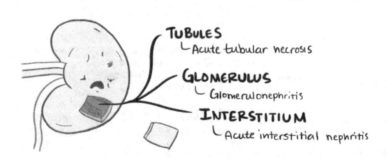

# Lupus nephritis

osmosis.org/learn/lupus_nephritis

The term *lupus* refers to systemic lupus erythematosus, *nephr-* refers to the nephron, the Greek word for kidney, and *-itis* means inflammation, so lupus nephritis refers to inflammation of the kidney that results from having systemic lupus erythematosus **(Figure 27.1)**.

## PHYSIOLOGY

Lupus is an autoimmune disease in which the immune system attacks various parts of the body, including the skin, joints, lungs, heart, central nervous system, and, of course, the kidneys. In fact, about half of all individuals with lupus develop some form of lupus nephritis **(Figure 27.2)**.

**Figure 27.1**

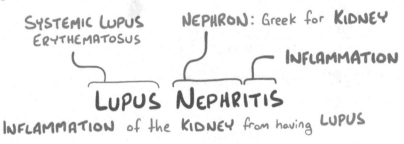

**Figure 27.2**

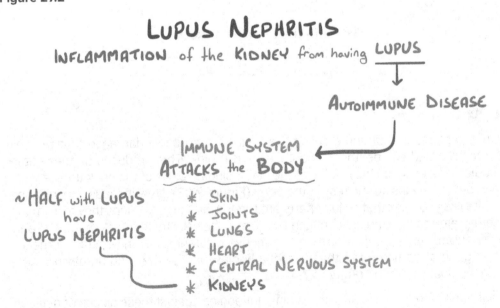

**Figure 27.3**

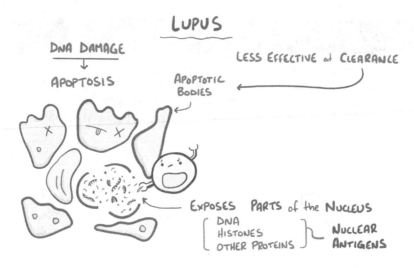

LUPUS

DNA DAMAGE
↓
APOPTOSIS

APOPTOTIC BODIES

LESS EFFECTIVE at CLEARANCE

EXPOSES PARTS of the NUCLEUS
[ DNA
HISTONES
OTHER PROTEINS ] NUCLEAR ANTIGENS

**Figure 27.4**

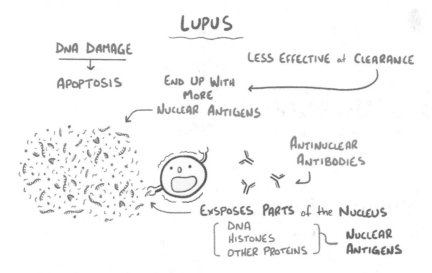

LUPUS

DNA DAMAGE
↓
APOPTOSIS

END UP WITH MORE NUCLEAR ANTIGENS

LESS EFFECTIVE at CLEARANCE

ANTINUCLEAR ANTIBODIES

EXSPOSES PARTS of the NUCLEUS
[ DNA
HISTONES
OTHER PROTEINS ] NUCLEAR ANTIGENS

## PATHOLOGY

In lupus, what happens is that some cells have their DNA so badly damaged that the cell undergoes programmed cell death, or apoptosis, and it dies. This produces all these little apoptotic bodies, and exposes the insides of the cell, including parts of the nucleus, like DNA, histones, and other proteins, to the rest of the body **(Figure 27.3)**. Now in lupus, the immune system is more likely to think that cellular parts are foreign, or antigens. Since they're from the nucleus, they're referred to as nuclear antigens, and immune cells try to attack them. Not only that, though: individuals with lupus have less effective clearance, which essentially means they aren't as good at getting rid of the apoptotic bodies, and so they end up having more nuclear antigens floating around **(Figure 27.4)**.

So as a result of all of this, B-cells start producing antibodies against these pieces of nucleus, which are called antinuclear antibodies. These antinuclear antibodies bind to nuclear antigens, forming antigen-antibody complexes, which drift away in the blood and deposit in various places including the kidneys. These immune complexes can then initiate an inflammatory reaction, which is known as a Type III hypersensitivity reaction (Figure 27.5).

**Figure 27.5**

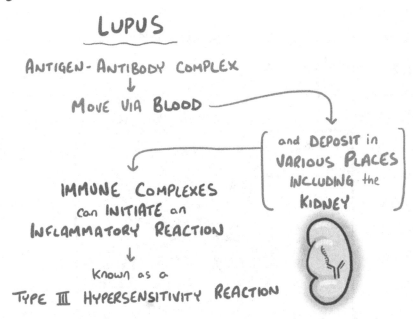

LUPUS

ANTIGEN - ANTIBODY COMPLEX
↓
MOVE VIA BLOOD

and DEPOSIT in
VARIOUS PLACES
INCLUDING the
KIDNEY

IMMUNE COMPLEXES
can INITIATE an
INFLAMMATORY REACTION
↓
Known as a
TYPE III HYPERSENSITIVITY REACTION

## CLASSIFICATION OF LUPUS NEPHRITIS

Lupus nephritis is classified into various types depending on the exact site of these immune complexes and subsequent inflammatory reaction. The most common site of deposition is just underneath the capillary wall, also known as the endothelium, but deposits can also be within the Bowman's space of the nephron, the basement membrane, or near the mesangial cells. The extent of inflammation within the kidney can be focal, involving nephrons in just one area, or diffuse, involving almost all of the nephrons in both kidneys **(Figure 27.6)**.

In the majority of cases, lupus nephritis presents as a nephrotic syndrome, which means that the damage to the nephron allows plasma proteins to get into the urine, which causes proteinuria of typically greater than 3.5 grams per day. An important protein in the blood is albumin, and so when it starts leaving the blood, people get hypoalbuminemia, or low albumin in the blood. With less protein in the blood the oncotic pressure falls, which lowers the overall osmotic pressure, which drives water *out* of the blood vessels and into the tissues, called edema. Finally, it's thought that as a result of either losing albumin or losing some protein or proteins that inhibit the synthesis of lipids, or fat, you get increased levels of lipids in the blood, called hyperlipidemia.

Just like the proteins, these lipids can also get into the urine, causing lipiduria. These are the hallmarks of nephrotic syndrome: proteinuria, hypoalbuminemia, edema, hyperlipidemia, and lipiduria **(Figure 27.7)**.

However, in some cases, lupus nephritis can present as a nephritic syndrome, which means that the damage to the nephron ends up allowing red blood cells to filter into the urine, which causes hematuria, or blood in the urine **(Figure 27.8)**.

The location of the lesions and the extent of kidney injury often predicts whether the general presentation will be nephrotic or nephritic, but it's far from exact **(Figure 27.9)**.

**Figure 27.6**

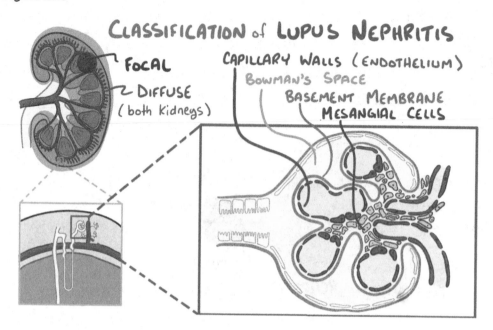

# CLASSIFICATION of LUPUS NEPHRITIS

FOCAL

DIFFUSE (both kidneys)

CAPILLARY WALLS (ENDOTHELIUM)
BOWMAN'S SPACE
BASEMENT MEMBRANE
MESANGIAL CELLS

**Figure 27.7**

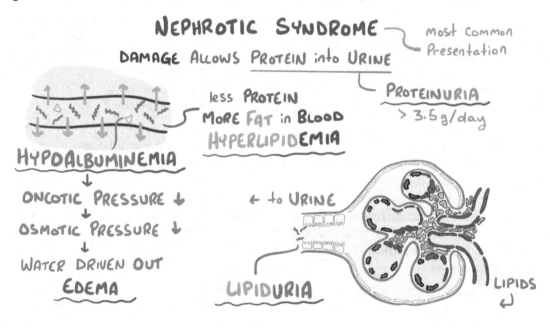

# NEPHROTIC SYNDROME
most common presentation

DAMAGE ALLOWS PROTEIN into URINE

less PROTEIN
MORE FAT in BLOOD
HYPERLIPIDEMIA

PROTEINURIA
> 3.5 g/day

HYPOALBUMINEMIA
↓
ONCOTIC PRESSURE ↓
↓
OSMOTIC PRESSURE ↓
↓
WATER DRIVEN OUT
EDEMA

← to URINE

LIPIDURIA

LIPIDS
↙

**Figure 27.8**

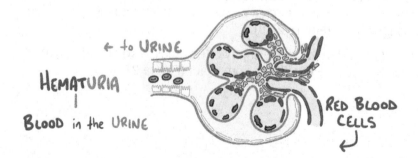

← to URINE

HEMATURIA

BLOOD in the URINE

RED BLOOD CELLS

**Figure 27.9**

the **LOCATION** of **LESIONS** & **EXTENT** of **KIDNEY INJURY** **PREDICTS**

**NEPHROTIC** vs. **NEPHRITIC** **SYNDROME**

KIND OF...

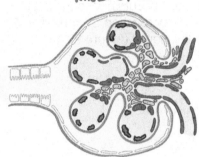

## DIAGNOSIS

This brings us to the diagnosis of lupus nephritis, which typically requires a kidney biopsy. Deposition of immune complexes in the Bowman's space results in a characteristic crescent-shaped swelling of the area and deposition in the basement membrane can cause thickening of the structure, giving rise to a "wire-loop" pattern. It's also possible to look for the presence of immune markers like complement proteins and immunoglobulins in the glomerulus by staining them with fluorescent markers **(Figure 27.10)**.

**Figure 27.10**

Can also look for **IMMUNE MARKERS** with **FLUORESCENCE MICROSCOPY**

**DIAGNOSIS** ⊃ typically requires a **BIOPSY**

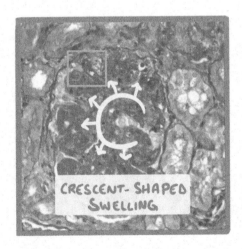

CRESCENT-SHAPED SWELLING

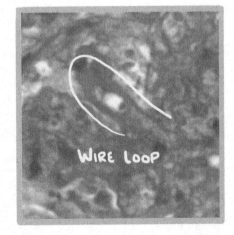

WIRE LOOP

## TREATMENT

Lupus nephritis is treated the same way that lupus is treated: by suppressing the immune system. This is often done with corticosteroids as well as specific medications like mycophenolate and cyclophosphamide.

## SUMMARY

All right, quick recap: lupus nephritis is inflammation of the kidneys caused by lupus, and it can present as a nephrotic or nephritic syndrome. It occurs due to the deposition the immune complexes in the nephron, a Type III hypersensitivity reaction, and the resulting inflammation causes damage that can be detected on a kidney biopsy **(Figure 27.11)**.

**Figure 27.11**

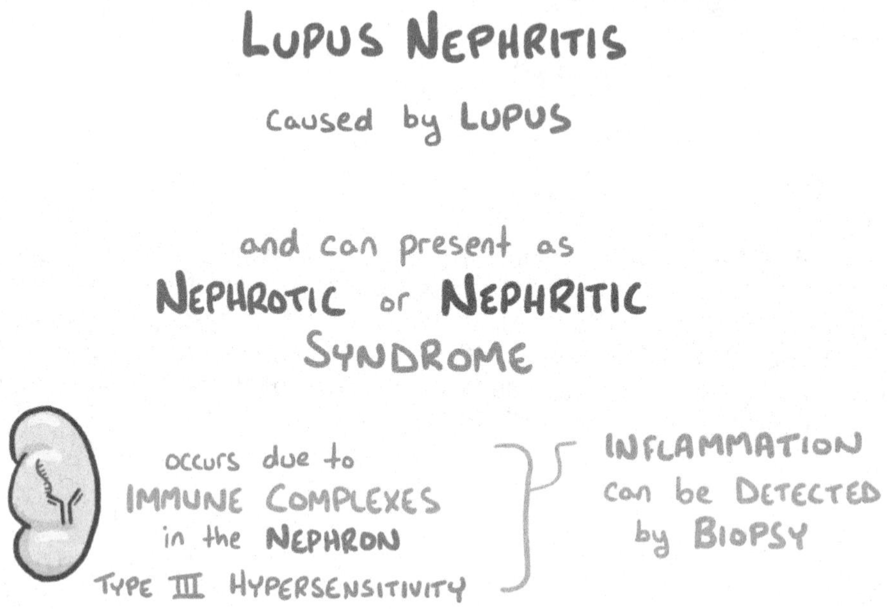

# LUPUS NEPHRITIS

Caused by LUPUS

and can present as
# NEPHROTIC or NEPHRITIC
## SYNDROME

occurs due to
IMMUNE COMPLEXES
in the NEPHRON

TYPE III HYPERSENSITIVITY

INFLAMMATION
can be DETECTED
by BIOPSY

# Medullary sponge kidney

osmosis.org/learn/medullary_sponge_kidney

**M**edullary sponge kidney, also known as Cacchi-Ricci disease, is a congenital disease where the medullary part of the kidney, which is deeper inside the kidney, is loaded with fluid-filled cysts, giving the kidney the appearance of a sponge **(Figure 28.1)**.

## PHYSIOLOGY

Now, the kidney can be divided into the cortex, which is the outer layer, and the medulla, which is the layer below that. Kidneys contain millions of tiny nephrons which filter the blood, and each of these is like a little tube receiving blood on one end in the cortex. From there, the nephron dips into the medulla, then goes back out into the cortex, and finally dips back into the medulla a second time to connect to the collecting ducts that gather up all of the urine. Not every nephron has this exact structure, but a lot of them do **(Figure 28.2)**.

**Figure 28.1**

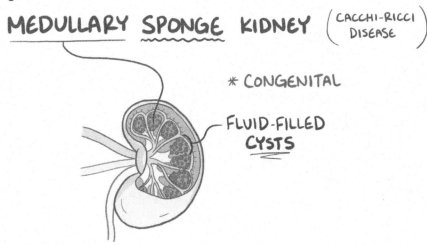

**Figure 28.2**

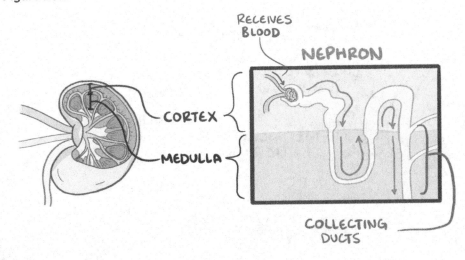

**Figure 28.3**

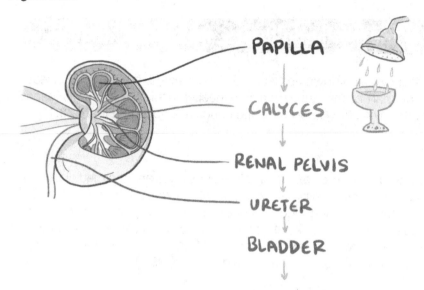

**Figure 28.4**

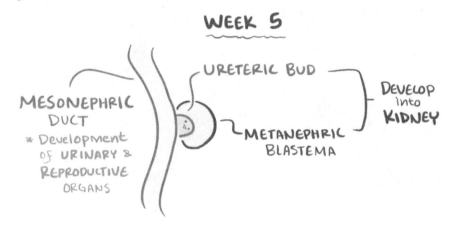

**Figure 28.5**

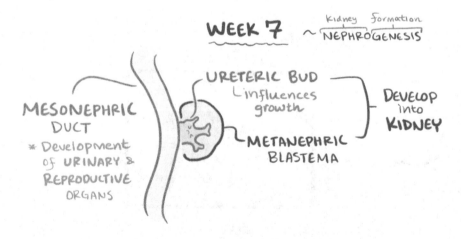

**Figure 28.6**

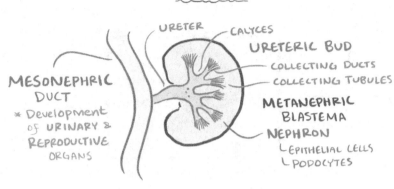

**Figure 28.7**

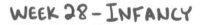

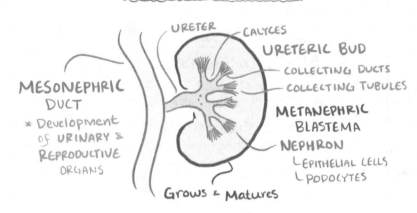

From there, the urine drains through the papilla, which is an inverted cone shaped pyramid, that, like a shower head, pours urine into the calyces. These get their name from the latin -calix, which means large cup, like a Roman chalice. From there, it enters the renal pelvis, which funnels the urine into the ureter, then to the bladder, and then it finally leaves the body through the urethra **(Figure 28.3)**.

Now, medullary sponge kidney has to do with the development of the kidney. So, during fetal development, first off you've got this structure called the mesonephric duct that's involved in development of urinary and reproductive organs, and during the fifth week of gestation, a little guy called the ureteric bud starts pushing its way into another structure called the metanephric blastema, and together, these two little embryologic structures go on to develop into a kidney **(Figure 28.4)**.

At about the seventh week, nephrogenesis, or formation of the kidneys, starts under the influence of that ureteric bud **(Figure 28.5)**. By about twenty weeks, the ureteric bud has formed the ureters, the renal calyces, collecting ducts, and collecting tubules, while the metanephric blastema develops into the nephron itself, which includes the epithelial cells and the podocytes of Bowman's capsule **(Figure 28.6)**. In the third trimester and throughout infancy, the kidneys continue to grow and mature **(Figure 28.7)**.

**Figure 28.8**

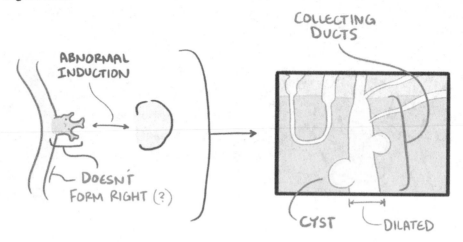

ABNORMAL INDUCTION

DOESN'T FORM RIGHT (?)

COLLECTING DUCTS

CYST — DILATED

**Figure 28.9**

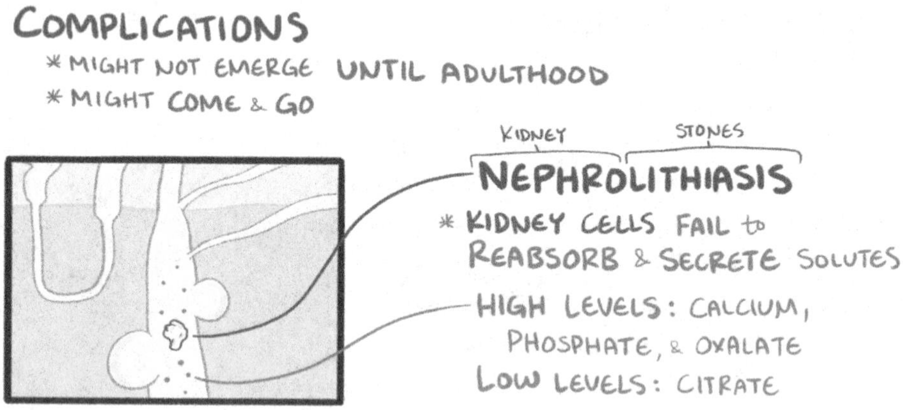

## COMPLICATIONS
* MIGHT NOT EMERGE UNTIL ADULTHOOD
* MIGHT COME & GO

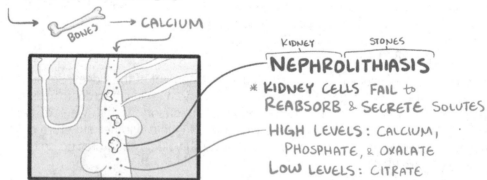

KIDNEY STONES

### NEPHROLITHIASIS
* KIDNEY CELLS FAIL to REABSORB & SECRETE SOLUTES

HIGH LEVELS: CALCIUM, PHOSPHATE, & OXALATE
LOW LEVELS: CITRATE

**Figure 28.10**

## METABOLIC ACIDOSIS

BONES → CALCIUM

KIDNEY STONES

### NEPHROLITHIASIS
* KIDNEY CELLS FAIL to REABSORB & SECRETE SOLUTES

HIGH LEVELS: CALCIUM, PHOSPHATE, & OXALATE
LOW LEVELS: CITRATE

**Figure 28.11**

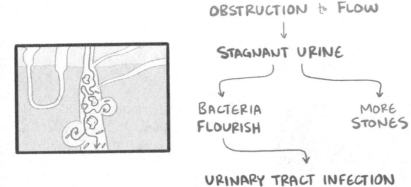

OBSTRUCTION to FLOW
↓
STAGNANT URINE

BACTERIA FLOURISH

MORE STONES

URINARY TRACT INFECTION

## PATHOLOGY

Although the causes aren't completely known, it's thought that medullary sponge kidney is a result of some sort of abnormal induction of the metanephric blastema by the ureteric bud. This failure might be the fault of the mesonephric duct not forming right, or the ureteric bud not forming right, or both. Whatever the case, in medullary sponge kidney, the hallmark features are dilated collecting ducts, meaning they're enlarged, and small cysts that form around the collecting ducts **(Figure 28.8)**.

Even though medullary sponge kidney is present at birth, sometimes complications don't emerge until adulthood, and even then, they might come and go. The most common one is nephrolithiasis, or developing kidney stones, which are made of calcium phosphate or calcium oxalate. These form in the collecting ducts and surrounding tissue, and these result mostly from a failure of kidney cells to properly reabsorb or secrete solutes, which ultimately results in stone formation. For example, there may be a high level of calcium, phosphate, and oxalate in the urine, all of which are not very soluble. In addition, there may be low levels of substances like citrate in the urine that would normally increase their solubility **(Figure 28.9)**.

Making matters worse, medullary sponge kidney can lead to metabolic acidosis, which can cause calcium to leach out of the bones, raising the amount of calcium that gets filtered through the kidneys **(Figure 28.10)**.

Together, the kidney stones and cysts obstruct urine flow, creating pockets of stagnant urine. Those stagnant pools of urine allow more time for solutes to precipitate and crystallize into stones, creating a vicious cycle of stone formation. Ultimately, a kidney that is full of cysts and stones with areas of stagnant urine also invites bacteria to flourish, resulting in kidney infections **(Figure 28.11)**.

## SYMPTOMS

So, the symptoms are related to these complications: kidney stones tend to cause bouts of extreme pain and blood in the urine from tissue damage, and urinary tract infections can cause fevers as well as pain.

## DIAGNOSIS

Medullary sponge kidney is usually diagnosed by medical imaging. For example, an intravenous pyelograms is a type of X-ray that uses contrast to show the enlargement and hyperdensity of the collecting ducts and cysts. These tend to show a classic "feathered" appearance of the ducts at the interface of the papilla and calyx **(Figure 28.12)**.

**Figure 28.12**

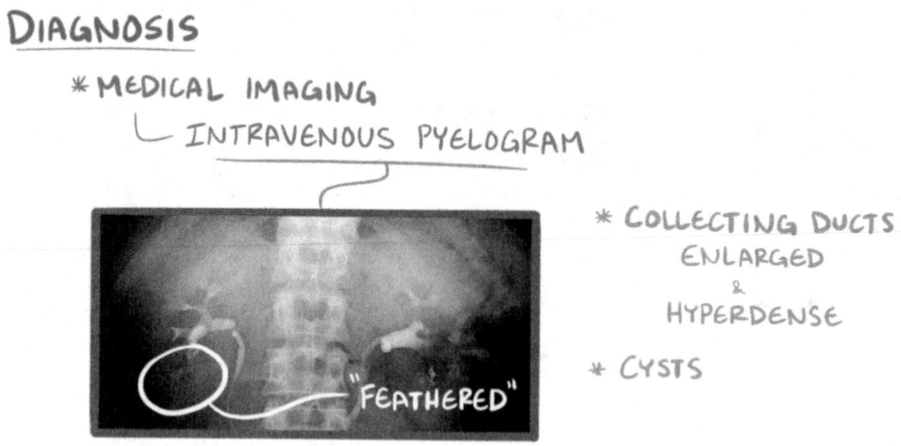

## DIAGNOSIS

\* MEDICAL IMAGING
　└ INTRAVENOUS PYELOGRAM

\* COLLECTING DUCTS
ENLARGED
&
HYPERDENSE

\* CYSTS

"FEATHERED"

## TREATMENT

Treatment of medullary sponge kidney might target preventing stones from forming, which includes keeping an individual well hydrated, taking citrate supplements to make calcium more soluble, and taking bicarbonate supplements to prevent calcium from being leached out of the bones. If small stones develop, they can be broken down with focused shockwaves or surgically removed before they get bigger. Finally, complications like urinary tract infections can be managed with antibiotics.

## SUMMARY

All right, as a quick recap: medullary sponge kidney is a congenital disorder where the medulla is full of large collecting ducts as well as cysts. To make matters worse, the nephrons can become dysfunctional, allowing high levels of calcium, phosphate, and oxalate in the urine, which can precipitate out and form kidney stones. Together, these cysts and stones can predispose an individual to getting infections **(Figure 28.13)**.

**Figure 28.13**

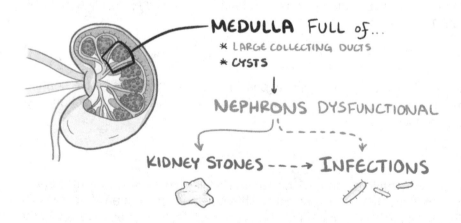

MEDULLARY SPONGE KIDNEY
\* CONGENITAL DISORDER \*

MEDULLA FULL of...
\* LARGE COLLECTING DUCTS
\* CYSTS
↓
NEPHRONS DYSFUNCTIONAL

KIDNEY STONES ----→ INFECTIONS

# Membranoproliferative glomerulonephritis

osmosis.org/learn/membranoproliferative_glomerulonephritis

**M**embranoproliferative glomerulonephritis, or MPGN, is a kidney disease triggered by immune deposits that end up in the walls of the glomerulus, which are the tufts of capillaries where blood is filtered. These deposits lead to inflammation and result in structural changes to the glomerulus, causing a decrease in kidney function that commonly presents as a nephrotic syndrome **(Figure 29.1)**.

## PHYSIOLOGY

But what exactly is nephrotic syndrome? Well, usually the glomerulus only lets small molecules, like sodium and water, move from the blood into the kidney nephron, where it eventually makes its way into the urine. But with nephrotic syndromes, the glomeruli are damaged and they become more permeable, so they start letting plasma proteins come across from the blood to the nephron and then into the urine, which causes *proteinuria*, typically at a level greater than 3.5 grams per day.

An important protein in the blood is albumin, and so when it starts leaving the blood, people get *hypoalbuminemia*, which means low albumin in the blood. With less protein in the blood, the oncotic pressure falls, lowering the overall osmotic pressure, which then drives water *out* of the blood vessels and into the tissues and leading to *edema*.

Finally, it's thought that as a result of either losing albumin or losing some protein or proteins that inhibit the synthesis of lipids, or fat, you get increased levels of lipids in the blood, which is called *hyperlipidemia*.

Just like the proteins, these lipids can also get into the urine, causing *lipiduria*. And those are the hallmarks of nephrotic syndrome: proteinuria, hypoalbuminemia, edema, hyperlipidemia, and lipiduria.

**Figure 29.1**

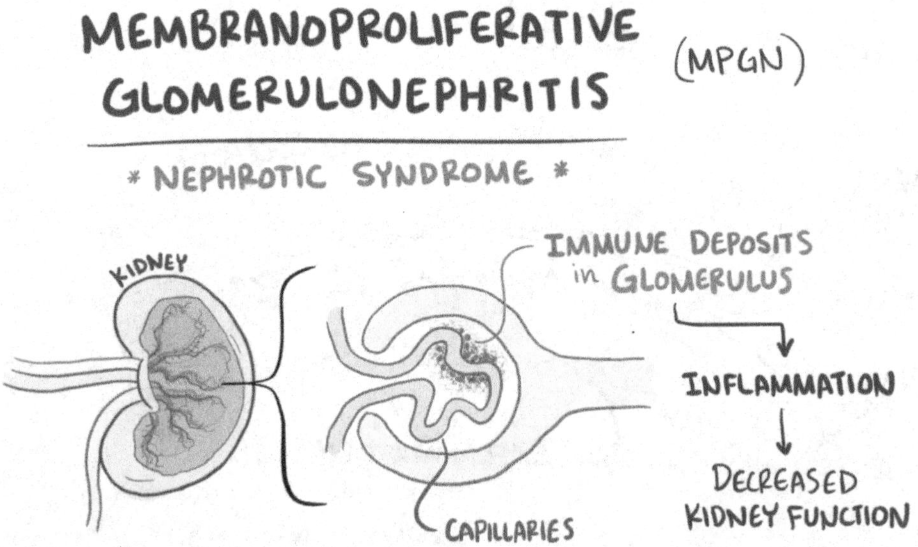

MEMBRANOPROLIFERATIVE GLOMERULONEPHRITIS (MPGN)

* NEPHROTIC SYNDROME *

KIDNEY

IMMUNE DEPOSITS in GLOMERULUS

INFLAMMATION

DECREASED KIDNEY FUNCTION

CAPILLARIES

**Figure 29.2**

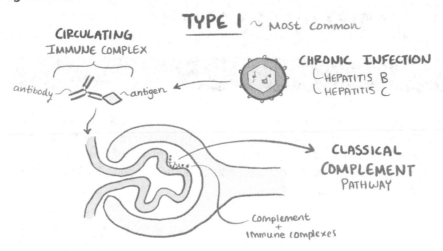

**Figure 29.3**

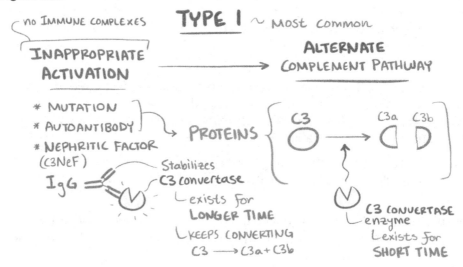

**Figure 29.4**

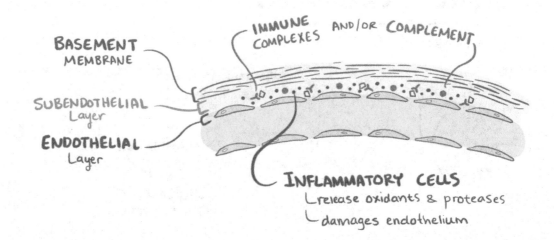

Figure 29.5

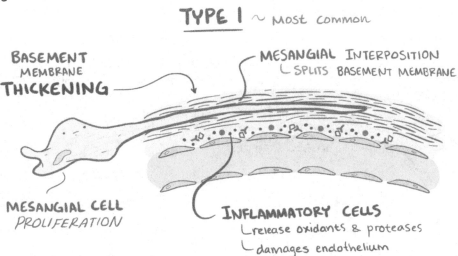

## PATHOLOGY

Okay, so membranoproliferative glomerulonephritis is a type of nephrotic syndrome. But how exactly do these glomeruli start letting plasma proteins like albumin through? Well, there are actually three types of MPGN, so let's go them through one by one. Type I MPGN is the most common form, and it usually starts in one of two ways. The first way involves circulating immune complexes, made up of antigens and antibodies. These might form, for example, because antigens released from a chronic infection, like hepatitis B or hepatitis C, might get bound by antibodies in the blood. Over time, many of these immune complexes might find their way to the glomerulus, where they cause an activation of the classical complement pathway, leading to complement protein deposition right alongside the immune complex deposits **(Figure 29.2)**.

The second way MGPN starts involves the inappropriate activation of the alternative pathway of complement. Specifically, with this pathway, C3 is converted to C3a and C3b by the enzyme C3 convertase. Inappropriate activation could mean a mutation in or autoantibody against proteins that regulate this process. On the flip side, since C3 convertase usually only exists for a short time, there could also be inappropriate activation if there is an IgG antibody that actually *binds* to C3 convertase, which makes the C3 convertase more stable, causing it to exist for *longer* periods of time, which means it keeps on converting C3 to C3a and C3b. This special IgG autoantibody is called "nephritic factor" (or C3NeF), and it's responsible for some of the cases of Type I MPGN. Because in this situation there's inappropriate activation of complement, there are no immune complex deposits with the complement deposits **(Figure 29.3)**.

Either way, the actual mutation or autoantibody triggering of all this trouble isn't always known. What is known, though, is that the immune complexes and/or complement deposits end up in the subendothelium, meaning between the endothelial layer and the basement membrane of the glomerular capillaries. These immune deposits recruit inflammatory cells to that area, which then release oxidants and proteases that damage the capillary wall **(Figure 29.4)**.

In addition to all of this, that inflammation triggers the thickening of the basement membrane, which also triggers the mesangial cells of the glomerulus to proliferate, or divide, and reach through the thick basement membrane with their cytoplasmic arms **(Figure 29.5)**.

**Figure 29.6**

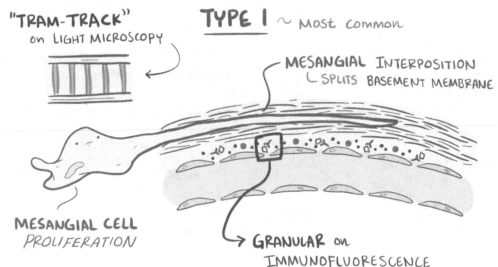

"TRAM-TRACK" on LIGHT MICROSCOPY

TYPE I ~ Most common

MESANGIAL INTERPOSITION
└ SPLITS BASEMENT MEMBRANE

MESANGIAL CELL PROLIFERATION

GRANULAR on IMMUNOFLUORESCENCE

**Figure 29.7**

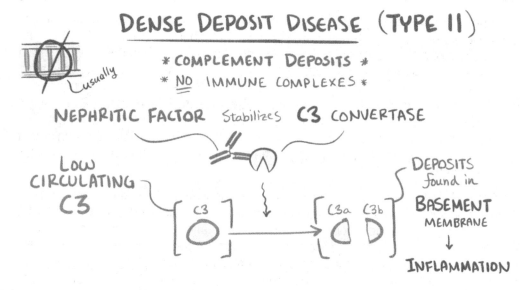

DENSE DEPOSIT DISEASE (TYPE II)

usually

* COMPLEMENT DEPOSITS *
* NO IMMUNE COMPLEXES *

NEPHRITIC FACTOR  Stabilizes  C3 CONVERTASE

LOW CIRCULATING C3

C3 → C3a C3b

DEPOSITS found in BASEMENT MEMBRANE
↓
INFLAMMATION

**Figure 29.8**

TYPE III

* IMMUNE COMPLEXES *
* COMPLEMENT *

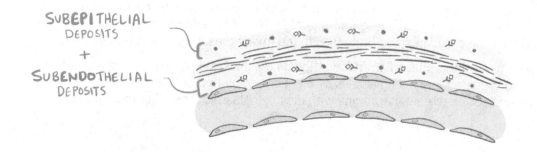

SUBEPITHELIAL DEPOSITS
+
SUBENDOTHELIAL DEPOSITS

This process is called mesangial interposition, and it sometimes causes the basement membrane to split around the mesangial cell, forming a duplication of the basement membrane and a "tram-track" appearance on light microscopy. Also, because of the immune complexes, the glomeruli also appear granular on immunofluorescence **(Figure 29.6)**.

Okay, so Type II MPGN generally involves only complement deposits and does not involve immune complexes. It's actually now classified as its own separate disease, dense deposit disease. The leading causal mechanism of Type II MPGN is the same IgG autoantibody, nephritic factor, that we talked about in Type I. Now, though, this mechanism is responsible for nearly all of the cases of MPGN II. Once again, this nephritic factor stabilizes the C3 convertase and allows it to keep on converting C3 to C3a and C3b. In this case, complement deposits in the basement membrane, as opposed to in the subendothelium as in Type I, which leads to inflammation in the basement membrane and low circulating levels of C3. Most cases of dense deposit disease don't show the same tram-track pattern, and it's not quite clear how these complement abnormalities induce changes in the glomeruli **(Figure 29.7)**.

Finally, we've got Type III MPGN, but this kind is shrouded in even more mystery. This type seems also to be an immune complex and complement disease like Type I, but, in addition to deposits in the subendothelial space, there also seems to be deposits in the sub*epi*thelial space, though again, many of the mechanisms leading to glomerular changes aren't well understood **(Figure 29.8)**.

## SYMPTOMS

Regardless of the differences between these three types of MPGN, they can all present as nephrotic syndrome, usually characterized by proteins in the urine, but in addition to this they can also present as nephrotic syndrome, since they all also involve some sort of inflammation. The characteristic findings are: hematuria, blood in the urine; oliguria, abnormally low production of urine; azotemia, increased nitrogen-containing compounds in the blood; and hypertension.

## TREATMENT

For treatment, sometimes steroids may be given to suppress the immune system, although responses have been inconsistent. All three types of MPGN can progress to chronic renal failure **(Figure 29.9)**.

**Figure 29.9**

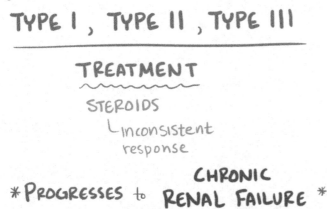

## SUMMARY

All right, to recap: Type I MPGN is caused by either immune complex or complement deposits in the subendothelium; Type II MPGN, or dense deposit disease, is when complement deposits are found in the basement membrane; and Type III MPGN is where immune complexes or complement deposits are found in the sub-epithelium as well as possibly the subendothelium. All three typically lead to nephrotic symptoms, but occasionally to nephritic symptoms as well **(Figure 29.10)**.

**Figure 29.10**

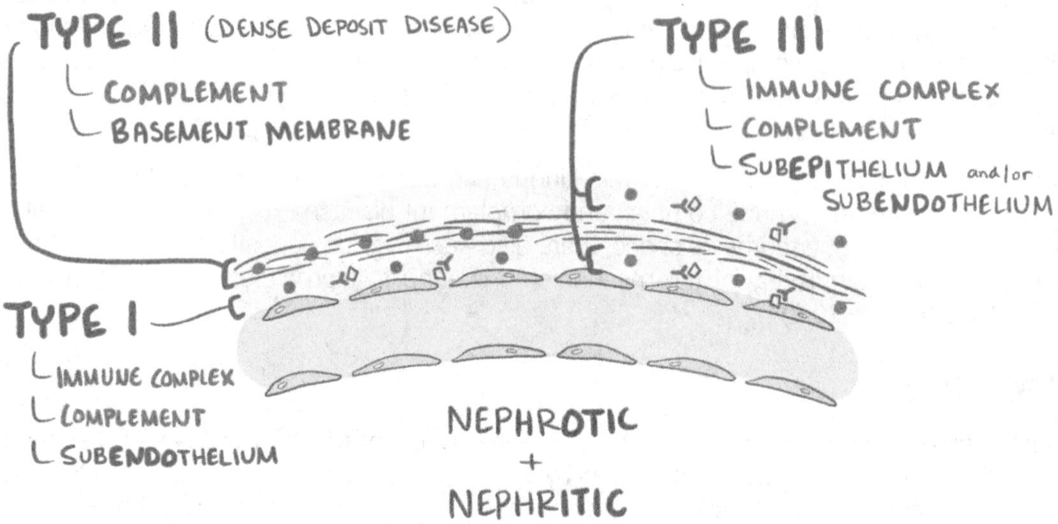

TYPE II (DENSE DEPOSIT DISEASE)
- COMPLEMENT
- BASEMENT MEMBRANE

TYPE III
- IMMUNE COMPLEX
- COMPLEMENT
- SUBEPITHELIUM and/or SUBENDOTHELIUM

TYPE I
- IMMUNE COMPLEX
- COMPLEMENT
- SUBENDOTHELIUM

NEPHROTIC
+
NEPHRITIC

# Membranous glomerulonephritis (membranous nephropathy)

osmosis.org/learn/membranous_glomerulonephritis

**M**embranous glomerulonephritis, also known as membranous nephropathy, is where the glomerular basement membrane, or GBM, which lines the glomeruli in the kidney, becomes inflamed and damaged. This results in increased permeability and proteins being able to filter through into the urine, causing nephrotic syndrome **(Figure 30.1)**.

## PHYSIOLOGY

But what exactly is nephrotic syndrome? Well, usually the glomerulus only lets small molecules, like sodium and water, move from the blood into the kidney nephron, where they eventually make their way into the urine. But with nephrotic syndromes, the glomeruli are damaged and they become more permeable, so they start letting plasma proteins come across from the blood to the nephron and then into the urine, which causes *proteinuria*, typically at a level greater than 3.5 grams per day **(Figure 30.2)**.

**Figure 30.1**

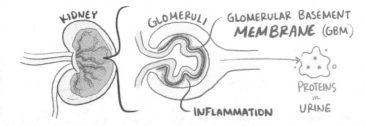

**Figure 30.2**

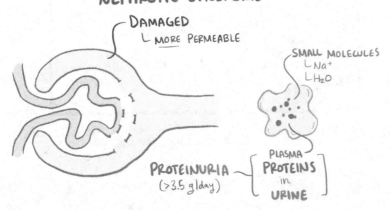

**Figure 30.3**

## NEPHROTIC SYNDROME

* PROTEINURIA *
(>3.5 g/day)

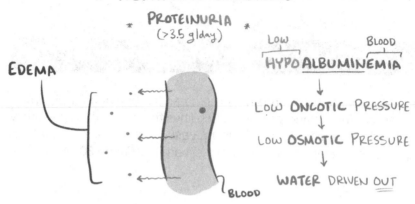

EDEMA

Low _____ BLOOD
HYPOALBUMINEMIA
↓
LOW ONCOTIC PRESSURE
↓
LOW OSMOTIC PRESSURE
↓
WATER DRIVEN OUT

BLOOD

---

**Figure 30.4**

## NEPHROTIC SYNDROME

* PROTEINURIA *
(>3.5 g/day)

* HYPOALBUMINEMIA *

* EDEMA *

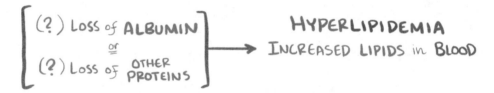

(?) LOSS of ALBUMIN
or
(?) LOSS of OTHER PROTEINS

→ HYPERLIPIDEMIA
INCREASED LIPIDS in BLOOD

---

**Figure 30.5**

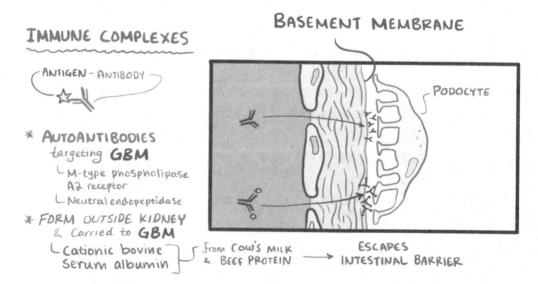

IMMUNE COMPLEXES

ANTIGEN – ANTIBODY

* AUTOANTIBODIES
targeting **GBM**
└ M-type phospholipase
A2 receptor
└ Neutral endopeptidase

* FORM OUTSIDE KIDNEY
& Carried to **GBM**
└ Cationic bovine
serum albumin ┤ from COW'S MILK
& BEEF PROTEIN → ESCAPES
INTESTINAL BARRIER

BASEMENT MEMBRANE

PODOCYTE

**Figure 30.6**

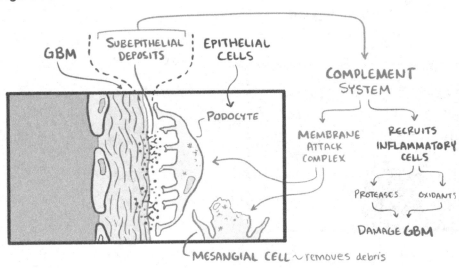

## PATHOLOGY

An important protein in the blood is albumin, and when it starts leaving the blood, this is called *hypo*albuminemia, or low albumin in the blood. With less protein in the blood, the oncotic pressure falls, lowering the overall osmotic pressure, which then drives water out of the blood vessels and into the tissues, a condition called *edema* **(Figure 30.3)**. Finally, it's thought that as a result of either losing albumin or losing some protein or proteins that inhibit the synthesis of lipids, or fat, you get increased levels of lipid in the blood, called *hyperlipidemia* **(Figure 30.4)**. Just like the proteins, these lipids can also get into the urine, causing *hyperlipiduria*. And those are the hallmarks of nephrotic syndrome: proteinuria, hypoalbuminemia, edema, hyperlipidemia, and hyperlipiduria.

All right, so with membranous glomerulonephritis, the basement membrane becomes damaged, which causes nephrotic syndrome. How does this happen, though? Well, ultimately this damage is caused by immune complexes, which are complexes composed of an antigen with an antibody bound to it. One way these complexes can form is as a result of autoantibodies directly targeting the glomerular basement membrane. Two major antigen targets that've been identified are the M-type phospholipase A2 receptor and neutral endopeptidase, which are both expressed on the podocyte surface, which means the cells that line the basement membrane. We know this because in a large proportion of cases, people with membranous glomerulonephritis have antibodies against these autoantigens in their bloodstream **(Figure 30.5)**.

Immune complexes, though, might also form outside of the kidney and then be carried through the bloodstream to the glomerulus and deposited in the basement membrane. One potential circulating antigen that's been identified is cationic bovine serum albumin, which is present in cow's milk and beef protein, and can escape the intestinal barrier, cause immune complex formation, and deposit in the GBM **(Figure 30.6)**.

Whether they bind directly to the GBM, or come from somewhere else, these immune complexes are called subepithelial deposits because they're sandwiched right between the epithelial cells or podocytes, and the GBM. These subepithelial deposits are thought to activate the complement system, which is a cascade of enzyme activation that ultimately produces the membrane attack complex that directly damages both the podocytes as well as mesangial cells, which are the cells that work to remove trapped residue and debris.

**Figure 30.7**

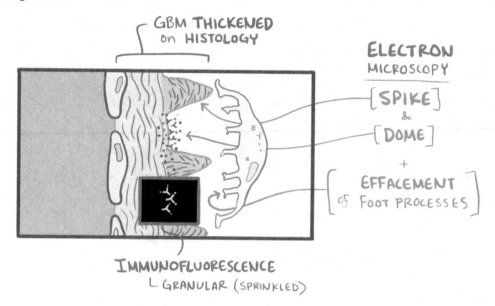

The immune reaction also recruits inflammatory cells that release proteases and oxidants that damage the basement membrane and cause it to become "leaky", allowing proteins to filter through into the urine, which causes the signs and symptoms of nephrotic syndrome.

## DIAGNOSIS

Over time, as a reaction to the immune deposits, GBM matrix is deposited in between the immune complexes, which makes the GBM appear thickened on histology. If you take a closer look on electron microscopy, you'll see that this pattern of GBM matrix on the subepithelial deposits creates a characteristic "spike and dome" pattern, and you also see effacement or flattening of the foot processes of the podocytes. Finally, on immunofluorescence, you'll see deposits of immune complexes, which appear as granular or sort of sprinkled throughout the GBM **(Figure 30.7)**.

**Figure 30.8**

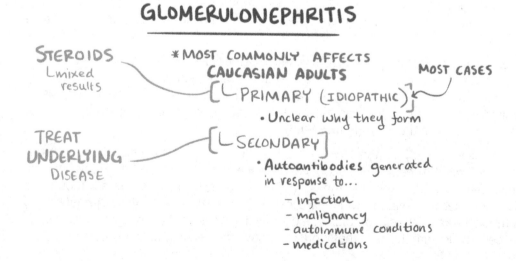

# CAUSES

Membranous glomerulonephritis most commonly affects Caucasian adults, and it can be primary, or idiopathic, meaning it's not quite clear why these complexes form, and this accounts for the vast majority of cases. The rest of cases, though, are secondary, and seem to arise from autoantibodies that are generated in response to another process like an infection, malignancies, autoimmune conditions, or medications.

# TREATMENT

If it *is* secondary to some other disease, then usually treatment starts by treating the underlying disease. If it's primary or idiopathic, then steroids are sometimes used, but they've been shown to have mixed results. If it goes untreated or the treatment is not successful, then membranous glomerulonephritis can progress to chronic renal failure **(Figure 30.8)**.

# SUMMARY

All right, as a quick recap: membranous glomerulonephritis is where immune complexes deposit in the GBM, causing a thickening of that GBM and a "spike and dome" appearance that leads to nephrotic syndrome **(Figure 30.9)**.

**Figure 30.9**

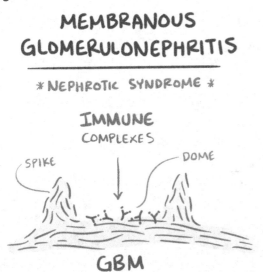

# Minimal change disease

osmosis.org/learn/minimal_change_disease

**M**inimal-change disease, sometimes called nil disease, affects the millions of the kidney's glomeruli, which are the specific parts of the kidney where small molecules are first filtered out of blood and into the urine. Specifically, it's a type of nephrotic syndrome; in fact, it's the most common nephrotic syndrome seen in children **(Figure 31.1)**.

## PHYSIOLOGY

But what exactly is nephrotic syndrome? Well, usually the glomerulus only lets small molecules—like sodium and water—move from the blood into the kidney nephron, where it eventually make its way into the urine. But with nephrotic syndromes, the glomeruli are damaged and they become *more* permeable, so they start letting plasma proteins come across from the blood to the nephron and then into the urine, which causes *proteinuria* at a level that's typically greater than 3.5 grams per day **(Figure 31.2)**.

**Figure 31.1**

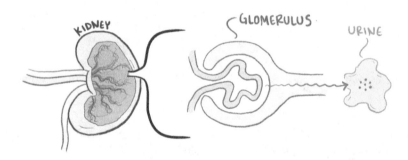

MINIMAL-CHANGE DISEASE
(NIL DISEASE)

MOST COMMON NEPHROTIC SYNDROME IN CHILDREN

**Figure 31.2**

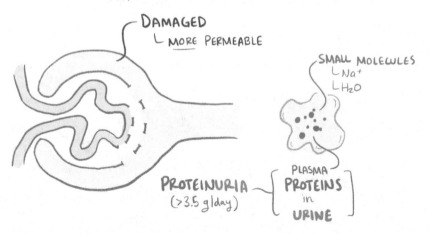

NEPHROTIC SYNDROME

**Figure 31.3**

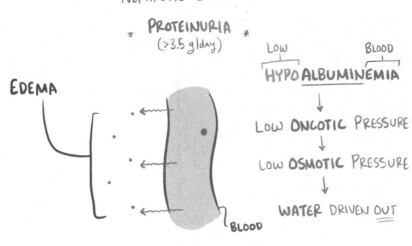

NEPHROTIC SYNDROME

* PROTEINURIA *
(>3.5 g/day)

EDEMA

HYPO ALBUMINEMIA
Low        Blood

↓

Low ONCOTIC PRESSURE

↓

Low OSMOTIC PRESSURE

↓

WATER DRIVEN OUT

BLOOD

**Figure 31.4**

NEPHROTIC SYNDROME

* PROTEINURIA *
(>3.5 g/day)

* HYPO ALBUMINEMIA *

* EDEMA *

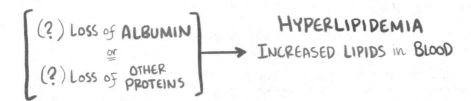

[ (?) LOSS of ALBUMIN
or
(?) LOSS of OTHER PROTEINS ]  →  HYPERLIPIDEMIA
INCREASED LIPIDS in BLOOD

**Figure 31.5**

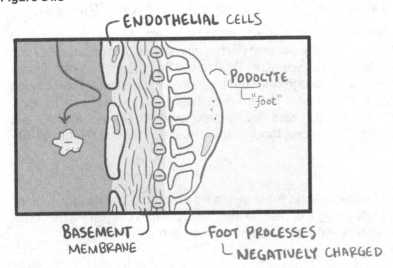

ENDOTHELIAL CELLS

PODOCYTE
"foot"

BASEMENT MEMBRANE

FOOT PROCESSES
NEGATIVELY CHARGED

**Figure 31.6**

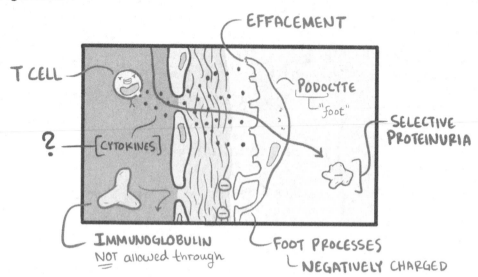

## PATHOLOGY

An important protein in the blood is albumin, and so when it starts leaving the blood, people get *hypoalbuminemia*, or low albumin in the blood. With less protein in the blood the oncotic pressure falls, which lowers the overall osmotic pressure, which then drives water out of the blood vessels and into the tissues, a condition called *edema* (**Figure 31.3**).

Finally, it's thought that as a result of either losing albumin or losing some protein or proteins that inhibit the synthesis of lipids, or fat, you get increased levels of lipids in the blood, called *hyperlipidemia*. Just like the proteins, these lipids can also get into the urine, causing *lipiduria*. And those are the hallmarks of nephrotic syndrome: proteinuria, hypoalbuminemia, edema, hyperlipidemia, and lipiduria (**Figure 31.4**).

Okay, so minimal change disease is a type of nephrotic syndrome, but how exactly do those glomeruli start letting plasma proteins like albumin through?

Well, usually in the glomerulus, you've got your endothelial cells lining the capillaries, then the basement membrane, and then the podocytes, which are the cells that have these long tentacle-like projections, called foot processes. This is also why they're called *podo*cytes since *podo-* refers to the foot. The foot processes have a negatively charged coat that helps repel negatively charged molecules like albumin, thereby acting as a charge barrier (**Figure 31.5**).

Although not completely known, it's thought that with minimal change disease, the T-cells in the blood release cytokines that specifically damage the foot processes of the podocytes and and flatten them out in a process called *effacement*. This means that there's less of a charge barrier, and albumin is allowed to slip through from the blood into the nephron. Even though albumin goes through, other larger proteins, like immunoglobulin, aren't allowed through, and so with minimal change disease there's *selective proteinuria*. The exact identity and mechanism of these ominous T-cell cytokines, though, still remains a mystery (**Figure 31.6**).

## CAUSES

As far as causes of minimal change goes, in most cases it's idiopathic, meaning the cause is unknown. One interesting clue, though, is that it's associated with Hodgkin's lymphoma, possibly because of the general increase in cytokine production in that disease.

## DIAGNOSIS

Diagnosing minimal-change disease can be kind of tricky. With only light microscopy and H&E stain, you can't see the foot process effacement, so it seems as if there's *no change* to the glomerulus, hence the names "minimal-change" and "nil" disease. With electron microscopy, though, you can see effacement of foot processes. Also, immunofluorescence with minimal-change disease is usually negative, since the damage is due to cytokines, not immune-complex deposition.

## TREATMENT

Treatment of minimal-change disease is typically corticosteroid therapy, to which about 90% of children respond very well. Adults also respond well to corticosteroid therapy, but their response is generally slower. In both cases, though, there's a potential for relapse.

## SUMMARY

All right, as a short recap: minimal change disease is a nephrotic syndrome thought to be caused by cytokine damage to the foot processes of the podocytes in the glomeruli of the kidney **(Figure 31.7)**.

**Figure 31.7**

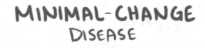

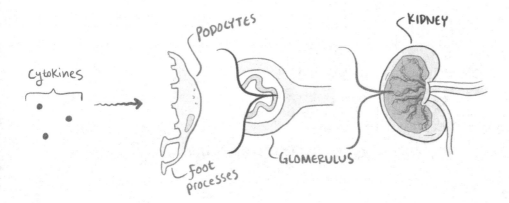

# Multicystic dysplastic kidney

osmosis.org/learn/multicystic_dysplastic_kidney

**M**ulticystic dysplastic kidney, or MCDK, is a congenital disease where one or both kidneys don't form quite right. Specifically, this causes them to not drain urine properly, which results in urine building up in the kidneys and forming multiple fluid-filled sacs called cysts **(Figure 32.1)**

## PHYSIOLOGY

All right, so during fetal development, you've got this structure called the mesonephric duct, which is involved in the development of urinary and reproductive organs. Meanwhile, during the fifth week of gestation, a little guy called the ureteric bud starts pushing its way into another structure called the metanephric blastema, and together, these two little embryologic structures go on to develop into a kidney. At about the seventh week, nephrogenesis, or formation of the kidneys, starts under the influence of that ureteric bud **(Figure 32.2)**.

**Figure 32.1**

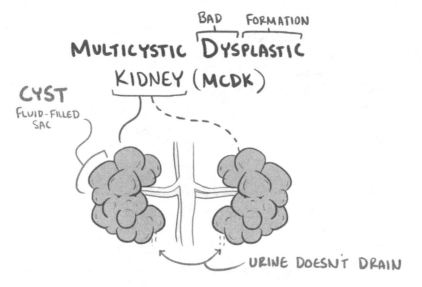

**Figure 32.2**

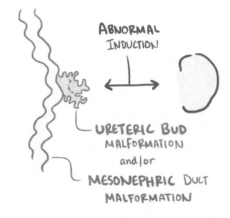

**Figure 32.3**

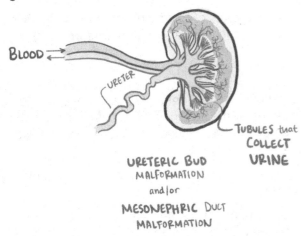

BLOOD ⇄

URETER

TUBULES that COLLECT URINE

URETERIC BUD MALFORMATION
and/or
MESONEPHRIC DUCT MALFORMATION

**Figure 32.4**

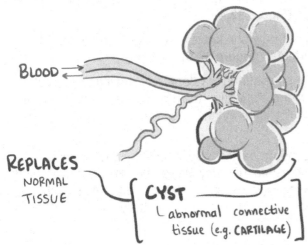

BLOOD ⇄

REPLACES NORMAL TISSUE

CYST
└ abnormal connective tissue (e.g. CARTILAGE)

**Figure 32.5**

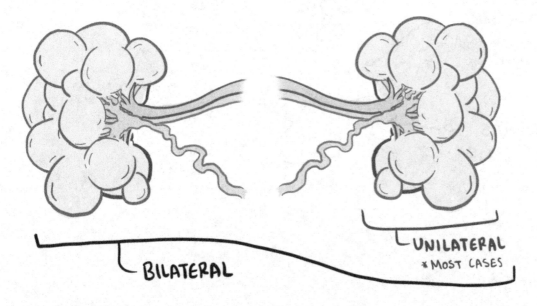

URETER

BILATERAL

UNILATERAL
* MOST CASES

By about twenty weeks, the ureteric bud has formed the ureters, the renal calyces, collecting ducts, and collecting tubules, while the metanephric blastema develops into the nephron itself, which includes the epithelial cells and the podocytes of Bowman's capsule. In the third trimester and throughout infancy, the kidneys continue to grow and mature (**Figure 32.3**).

## CAUSES

Although the cause of MCDK is not completely known, it's thought to be a result of some sort of abnormal induction of the metanephric blastema by the ureteric bud. This failure might be the fault of the mesonephric duct not forming right, or the ureteric bud not forming right, or both.

Regardless of the cause of failure, the ureteric bud is supposed to go on to form the ureters as well as the rest of the tubules that branch out to collect urine.

So, as blood starts coming in to be filtered, and urine starts getting produced, a failure to properly develop into these urine-collecting tubules means that the urine has nowhere to go. So, it builds up in the kidneys and forms these fluid-filled cysts that are composed of abnormal connective tissue—especially cartilage—that actually replaces normal kidney tissue and decreases the kidney's ability to function (**Figure 32.4**).

Most cases are unilateral, meaning they affect only one kidney, although sometimes MCDK might be bilateral, where both kidneys are affected (**Figure 32.5**).

MCDK is usually a sporadic condition that happens during development, and it does not follow a clear inheritance pattern. This is an important distinction from polycystic kidney disease, a similar cystic kidney disease that's familial, meaning inherited, and, it's typically passed through autosomal dominant inheritance.

Having said that, there are some genetic syndromes, like papillorenal syndrome, that have been associated with MCDK, as well as some genes that may play a role, like EYA1, SIX1, and the PAX2 gene. Certain prescription drugs taken for maternal hypertension, like ACE inhibitors, as well as illicit drugs like cocaine, have also been implicated as potentially causing MCDK in the developing fetus (**Figure 32.6**).

**Figure 32.6**

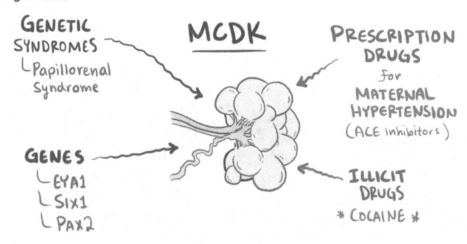

## TREATMENT

If only one kidney's been affected and the other's functioning normally, the remaining kidney might be able to preserve overall kidney function **(Figure 32.7)**. If MCDK is bilateral and mild, the newborn may need dialysis and/or a kidney transplant, but newborns with severe bilateral MCDK usually don't survive **(Figure 32.8)**.

## SUMMARY

All right, so as a quick recap: multicystic dysplastic kidney is a type of non-inherited congenital kidney disease where the ureteric bud fails to develop properly, resulting in a buildup of urine and the formation of cysts **(Figure 32.9)**.

**Figure 32.7**

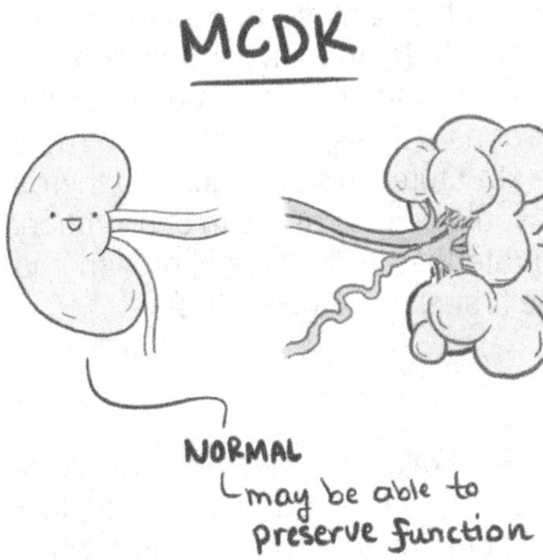

MCDK

NORMAL
└ may be able to
preserve function

**Figure 32.8**

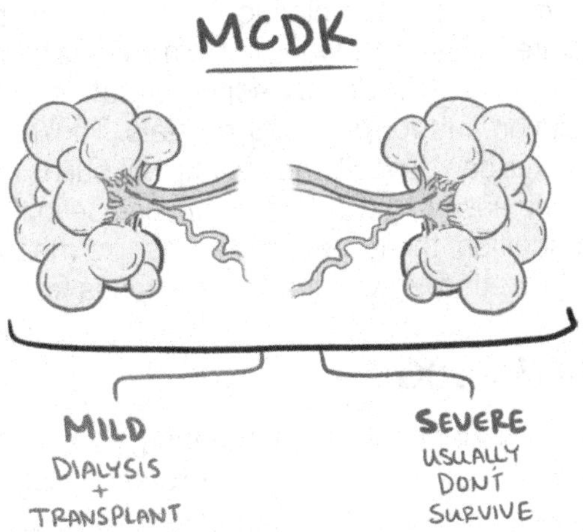

MCDK

MILD
DIALYSIS
+
TRANSPLANT

SEVERE
USUALLY
DON'T
SURVIVE

**Figure 32.9**

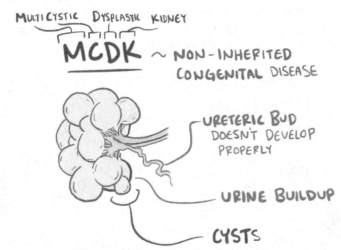

MULTICYSTIC DYSPLASTIC KIDNEY

MCDK ~ NON-INHERITED
CONGENITAL DISEASE

┌ URETERIC BUD
DOESN'T DEVELOP
PROPERLY

URINE BUILDUP

CYSTS

# Nephrolithiasis (kidney stones)

With nephrolithiasis, *nephro-* refers to the kidneys, and *-lithiasis* means stone, so nephrolithiasis means kidney stones, which are sometimes also referred to as renal calculi or urolithiasis. Kidney stones form when solutes in the urine precipitate out and crystalize, and although they most commonly form in the kidneys themselves, they can also form in the ureters, the bladder, or the urethra **(Figure 33.1)**.

## PHYSIOLOGY

Now, urine's a combination of water, which acts as a solvent, and all sorts of particles, or solutes. In general, when certain solutes become too concentrated in the solvent, they become *supersaturated*. Urinary supersaturation of certain solutes results in precipitation out of the solution and formation of crystals. Those crystals then act as a *nidus*, or place where more solutes can deposit and over time it builds up a crystalline structure. This can happen if there's an increase in the solute or a *decrease* in the solvent, as would be the case with dehydration. In addition, there are substances like magnesium and citrate that inhibit crystal growth and aggregation, preventing kidney stones from forming in the first place **(Figure 33.2)**.

## PATHOLOGY

In the majority of cases, the inorganic precipitate is calcium oxalate, formed by a positively charged calcium ion binding to a negatively charged oxalate ion, that results in a black or dark brown colored stone that is radio-opaque on an X-ray, meaning that it shows up as a white spot **(Figure 33.3)**.

Sometimes, instead of oxalate, the calcium binds a negatively charged phosphate group to form calcium phosphate stones which are dirty white in color and alsop radiopaque on an X-ray. Calcium oxalate crystals are more likely to form in acidic urine, whereas calcium phosphate crystals are more likely to form in alkaline urine **(Figure 33.4)**.

**Figure 33.1**

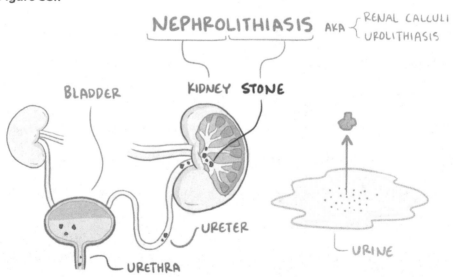

**Figure 33.2**

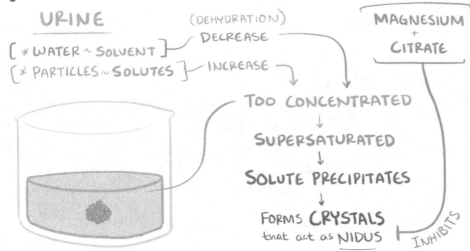

URINE
[ * WATER ~ SOLVENT ]  (DEHYDRATION) DECREASE
[ * PARTICLES ~ SOLUTES ]  INCREASE

MAGNESIUM + CITRATE

TOO CONCENTRATED
↓
SUPERSATURATED
↓
SOLUTE PRECIPITATES
↓
FORMS **CRYSTALS** that act as NIDUS

INHIBITS

**Figure 33.3**

(MOST COMMON)
## CALCIUM OXALATE

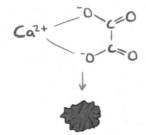

$Ca^{2+}$

* BLACK / DARK BROWN
* RADIOPAQUE on X-RAY

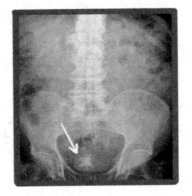

**Figure 33.4**

(MOST COMMON)
## CALCIUM OXALATE

$Ca^{2+}$

* BLACK / DARK BROWN
* RADIOPAQUE on X-RAY
* forms in **ACIDIC** urine

## CALCIUM PHOSPHATE

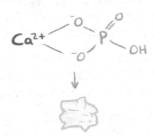

$Ca^{2+}$

* DIRTY WHITE
* RADIOPAQUE on X-RAY
* forms in **ALKALINE** urine

**Figure 33.5**

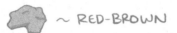

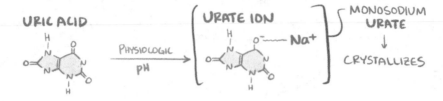

URIC ACID STONES

~ RED-BROWN

* RADIOLUCENT ~ TRANSPARENT to X-RAYS

URIC ACID → (PHYSIOLOGIC pH) → [ URATE ION —Na+ ] → MONOSODIUM URATE ↓ CRYSTALLIZES

**Figure 33.6**

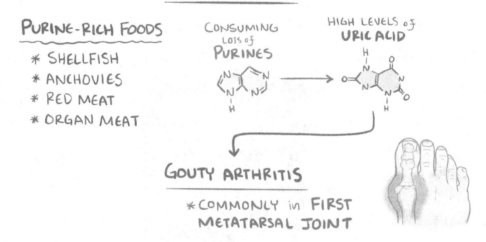

URIC ACID STONES

PURINE-RICH FOODS
* SHELLFISH
* ANCHOVIES
* RED MEAT
* ORGAN MEAT

CONSUMING LOTS of PURINES → HIGH LEVELS of URIC ACID

GOUTY ARTHRITIS
* COMMONLY in FIRST METATARSAL JOINT

## CAUSES

The exact reason why these stones form is usually unknown, but there are some known risk factors, like hypercalcemia and hypercalciuria, or having too much calcium in the blood and urine, respectively. Hypercalcemia can result from increased calcium absorption in the gastrointestinal tract as well as hormonal causes like primary hyperparathyroidism. Hypercalciuria can result from impaired renal tubular reabsorption of calcium, which leaves a lot of calcium behind in the tubule.

For the calcium oxalate stones, hyperoxaluria is a risk factor as well, and it can be due to a genetic defect that increases oxalate excretion, a defect in liver metabolism, or a diet heavy in oxalate-rich foods like rhubarb, spinach, chocolate, nuts, and beer.

There are also uric acid stones, which are red-brown in color and radiolucent under an X-ray, meaning that they're transparent to X-rays and don't show up very well. At a physiologic pH, uric acid loses a proton and becomes a urate ion, which then binds sodium, forming monosodium urate, which then crystallizes and ultimately forms uric acid stones **(Figure 33.5)**.

Since uric acid is a breakdown product of purines, a very common reason for high levels of uric acid is consuming lots of purines. Purine-rich foods include shellfish, anchovies, red meat or organ meat. High levels of uric acid can also cause gouty arthritis, most commonly in the first metatarsal joint, which is the base of the big toe **(Figure 33.6)**.

**Figure 33.7**

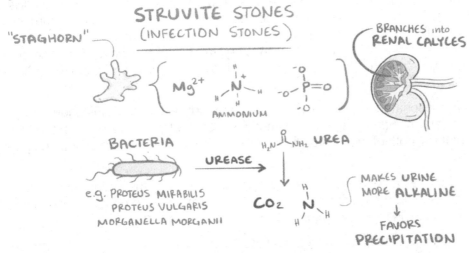

STRUVITE STONES (INFECTION STONES)

"STAGHORN"

$Mg^{2+}$ AMMONIUM $P=O$

BRANCHES into RENAL CALYCES

BACTERIA

e.g. PROTEUS MIRABILIS
PROTEUS VULGARIS
MORGANELLA MORGANII

UREASE

$H_2N$ UREA $NH_2$

$CO_2$ N

MAKES URINE MORE ALKALINE
↓
FAVORS PRECIPITATION

**Figure 33.8**

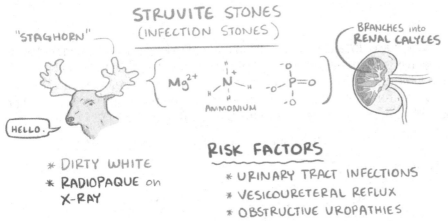

STRUVITE STONES (INFECTION STONES)

"STAGHORN"

$Mg^{2+}$ AMMONIUM $P=O$

BRANCHES into RENAL CALYCES

HELLO.

* DIRTY WHITE
* RADIOPAQUE on X-RAY

RISK FACTORS

* URINARY TRACT INFECTIONS
* VESICOURETERAL REFLUX
* OBSTRUCTIVE UROPATHIES

**Figure 33.9**

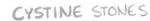
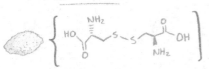

CYSTINE STONES

* YELLOW or LIGHT PINK
* RADIOPAQUE on X-RAY

**Figure 33.10**

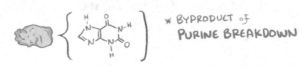

XANTHINE STONES

* BYPRODUCT of PURINE BREAKDOWN

* RED-BROWN
* RADIOLUCENT on X-RAY

A fourth type are struvite stones, sometimes called infection stones, which are a composite mix of magnesium, ammonium, and phosphate. These form when bacteria like *Proteus mirabilis*, *Proteus vulgaris*, and *Morganella morganii* use the enzyme urease to split urea into ammonia and carbon dioxide. The ammonia makes the urine more alkaline and favors precipitation of magnesium, ammonium, and phosphate into jagged crystals called "staghorns" because they often branch into the several of the renal calyces and look like the horns of a staghorn deer **(Figure 33.7)**.

Like the calcium phosphate stones, struvite stones are dirty white and radiopaque under an X-ray. Risk factors include urinary tract infections along with vesicoureteral reflux and obstructive uropathies, both of which are also risk factors for urinary tract infections **(Figure 33.8)**.

A tiny minority of stones are cystine stones that are composed of the amino acid cystine, which sometimes leaks into the urine to crystalize and form a yellow or light pink colored stone that is radiopaque under X-ray **(Figure 33.9)**.

Finally, there are some rare stones made of xanthine, which, just like uric acid, is a byproduct of purine breakdown. These stones, also like uric acid stones, are red-brown in color and radiolucent under an X-ray **(Figure 33.10)**.

## SYMPTOMS

Kidney stones can cause dull or localized flank pain in the mid to lower back on both sides, as well as renal colic, which is a sharp pain and is a bit of a misnomer because the pain is usually constant rather than intermittent. The pain is caused by the dilation, stretching, and spasm caused by obstruction of the ureter, and is typically worse at the ureteropelvic junction and down the ureter, subsiding once the stone gets to the bladder **(Figure 33.11)**.

Stones that are less than 5 mm across are usually passed within hours.

**Figure 33.11**

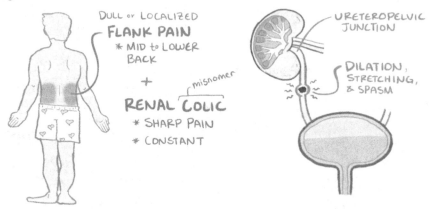

## DIAGNOSIS

Diagnosis involves a history and physical exam, as well as imaging studies like ultrasound and CT scans, and, finally, urinalysis because it might show microscopic or gross hematuria or blood in the urine.

## TREATMENT

Treatment or management includes hydrating an individual to reverse the process of precipitation. Also, medications might be given to help reduce pain, to reduce stone formation, like potassium citrate, and to help stones pass through, like alpha adrenergic blockers and calcium channel blockers. Also, shockwave lithotripsy might be used, which is a noninvasive treatment that uses high-intensity acoustic pulses that travel through the body to break up the kidney stones. Finally, surgery and stent placement might be needed for larger stones.

## SUMMARY

All right, as a quick recap: nephrolithiasis is the formation of kidney stones, which form when solutes precipitate out into crystals in the urine. The most common type of stones are calcium oxalate stones, though other types include uric acid stones and struvite stones **(Figure 33.12)**.

**Figure 33.12**

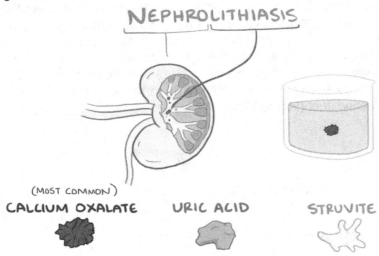

NEPHROLITHIASIS

(MOST COMMON)
CALCIUM OXALATE          URIC ACID          STRUVITE

# Nephronophthisis & medullary cystic kidney disease

osmosis.org/learn/medullary_cystic_kidney_disease

Nephronophthisis, which means "nephron wasting," and medullary cystic kidney disease, which refers to fluid-filled sacs in the medulla, are two kidney diseases that share some similar features: they're both genetic, they both affect the nephrons, and both can lead to kidney cysts and renal failure over time (Figure 34.1).

## PHYSIOLOGY

To help understand these diseases, let's first take a zoomed-in look at a nephron and talk about how it works. So, the outer layer of the kidney is called the cortex, and this is where the glomeruli live. The glomeruli are where blood is initially filtered into the nephron, as well as the proximal convoluted tubule, where some of the filtered substances are reabsorbed back into the body. The filtered substances, or filtrate, that don't get reabsorbed then move down through the medulla via the descending and then ascending parts of the loop of Henle. The filtrate then goes back to the cortex briefly in the distal convoluted tubule, and then returns back to the medulla in the collecting duct (Figure 34.2).

**Figure 34.1**

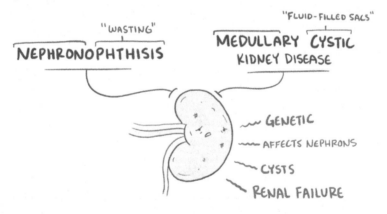

**Figure 34.2**

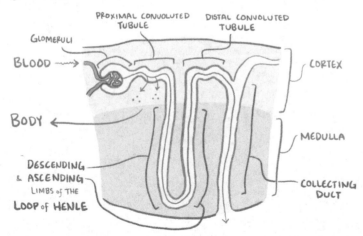

**Figure 34.3**

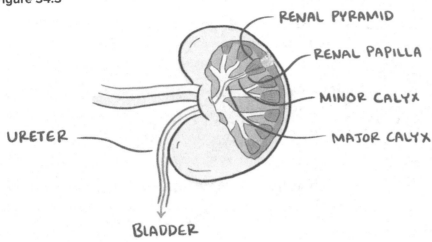

**Figure 34.4**

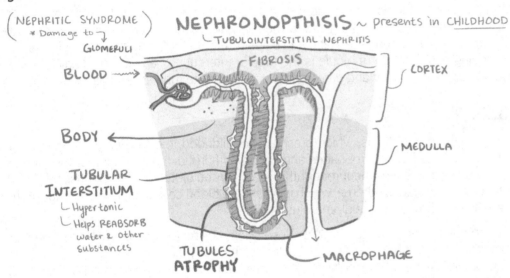

**Figure 34.5**

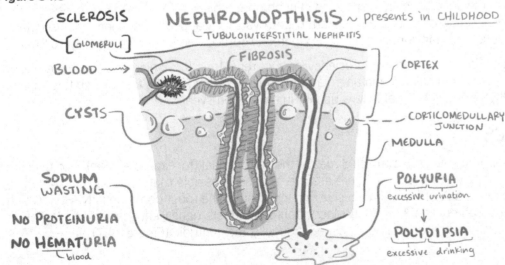

**Figure 34.6**

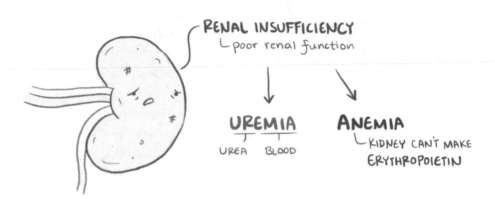

NEPHRONOPTHISIS ~ presents in CHILDHOOD
└ TUBULOINTERSTITIAL NEPHRITIS

RENAL INSUFFICIENCY
└ poor renal function

UREMIA
├─┬─┤
UREA  BLOOD

ANEMIA
└ KIDNEY CAN'T MAKE
ERYTHROPOIETIN

Zooming back out a bit, the collecting ducts in each region of the kidney, called renal pyramids, converge on the renal papilla, dumping fully formed urine into a minor calyx. This urine goes into the major calyx, before entering the ureter and bladder **(Figure 34.3)**. Zooming back in, we see that surrounding each nephron's tubule is the tubular interstitium, a hypertonic environment optimized to help resorb water and other substances from the tubules **(Figure 34.4)**.

## PATHOLOGY

All right, so in nephronophthisis, which presents in childhood, the tubules atrophy and the interstitium is infiltrated by macrophages and becomes fibrotic. Inflammation of the tubules and the interstitium qualifies nephronophthisis as a tubulointerstitial nephritis, but don't confuse this with nephritic syndrome, which is where red blood cells and protein escape in the urine as a result of damage to the glomerulus.

In nephronophthisis, the affected tubules lose their ability to concentrate the urine by reabsorbing water and other substances back into the body, so urine ends up being more dilute than usual. This leads to polyuria, excessive urination, and therefore polydipsia, or excessive drinking **(Figure 34.5)**. Sodium wasting also happens, which is where excess sodium is excreted in the urine, but proteinuria or proteins in the urine as well as hematuria or blood in the urine typically aren't seen in nephronophthisis. As the disease progresses, the glomeruli can become sclerosed, or scarred, and cysts may appear in the medulla, particularly in the corticomedullary junction, which is where the cortex meets the medulla **(Figure 34.6)**.

Over time, this leads to renal insufficiency, or poor renal function, which can cause uremia, or too much urea in the blood, and anemia from a failure of the kidneys to make erythropoietin. Eventually, this leads to renal failure, usually in the teenage years.

## CAUSES

Nephronophthisis is broken into subtypes by the age of onset (for example, infantile or juvenile) or by the gene that's mutated. There are over a dozen possible mutated genes, all of which are inherited in an autosomal recessive fashion, though the most common is NPHP1, which codes for nephrocystin 1 protein. Most nephronophthisis genes encode for and therefore affect proteins in primary cilia or a related organelle, the centriole **(Figure 34.7)**.

**Figure 34.7**

# NEPHRONOPTHISIS

## SUBTYPES
└ AGE of ONSET
  e.g. Infantile, juvenile
└ GENE MUTATION
  • Autosomal recessive
  • Most common ~ NPHP1
  • USUALLY AFFECTS
    └ PRIMARY CILIA
    └ CENTRIOLE

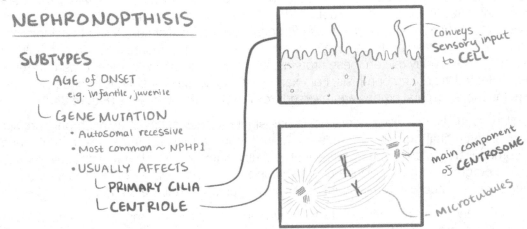

conveys Sensory input to CELL

main component of CENTROSOME

Microtubules

**Figure 34.8**

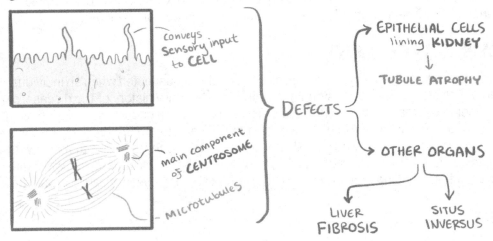

conveys Sensory input to CELL

main component of CENTROSOME

Microtubules

DEFECTS

→ EPITHELIAL CELLS lining KIDNEY
  ↓
  TUBULE ATROPHY

→ OTHER ORGANS

LIVER FIBROSIS

SITUS INVERSUS

**Figure 34.9**

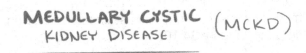

# MEDULLARY CYSTIC (MCKD)
## KIDNEY DISEASE

\* SIMILAR CHANGES to NEPHRONOPHTHISIS

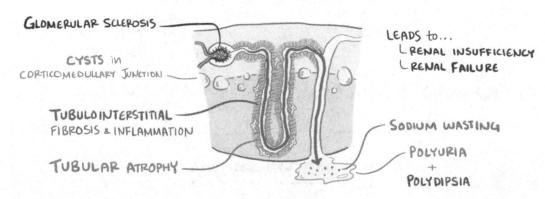

GLOMERULAR SCLEROSIS

CYSTS in CORTICOMEDULLARY JUNCTION

TUBULOINTERSTITIAL FIBROSIS & INFLAMMATION

TUBULAR ATROPHY

LEADS to...
└ RENAL INSUFFICIENCY
└ RENAL FAILURE

SODIUM WASTING

POLYURIA
+
POLYDIPSIA

Primary cilia are present on almost every human cell. These tiny appendages project outside the cell and convey sensory input to the inside of the cell. The centriole is the main component of the centrosome, and it helps organize the mitotic spindle and microtubules during cell division. When there are defects in these structures, the epithelial cells lining the kidney are seriously affected, leading to the tubule atrophy seen in nephronophthisis. Primary cilia in other parts of the body rely on these proteins, too, which explains why other organ systems can be affected in nephronophthisis. For example, it can cause liver fibrosis or situs inversus, where the major visceral organs are reversed from their normal positions **(Figure 34.8)**.

Medullary cystic kidney disease, or MCKD, has similar kidney changes as nephronophthisis, like tubulointerstitial fibrosis and inflammation, tubular atrophy, cysts in the medulla and corticomedullary junction, and eventually glomerular sclerosis. MCKD's also clinically similar too, with progression from polyuria and polydipsia due to poor urine concentration and salt wasting, and eventually to renal insufficiency and renal failure **(Figure 34.9)**.

 Some differences are that MCKD starts in adulthood, and doesn't have symptoms in other organs except for hyperuricemia, which is due to a failure to excrete uric acid and causes gout. Also, there are two types of medullary cystic kidney disease: one is called MCKD1, which is caused by mutations in the MUC1 gene, and the other is called MCKD2, which is caused by mutations in the UMOD gene. Both of these conditions are autosomal dominant.

## DIAGNOSIS & TREATMENT

Nephronophthisis and medullary cystic kidney disease might be suspected when an individual has polyuria or polydipsia as an early symptom, or if there's a family history of the disease, or if there is a finding on imaging like kidney cysts. To confirm the diagnosis, a renal biopsy or genetic testing can be done. Based on the severity of the disease, treatment primarily involves dialysis and kidney transplant. Having said all that, it's important to remember that renal cysts can be caused by a lot of other diseases, and they can also just be simple renal cysts, which are a common, age-related finding that tend to be in the cortex and don't usually cause problems.

## SUMMARY

All right, to recap: nephronophthisis and medullary cystic kidney disease are genetic disorders that affect the renal tubules and interstitium and can lead to cysts and renal failure. Nephronophthisis presents in childhood, is autosomal recessive, and can involve other organs, whereas medullary cystic kidney disease presents later on, is autosomal dominant, and affects only the kidney **(Figure 34.10)**.

**Figure 34.10**

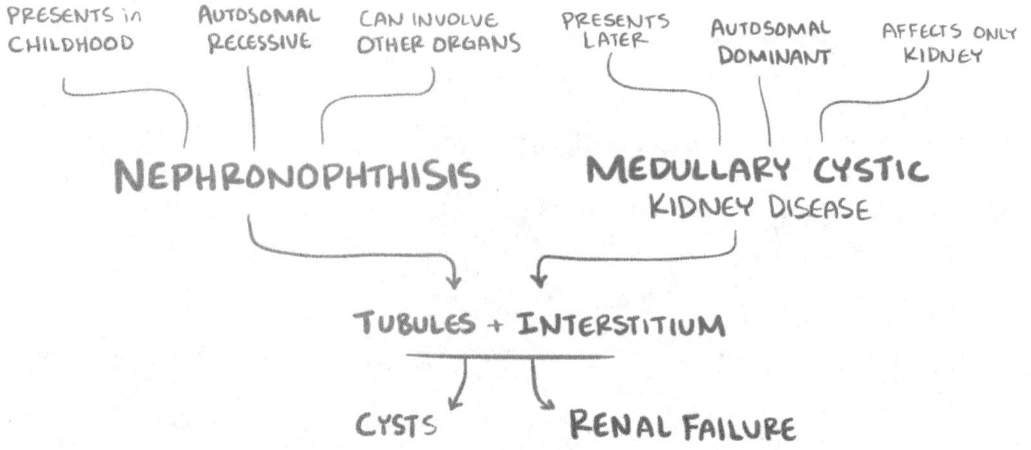

# Neurogenic bladder

osmosis.org/learn/neurogenic_bladder

**W**ith neurogenic bladder, *neurogenic* refers to a condition that arises from the nervous system, so neurogenic bladder is typically some difficulty emptying the bladder normally, and this is the result of damage to either the peripheral nerves, brain, or spinal cord **(Figure 35.1)**.

## PHYSIOLOGY

Normally, urine is held in the bladder, which receives urine from two ureters coming down from the kidneys; then, that urine leaves the bladder through the urethra. As urine flows from the kidney through the ureters and into the bladder, the bladder starts to expand into the abdomen. The bladder is able to expand and contract because it's wrapped in a muscular layer, called the detrusor muscle, and then lining the bladder itself is a layer of transitional epithelium containing umbrella cells. These umbrella cells get their name because they physically stretch out as the bladder fills, just like an umbrella opening in slow-motion. In a grown adult, the bladder can expand to hold about 750 ml. This is usually slightly less in women than in men because the uterus crowds the bladder out a bit **(Figure 35.2)**.

**Figure 35.1**

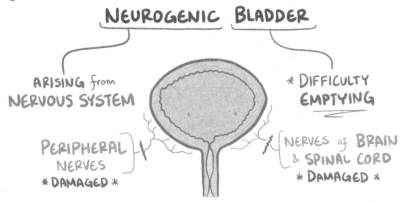

**Figure 35.2**

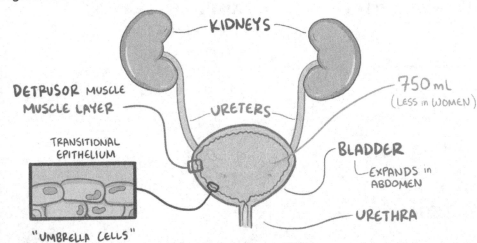

**Figure 35.3**

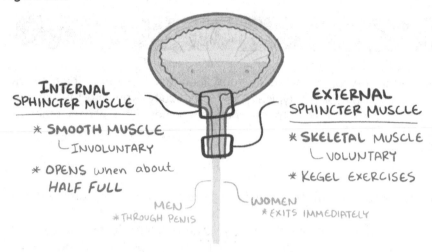

INTERNAL SPHINCTER MUSCLE
* SMOOTH MUSCLE
  └ INVOLUNTARY
* OPENS when about HALF FULL

EXTERNAL SPHINCTER MUSCLE
* SKELETAL MUSCLE
  └ VOLUNTARY
* KEGEL EXERCISES

MEN
* THROUGH PENIS

WOMEN
* EXITS IMMEDIATELY

**Figure 35.4**

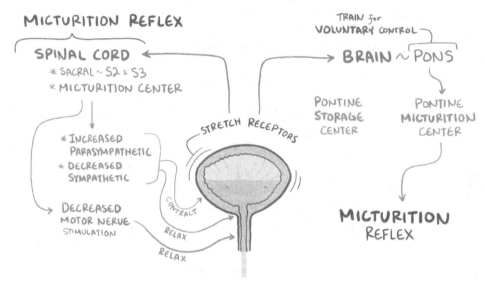

MICTURITION REFLEX

SPINAL CORD
* SACRAL ~ S2 & S3
* MICTURITION CENTER

* INCREASED PARASYMPATHETIC
* DECREASED SYMPATHETIC

DECREASED MOTOR NERVE STIMULATION

CONTRACT

RELAX

RELAX

STRETCH RECEPTORS

TRAIN for VOLUNTARY CONTROL

BRAIN ~ PONS

PONTINE STORAGE CENTER

PONTINE MICTURITION CENTER

MICTURITION REFLEX

**Figure 35.5**

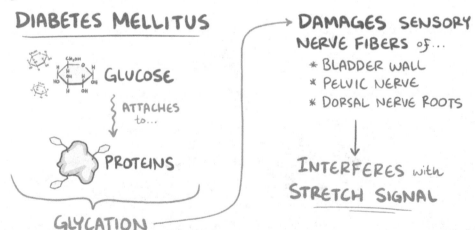

DIABETES MELLITUS

GLUCOSE

ATTACHES to...

PROTEINS

GLYCATION

DAMAGES SENSORY NERVE FIBERS of...
* BLADDER WALL
* PELVIC NERVE
* DORSAL NERVE ROOTS

INTERFERES with STRETCH SIGNAL

Okay, so when the urine is collecting in the bladder, there are basically two "doors" that are shut and holding that urine in. The first door is the internal sphincter muscle, which is made of smooth muscle and is under involuntary control, meaning that it opens and closes automatically. Typically, the internal sphincter muscle opens up when the bladder is about half full. Now, the second door is the external sphincter muscle, and it's made of skeletal muscle and is under voluntary control, meaning that it opens and closes when a person wants it to do so. This is the reason that it's possible to stop urine midstream by tightening up that muscle, and this is called doing Kegel exercises. Once urine has passed through the external sphincter muscle, it exits the body. In women, the exit is generally immediate, and in men, the urine generally flows through the penis before it exits **(Figure 35.3)**.

So, when specialized nerves called "stretch receptors" in the bladder wall sense that the bladder is about half full, they send impulses to the spinal cord and the brain. More specifically, they signal to the sacral spinal cord at levels S2 and S3, known as the micturition center, and two locations in the pons, the pontine storage center and pontine micturition center. The spinal cord response is part of the micturition reflex, and it causes an increase in parasympathetic stimulation and decrease in sympathetic stimulation, making the detrusor muscle contract and the internal sphincter relax. It also decreases motor nerve stimulation to the external sphincter, allowing it to relax as well. At this point, urination would occur if not for the pons. The pons is the region of the brain that we train to voluntarily control urination.

If we want to delay urination, or hold it in, the pontine storage center overrides the micturition reflex, and when we want to urinate, the pontine micturition center allows for the micturition reflex to happen **(Figure 35.4)**.

## CAUSES

Now with neurogenic bladder, the exact pattern of symptoms depends on the nerve that is damaged. In diabetes mellitus, excess glucose levels in the blood attaches to various proteins, and this process is called glycation. Glycation can damage sensory nerve fibers in the bladder wall, in the pelvic nerve, or in the dorsal nerve roots entering the spinal cord, and all of this interferes with the initial stretch signal that gets sent out as the bladder fills **(Figure 35.5)**.

Another potential cause of neurogenic bladder is syphilis. This infection can eventually lead to tabes dorsalis, which is inflammation and scarring of those same little dorsal root nerves. In individuals with herpes, the virus takes up a home in the dorsal nerve roots for months to years, and it can also disrupt the sensory fibers that they carry within them. In both of these cases, this damage means that as the bladder fills to capacity and stretches, that sensory information is not received, and the bladder starts to overflow, drop by drop, out of the urethra. This is called overflow incontinence **(Figure 35.6)**.

**Figure 35.6**

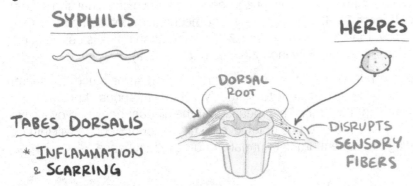

**Figure 35.7**

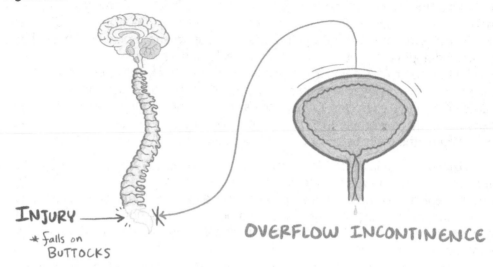

INJURY ──→
＊ falls on
BUTTOCKS

OVERFLOW INCONTINENCE

**Figure 35.8**

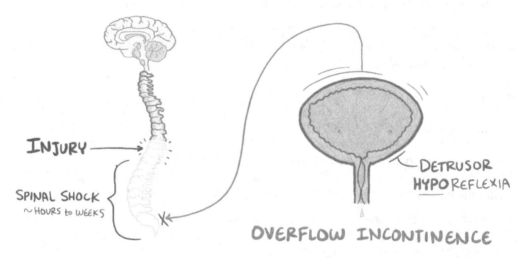

INJURY ──────→

SPINAL SHOCK {
~ HOURS to WEEKS

DETRUSOR
HYPO REFLEXIA

OVERFLOW INCONTINENCE

Now, as we know, that sensory information goes through the micturition center at the S2-S3 region of the spinal cord. If there's an injury to the spinal cord in that region—for example, if someone falls from a tree or ladder and lands on their buttocks—then that micturition reflex pathway is interrupted, and the individual can get overflow incontinence **(Figure 35.7)**.

Now, if there's a spinal cord injury above the sacral region, immediately afterward all of the reflexes below the injury will be suppressed. This phenomenon is known as spinal shock, and it can last hours to weeks **(Figure 35.8)**. Though the exact mechanism behind spinal shock isn't completely clear, we know that during spinal shock, the micturition reflex is suppressed, leading to detrusor hyporeflexia and overflow incontinence **(Figure 35.9)**.

Now, once the shock wears off, the micturition reflex will normally resume since the sacral region is intact. However, signals can't be sent to or received from the pons, which means there's no inhibitory pathway from the brain. This means that the bladder goes into overdrive mode, leading to detrusor *hyper*reflexia. At this point, even a tiny amount of urine will initiate the micturition reflex, leading to frequent urges to urinate, or urge incontinence.

**Figure 35.9**

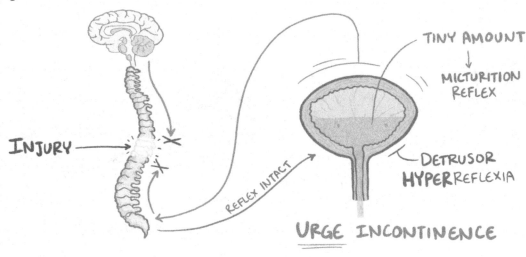

**Figure 35.10**

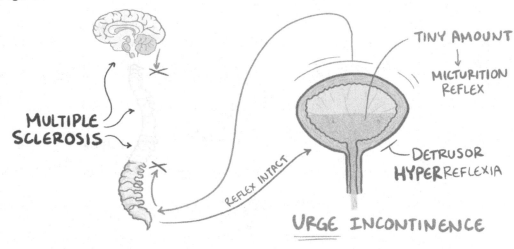

A similar pattern unfolds in multiple sclerosis, except in this case, it's the body's immune system that attacks the myelin sheath of the nerves in the brain and spinal cord. Once again, though, this can prevent the inhibitory signals from the brain from reaching the micturition reflex pathway, causing detrusor *hyper*reflexia and urge incontinence **(Figure 35.10)**.

If there are acute injuries to the brain, like a stroke, then we'll see a similar pattern as spinal injuries: an initial "shock" phase of detrusor hyporeflexia followed by detrusor hyperreflexia and urge incontinence **(Figure 35.11; Figure 35.12)**.

In chronic processes like a brain tumor or Parkinson's disease, there is usually no state of shock; instead, the body proceeds directly to detrusor hyperreflexia and urge incontinence **(Figure 35.13)**.

# DIAGNOSIS

Diagnosis can be done by measuring post-void residuals or the amount of urine left in the bladder after urination and the pressure and flow of urine.

**Figure 35.11**

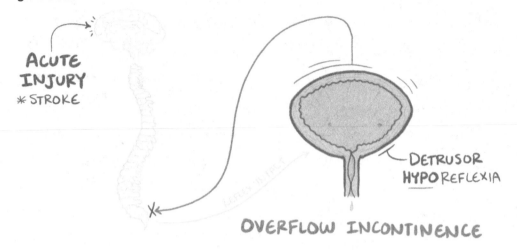

ACUTE
INJURY
* STROKE

REFLEX IS INTACT

DETRUSOR
**HYPO**REFLEXIA

OVERFLOW INCONTINENCE

**Figure 35.12**

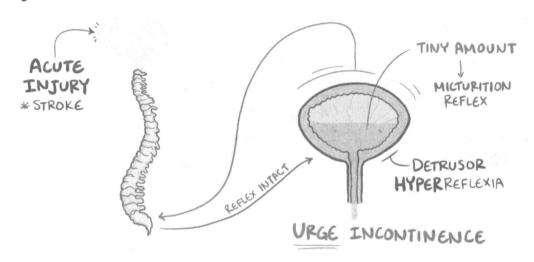

ACUTE
INJURY
* STROKE

TINY AMOUNT
↓
MICTURITION
REFLEX

REFLEX INTACT

DETRUSOR
**HYPER**REFLEXIA

URGE INCONTINENCE

**Figure 35.13**

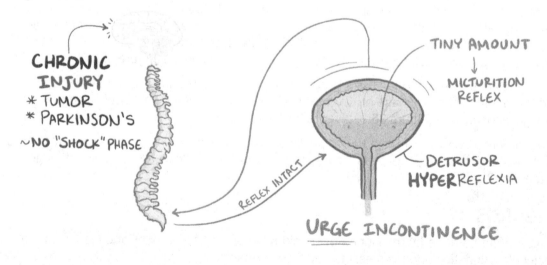

**CHRONIC
INJURY**
* TUMOR
* PARKINSON'S
~ NO "SHOCK" PHASE

TINY AMOUNT
↓
MICTURITION
REFLEX

REFLEX INTACT

DETRUSOR
**HYPER**REFLEXIA

URGE INCONTINENCE

## TREATMENT

To treat overflow incontinence, healthcare professionals put a catheter through the urethra in order to drain the urine. Urge incontinence can be relieved with anticholinergic drugs that help relax the detrusor muscle.

## SUMMARY

All right, as a quick recap: neurogenic bladder is where some form of nerve damage causes bladder dysfunction. This dysfunction could be overflow incontinence, where the bladder fills up to capacity and then dribbles out of the urethra, or urge incontinence, where an individual feels frequent urges to urinate **(Figure 35.14)**.

**Figure 35.14**

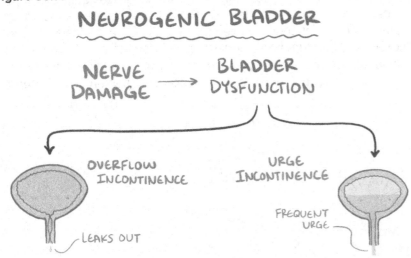

# Non-urothelial bladder cancers

osmosis.org/learn/bladder_cancer

**T**here are two types of bladder cancers: urothelial and non-urothelial types **(Figure 36.1)**. The urothelium is a special type of transitional cell epithelium that forms a stretchy, protective barrier in the bladder. The majority of primary bladder tumors are urothelial cell carcinomas, also known as transitional cell carcinomas, that obviously originate from the urothelium. Somewhat confusingly, non-urothelial tumors, like squamous cell carcinomas and adenocarcinomas, also often arise from the urothelium layer, but they're distinguished by the way that their cells differentiate **(Figure 36.2)**.

For example, the normal bladder surface is not normally lined with squamous epithelium, yet the cells in the urothelium can change shape and take on the flat, pancake-like appearance of squamous cells. This non-cancerous change is called squamous cell metaplasia. If these cells begin to grow unchecked, they can turn into a squamous cell carcinoma. These tumors typically pop up in multiple locations and show extensive keratinization, which is where the cytoplasm of the cells is filled with keratin, the same tough material in hair and nails **(Figure 36.3; Figure 36.4)**.

**Figure 36.1**

there are
### TWO TYPES of BLADDER CANCERS

UROTHELIAL
CELL CARCINOMAS

BLADDER!

NON-UROTHELIAL

**Figure 36.2**

there are
### TWO TYPES of BLADDER CANCERS

UROTHELIAL
CELL CARCINOMAS

MAJORITY of PRIMARY
BLADDER TUMORS

A.K.A. TRANSITIONAL
CELL CARCINOMAS

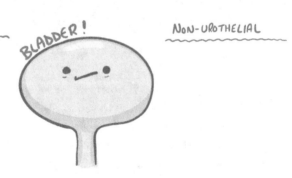

NON-UROTHELIAL

ALSO COME FROM THE
UROTHELIUM

\* SQUAMOUS CELL
CARCINOMAS

\* ADENOCARCINOMAS

UROTHELIUM: a type of TRANSITIONAL CELL
EPITHELIUM that forms a STRETCHY, PROTECTIVE BARRIER

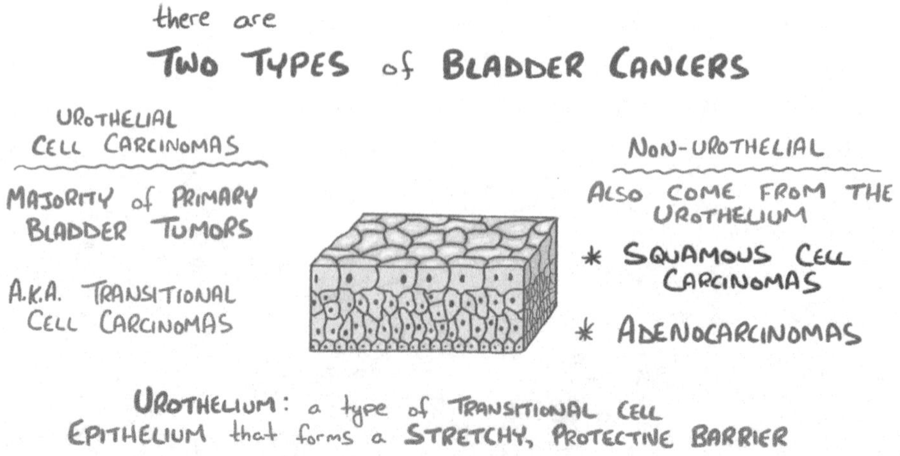

**Figure 36.3**

this is called
SQUAMOUS CELL
METAPLASIA
↑

cells of the UROTHELIUM
can take on a
FLAT, PANCAKE-LIKE
APPEARANCE of
SQUAMOUS CELLS

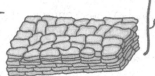

NORMAL BLADDER
is NOT LINED with
SQUAMOUS CELLS

UROTHELIUM: a type of TRANSITIONAL CELL
EPITHELIUM that forms a STRETCHY, PROTECTIVE BARRIER

**Figure 36.4**

## SQUAMOUS CELL CARCINOMA

this is called
SQUAMOUS CELL
METAPLASIA
↑

cells of the UROTHELIUM
can take on a
FLAT, PANCAKE-LIKE
APPEARANCE of
SQUAMOUS CELLS

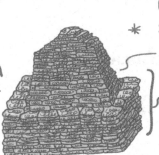

* TYPICALLY form in
  MULTIPLE LOCATIONS
* SHOW KERATIZATION
  like in HAIR & NAILS

NORMAL BLADDER
is NOT LINED with
SQUAMOUS CELLS

UROTHELIUM: a type of TRANSITIONAL CELL
EPITHELIUM that forms a STRETCHY, PROTECTIVE BARRIER

**Figure 36.5**

## SQUAMOUS CELL CARCINOMA

CHRONIC IRRITATION

* URINARY TRACT INFECTION
* KIDNEY STONES
* SCHISTOSOMA HAEMATOBIUM
  (a flatworm)

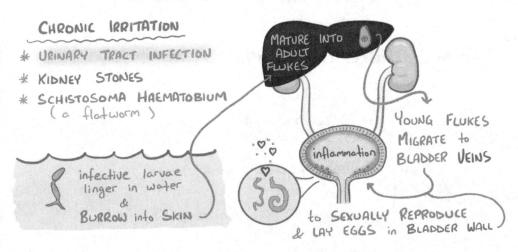

MATURE INTO
ADULT
FLUKES

YOUNG FLUKES
MIGRATE to
BLADDER VEINS

infective larvae
linger in water
&
BURROW into SKIN

inflammation

to SEXUALLY REPRODUCE
& LAY EGGS in BLADDER WALL

# PATHOLOGY

Squamous cell carcinomas typically arise in response to chronic irritation, like from recurrent urinary tract infections and long-standing kidney stones. Another cause common in some parts of the world, is an infection with *Schistosoma haematobium*, a type of flatworm. In this infection, the infective larvae linger in the water and then burrow into human skin when given the opportunity, travelling to the liver to mature into adult flukes. From there, young flukes migrate to the urinary bladder veins to sexually reproduce and lay eggs in the bladder wall. These eggs can get urinated out, but they also cause chronic inflammation in the bladder wall, which is how they lead to squamous cell carcinomas **(Figure 36.5)**.

Primary adenocarcinomas of the bladder are more rare, but unlike squamous cell carcinomas, they frequently metastasize. These are usually solitary and derive from glandular tissue, so they can often produce a lot of mucin. Adenocarcinomas are the main form of bladder tumors in patients with bladder exstrophy, which is where the bladder protrudes through a birth defect in the abdominal wall and partially or completely sits outside of the body. Adenocarcinomas can also develop in response to *Schistosoma haematobium* infections **(Figure 36.6)**.

Finally, it's worth noting that adenocarcinomas of the urachus are quite similar to bladder adenocarcinomas. The urachus is the fibrous tissue sitting at the dome of the bladder that serves as the remnant of the allantois, the canal that allows urine to flow from the fetal bladder into the amniotic sac **(Figure 36.7)**.

**Figure 36.6**

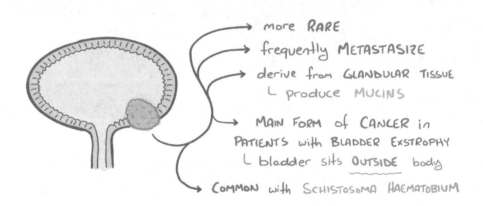

PRIMARY ADENOCARCINOMA

- more RARE
- frequently METASTASIZE
- derive from GLANDULAR TISSUE
  - └ produce MUCINS
- MAIN FORM of CANCER in PATIENTS with BLADDER EXSTROPHY
  - └ bladder sits OUTSIDE body
- COMMON with SCHISTOSOMA HAEMATOBIUM

**Figure 36.7**

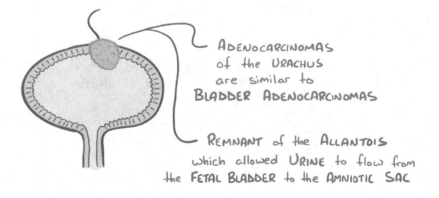

PRIMARY ADENOCARCINOMA

ADENOCARCINOMAS of the URACHUS are similar to BLADDER ADENOCARCINOMAS

REMNANT of the ALLANTOIS which allowed URINE to flow from the FETAL BLADDER to the AMNIOTIC SAC

**Figure 36.8**

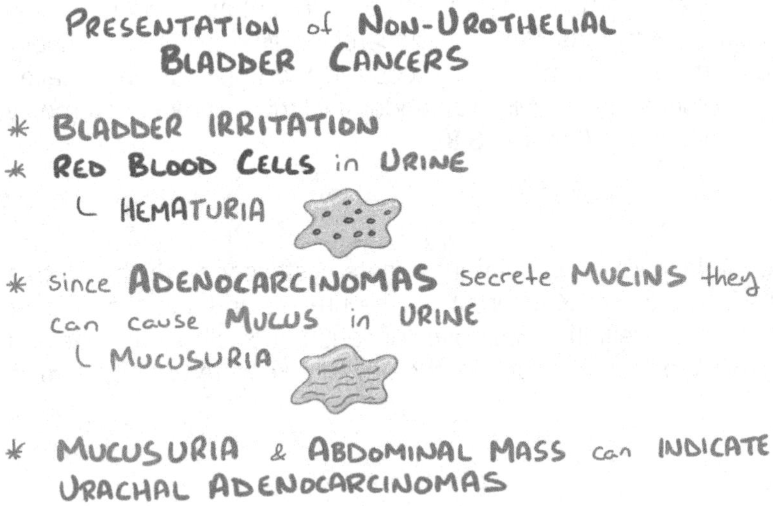

## PRESENTATION of NON-UROTHELIAL BLADDER CANCERS

* BLADDER IRRITATION
* RED BLOOD CELLS in URINE
   └ HEMATURIA

* since ADENOCARCINOMAS secrete MUCINS they can cause MUCUS in URINE
   └ MUCUSURIA

* MUCUSURIA & ABDOMINAL MASS can INDICATE URACHAL ADENOCARCINOMAS

**Figure 36.9**

## DIAGNOSIS

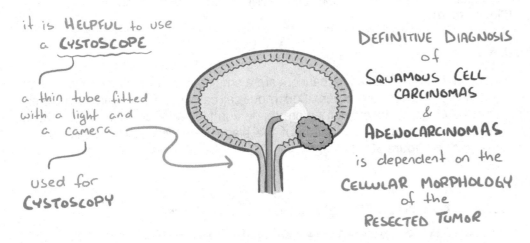

it is HELPFUL to use a CYSTOSCOPE

a thin tube fitted with a light and a camera

used for CYSTOSCOPY

DEFINITIVE DIAGNOSIS of SQUAMOUS CELL CARCINOMAS & ADENOCARCINOMAS is dependent on the CELLULAR MORPHOLOGY of the RESECTED TUMOR

**Figure 36.10**

## TREATMENT

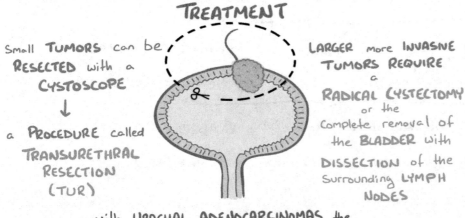

Small TUMORS can be RESECTED with a CYSTOSCOPE
↓
a PROCEDURE called TRANSURETHRAL RESECTION (TUR)

LARGER more INVASIVE TUMORS REQUIRE a RADICAL CYSTECTOMY or the complete removal of the BLADDER with DISSECTION of the surrounding LYMPH NODES

with URACHAL ADENOCARCINOMAS the BLADDER DOME, URACHAL LIGAMENT & UMBILICUS are removed

## SYMPTOMS

These non-urothelial bladder cancers typically present with bladder irritation and red blood cells in the urine, a condition called hematuria. Since adenocarcinomas often secrete mucin, these cancers can also cause an excess amount of mucus in the urine, which is called mucusuria. While relatively rare, mucusuria as well as an abdominal mass is most commonly associated with urachal adenocarcinomas **(Figure 36.8)**.

## DIAGNOSIS

To diagnose a cancer of the bladder, it's often helpful to use a cystoscope, which is a thin tube fitted with a light, and a camera that is inserted up the urethra and into the bladder during a procedure called cystoscopy. Definitive diagnoses of squamous cell carcinomas and adenocarcinomas is based mainly on the cellular morphology of a resected tumor **(Figure 36.9)**.

## TREATMENT

Small tumors can be resected with a cystoscope in a procedure called Transurethral Resection, or TUR. But larger, invasive tumors could require a radical cystectomy, which is the complete removal of the bladder along with dissection of the surrounding lymph nodes. With urachal adenocarcinomas, the bladder dome, urachal ligament, and umbilicus are all generally removed **(Figure 36.10)**.

## SUMMARY

All right, to recap: non-urothelial bladder cancers are a small subset of bladder cancers that confusingly, often arise from the urothelium. Squamous cell carcinomas are made completely of squamous cells, while adenocarcinomas are made completely of glandular cells. These cancers often arise due to chronic irritation of the bladder, especially from *Schistosoma haematobium* infection **(Figure 36.11)**.

Figure 36.11

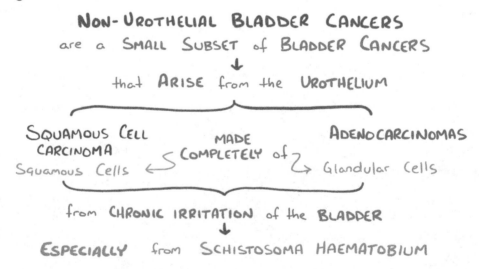

# Polycystic kidney disease

osmosis.org/learn/polycystic_kidney_disease

Polycystic kidney disease, or PKD, is a genetic disease in which the kidneys become filled with hundreds of cysts, or fluid-filled sacs, causing them to be larger than normal and to eventually stop functioning **(Figure 37.1)**.

## PHYSIOLOGY

These cysts develop in the cortex, or outer layer, as well as the medulla, or inner layer, of both kidneys. These cysts, which are lined with renal tubular epithelium, fill up with fluid and get larger and larger over time, making the kidneys much larger than normal. The blood vessels that feed neighboring healthy nephrons can get compressed by growing cysts, which literally starves them of oxygen. Poorly perfused kidneys respond by activating the renin-angiotensin-aldosterone system, which facilitates fluid retention and leads to hypertension **(Figure 37.2)**. Also, expanding cysts can compress the collecting system, causing urinary stasis. In some cases, this can lead to kidney stones **(Figure 37.3)**.

Additionally, destruction of the normal renal architecture can cause symptoms like flank pain and hematuria, or blood in the urine. Over time, as enough nephrons are affected, this leads to renal insufficiency and eventually renal failure **(Figure 37.4)**.

**Figure 37.1**

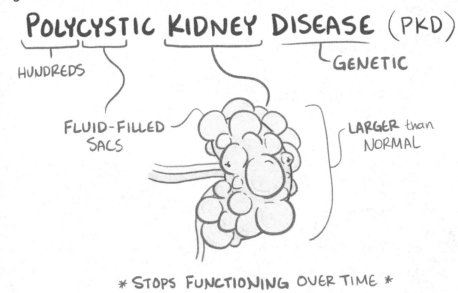

POLYCYSTIC KIDNEY DISEASE (PKD)

GENETIC

HUNDREDS

FLUID-FILLED SACS

LARGER than NORMAL

* STOPS FUNCTIONING OVER TIME *

## PATHOLOGY

Now, the first type of PKD is autosomal dominant PKD, or ADPKD, which used to be called adult PKD, since its symptoms usually manifest in adulthood. The first gene responsible for ADPKD is PKD1, which, when mutated, causes the more severe and earlier onset variety, and PKD2, which, when mutated, causes less severe disease and is also later in onset. *PKD1* and *PKD2* code for the polycystin 1 and polycystin 2 proteins, respectively, which are components of the primary cilium **(Figure 37.5)**.

**Figure 37.2**

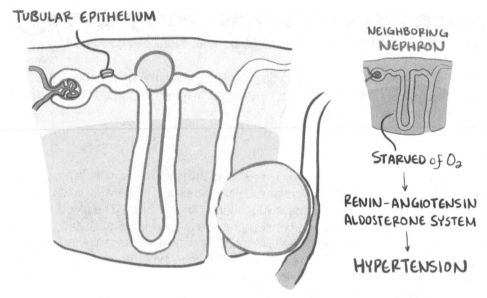

TUBULAR EPITHELIUM

NEIGHBORING NEPHRON

STARVED of $O_2$
↓
RENIN-ANGIOTENSIN ALDOSTERONE SYSTEM
↓
HYPERTENSION

**Figure 37.3**

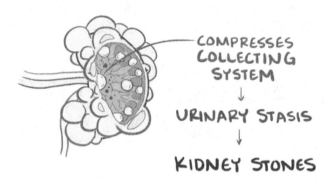

COMPRESSES COLLECTING SYSTEM
↓
URINARY STASIS
↓
KIDNEY STONES

**Figure 37.4**

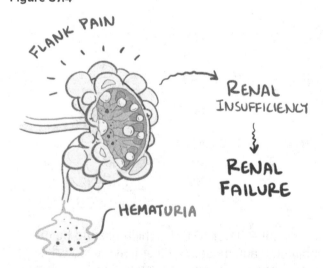

FLANK PAIN

RENAL INSUFFICIENCY
↓
RENAL FAILURE

HEMATURIA

**Figure 37.5**

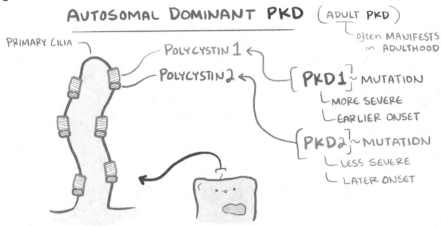

**Figure 37.6**

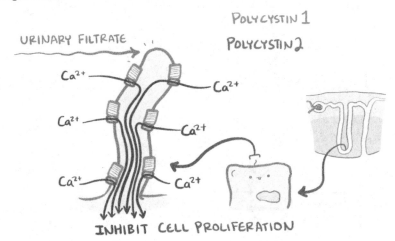

Now, the primary cilium is an appendage that sticks out from most cells in the body and receives developmentally important signals. More specifically, in the nephron, as the urinary filtrate flows by and cause it to bend, polycystin 1 and polycystin 2 respond by allowing calcium influx, which activates pathways in the cell that inhibit cell proliferation **(Figure 37.6)**.

If either component is absent, that signal to inhibit growth isn't received, and so cells proliferate abnormally and start to express proteins that cause water to be transported into the lumen of the cyst. This makes them get larger and larger, compressing the surrounding tissue more and more, and this is how the cysts develop and grow **(Figure 37.7; Figure 37.8)**.

As is expected for a dominant disease, a person who develops ADPKD would have inherited a single, heterozygous mutation in PKD1 or PKD2. This leaves one functional copy of the gene in every cell, and this turns out to actually produce enough polycystin 1 or polycystin 2 to prevent cyst formation **(Figure 37.9)**.

So, how do cysts occur, then? Well, it turns out that a random mutation in the remaining good copy of the gene is almost guaranteed to happen in some of the tubular cells as the kidney develops. This 'second hit' causes polycystin 1 or 2 to be absent, which is what impairs normal signalling through the cilium and leads to cyst formation. So, on the level of the person as a whole, ADPKD shows a pattern of dominant inheritance, but on the cellular level, it's technically a recessive trait **(Figure 37.10)**.

**Figure 37.7**

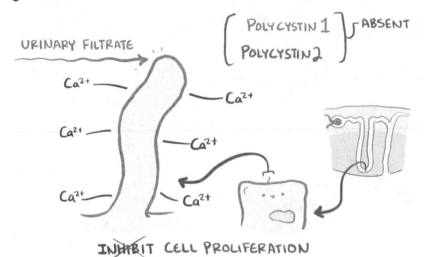

URINARY FILTRATE

$Ca^{2+}$ — ... — $Ca^{2+}$

$Ca^{2+}$ — ... — $Ca^{2+}$

$Ca^{2+}$ — ... — $Ca^{2+}$

$\begin{bmatrix} \text{POLYCYSTIN 1} \\ \text{POLYCYSTIN 2} \end{bmatrix}$ ABSENT

~~IN~~HIBIT CELL PROLIFERATION

**Figure 37.8**

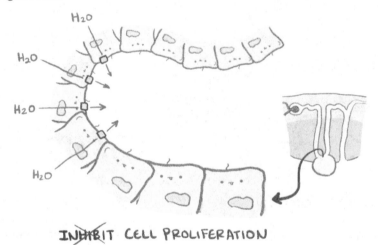

$H_2O$

$H_2O$

$H_2O$

$H_2O$

~~IN~~HIBIT CELL PROLIFERATION

**Figure 37.9**

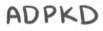

# ADPKD

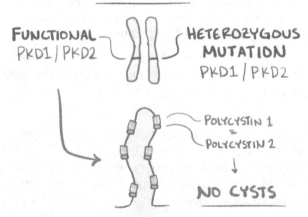

FUNCTIONAL
PKD1 / PKD2

HETEROZYGOUS
MUTATION
PKD1 / PKD2

POLYCYSTIN 1
&
POLYCYSTIN 2
↓
NO CYSTS

**Figure 37.10**

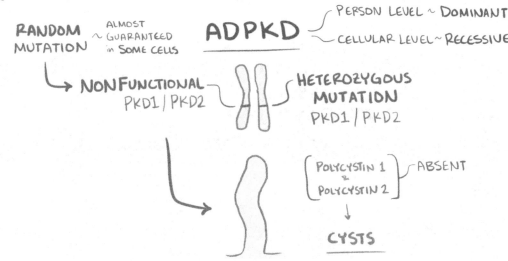

Polycystins are important in the kidney, but are developmentally important in other places of the body, too. Patients can have cysts that are typically benign pop up in the liver, seminal vesicles, and pancreas. The vasculature can also be affected: for example, individuals might develop aortic root dilation, which can lead to heart failure, and have berry aneurysms of the cerebral arteries, usually in the Circle of Willis. These aneurysms can have a thin wall, allowing them to rupture and develop into a subarachnoid hemorrhage **(Figure 37.11)**.

Autosomal recessive PKD, or ARPKD, used to be called infantile PKD, since symptoms usually manifest in infancy. ARPKD happens when someone inherits a mutation on both copies of the PKHD1 gene, which codes for the fibrocystin protein. Fibrocystin co-localizes with polycystin 2, where, although this largely unclear, it might be involved in the regulation pathway and calcium signaling described with ADPKD; therefore, it's thought that a similar mechanism might cause cyst formation in ARPKD **(Figure 37.12)**.

In any case, with ARPKD, this cyst formation can lead to renal failure even before birth. This means that the fetus has trouble producing urine, and, since amniotic fluid comes from fetal urine, fetuses with ARPKD can develop oligohydramnios, or low amniotic fluid. In fact, if enough amniotic fluid is missing, it can can cause Potter sequence. Without the amniotic fluid, the uterine walls actually compress the fetus, which causes physical developmental abnormalities, like club feet and a flattened nose. Another part of Potter sequence is pulmonary hypoplasia, or underdeveloped lungs, since the amniotic fluid is important in helping the lungs expand and develop normally. Underdeveloped lungs can cause respiratory insufficiency after birth, which ends up being fatal in a lot of cases of ARPKD **(Figure 37.13)**.

## DIAGNOSIS

For diagnosis, ARPKD is one of the many conditions that can be picked up via prenatal ultrasound, which could show bilaterally large kidneys with cysts and and oligohydramnios. ARPKD also causes congenital hepatic fibrosis, which over time can cause portal hypertension, or compromised blood flow through the portal venous system. Portal hypertension can cause esophageal varices, upper GI bleeds, hemorrhoids, and splenomegaly from blood being shunted through collateral veins.

**Figure 37.11**

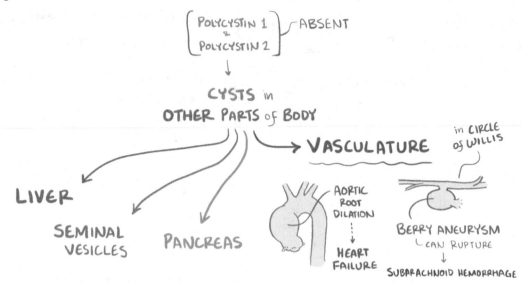

Polycystin 1 & Polycystin 2 — ABSENT

↓

CYSTS in OTHER PARTS of BODY

→ VASCULATURE — in CIRCLE of WILLIS

LIVER

SEMINAL VESICLES

PANCREAS

AORTIC ROOT DILATION ⤵ HEART FAILURE

BERRY ANEURYSM
└ CAN RUPTURE
↓
SUBARACHNOID HEMORRHAGE

**Figure 37.12**

## AUTOSOMAL RECESSIVE PKD (ARPKD)

*INFANTILE PKD ~ manifests in INFANCY

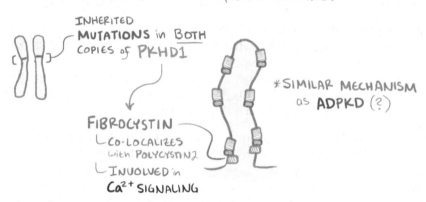

INHERITED MUTATIONS in BOTH COPIES of PKHD1

↓

FIBROCYSTIN
└ CO-LOCALIZES with POLYCYSTIN 2
└ INVOLVED in $Ca^{2+}$ SIGNALING

*SIMILAR MECHANISM as ADPKD (?)

**Figure 37.13**

## AUTOSOMAL RECESSIVE PKD (ARPKD)

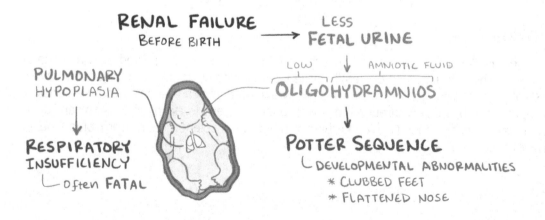

RENAL FAILURE BEFORE BIRTH → LESS FETAL URINE

PULMONARY HYPOPLASIA

LOW AMNIOTIC FLUID
OLIGOHYDRAMNIOS
↓
POTTER SEQUENCE

RESPIRATORY INSUFFICIENCY
└ often FATAL

└ DEVELOPMENTAL ABNORMALITIES
* CLUBBED FEET
* FLATTENED NOSE

**Figure 37.14**

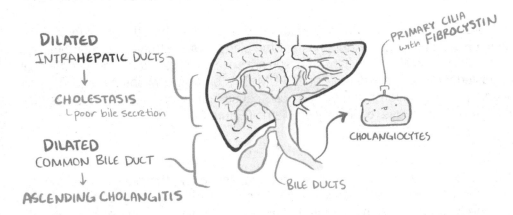

Since cholangiocytes, or the epithelial cells that line the bile ducts, also have primary cilia that express fibrocystin, ARPKD can also cause defects in the bile ducts that leads to dilation. Dilated intrahepatic ducts can cause cholestasis or poor bile secretion, and dilation of the common bile duct can lead to ascending cholangitis **(Figure 37.14)**.

## TREATMENT

The treatment of PKD is usually directed at specific symptoms and organ dysfunction. For example, for hypertension, medications like angiotensin converting enzyme inhibitors or angiotensin receptor blockers can be used to counteract activation of the renin-angiotensin-aldosterone system. Also, ursodiol is sometimes taken to help treat cholestasis because it slows down the rate at which cholesterol is absorbed by the intestines. In cases of kidney failure, dialysis or kidney transplant are sometimes needed. For individuals with portal hypertension, a portocaval shunt, which bypasses the liver by connecting the portal vein to the inferior vena cava, or, again, a liver transplant, might be needed.

## SUMMARY

All right, to recap: polycystic kidney disease is a genetic disorder in which the kidneys become filled with hundreds of cysts, causing them to be larger than normal and to fail over time. PKD comes in two varieties: autosomal dominant, which presents in adulthood, and autosomal recessive, which presents in infancy or even before birth **(Figure 37.15)**.

**Figure 37.15**

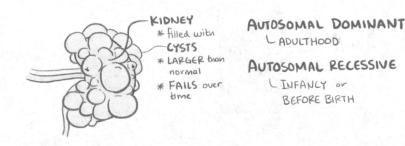

# Posterior urethral valve

osmosis.org/learn/posterior_urethral_valve

Posterior urethral valve, or PUV, is a congenital disorder in boys where the posterior urethra, which is the section of the urethra nearest the bladder, is obstructed by membranous folds, or flaps of tissue. These flaps of tissue are collectively referred to as a congenital obstructive posterior urethral membrane, or COPUM. This blockage means urine can't easily flow out, leading to a backup of urine, which can cause kidney problems, as well as less amniotic fluid, which can cause respiratory problems **(Figure 38.1)**.

## CAUSES

Although the cause of PUV isn't completely understood, it's thought that normal development of the male urethra is disrupted between weeks nine and fourteen of gestation. Normal development involves the Wolffian duct integrating with the posterior urethra, which results in thin mucosal folds called plicae colliculi. It's thought that PUV might result from abnormal integration of the Wolffian duct, resulting in large plicae colliculi that fuse anteriorly, making it more difficult for urine to flow through **(Figure 38.2)**.

**Figure 38.1**

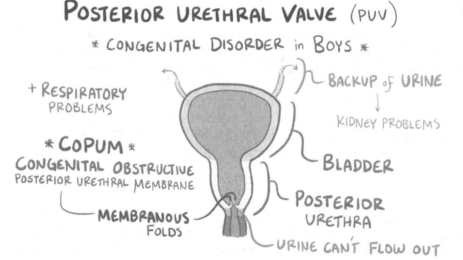

**Figure 38.2**

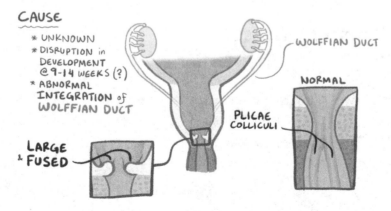

**Figure 38.3**

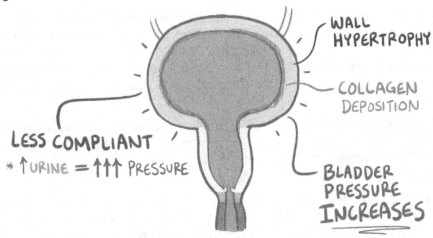

WALL HYPERTROPHY

COLLAGEN DEPOSITION

LESS COMPLIANT
* ↑URINE = ↑↑↑ PRESSURE

BLADDER PRESSURE INCREASES

**Figure 38.4**

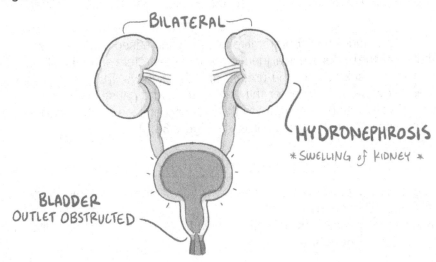

BILATERAL

HYDRONEPHROSIS
* SWELLING of KIDNEY *

BLADDER OUTLET OBSTRUCTED

**Figure 38.5**

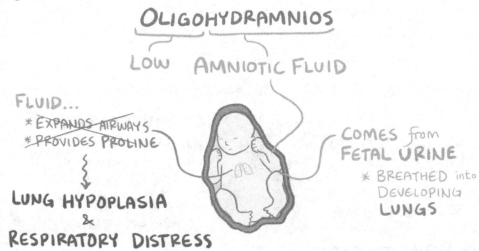

OLIGOHYDRAMNIOS

LOW AMNIOTIC FLUID

FLUID...
* EXPANDS AIRWAYS
* PROVIDES PROLINE
↓
LUNG HYPOPLASIA
&
RESPIRATORY DISTRESS

COMES from FETAL URINE
* BREATHED into DEVELOPING LUNGS

## SYMPTOMS

When urine can't easily flow out because of increased resistance from an obstruction, the intravesical pressure, or bladder pressure, starts to creep up. Holding urine under higher pressure leads to bladder wall hypertrophy and collagen deposition, both of which thicken the bladder wall. This thickening makes the bladder less compliant, meaning that small increases in urine volume causes large increases in bladder pressure, making the problem even worse **(Figure 38.3)**.

That high-pressure urine has nowhere to go but up to the ureters and eventually to the kidneys, causing hydronephrosis, which is the swelling of a kidney due to a buildup of urine. In PUV, since the bladder outlet is obstructed, the hydronephrosis is bilateral, meaning it affects both kidneys **(Figure 38.4)**.

Severe obstruction in utero can also lead to oligohydramnios, which is a low volume of amniotic fluid, since normally a significant proportion of amniotic fluid comes from fetal urine. Also, amniotic fluid normally gets breathed into the developing lungs, which helps expand the airways and also provides the amino acid proline, and both of these things are critical to normal lung development. Therefore, with less amniotic fluid, the lungs may not develop completely, which is called lung hypoplasia, and as a result, some newborns have respiratory distress **(Figure 38.5)**.

Another complication of PUV includes vesicoureteral reflux, since increased bladder pressure can also lead to dysfunction of the ureterovesical junction, where the ureters enter the bladder, resulting in the reflux of urine back up into the ureters and the kidneys. PUV also causes urinary stasis, which can allow bacteria to enter the urinary tract and cause a urinary tract infection. Over time, recurring infections and injury to the kidneys can lead to chronic kidney disease, which might progress to end-stage renal disease **(Figure 38.6)**.

## DIAGNOSIS

Often, PUV can be diagnosed by prenatal ultrasound, which can show a dilated bladder, thickened bladder wall, and bilateral hydronephrosis. If not found prenatally, postnatal diagnosis of PUV might be done by voiding cystourethrogram, or VCUG, which shows a dilated and elongated posterior urethra **(Figure 38.7)**.

**Figure 38.6**

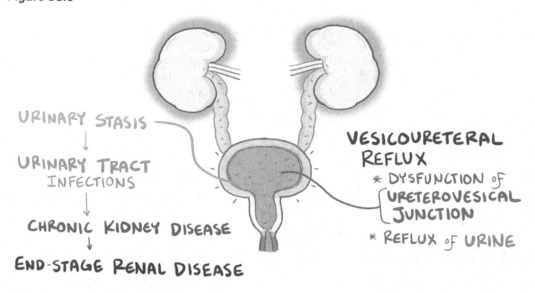

**Figure 38.7**

# DIAGNOSIS

* PRENATAL ULTRASOUND
  ∟ DILATED BLADDER
  ∟ BILATERAL HYDRONEPHROSIS

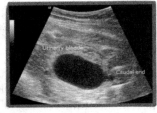

* VOIDING CYSTOURETHROGRAM (VCUG)
  ∟ DILATED & ELONGATED
     POSTERIOR URETHRA

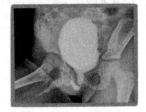

## TREATMENT

Treatment involves surgery and ablation of the membrane, which allows urine to flow through unobstructed. Prenatal surgery can be risky, so it's typically reserved for severe cases of oligohydramnios and possible lung hypoplasia. Postnatally, the standard surgery is transurethral catheter ablation.

## SUMMARY

All right, as a quick recap: posterior urethral valve, sometimes more descriptively referred to as a congenital obstructive posterior urethral membrane, is a congenital condition in boys where membranous folds obstruct the normal flow of urine. This leads to bladder outlet obstruction, which causes high bladder pressure, which can cause vesicoureteral reflux, which results in reflux of urine back up into the ureters and kidneys. That obstruction also leads to urinary stasis, which can lead to recurrent urinary tract infections and, eventually, chronic kidney disease **(Figure 38.8)**.

**Figure 38.8**

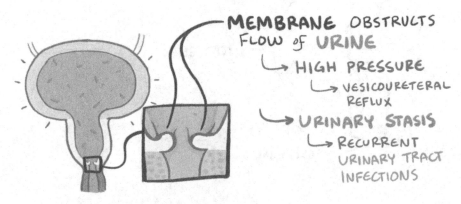

POSTERIOR URETHRAL VALVE
AKA CONGENITAL OBSTRUCTIVE POSTERIOR URETHRAL MEMBRANE

MEMBRANE OBSTRUCTS FLOW of URINE
∟ HIGH PRESSURE
   ∟ VESICOURETERAL REFLUX
∟ URINARY STASIS
   ∟ RECURRENT URINARY TRACT INFECTIONS

# Postrenal acute kidney injury

osmosis.org/learn/kidney_stones

**A**cute kidney injury, or AKI, is when the kidney isn't functioning at 100%, and this decrease in function develops relatively quickly, typically over a few days. Actually, AKI used to be known as acute renal failure, or ARF, but AKI is a broader term that also includes subtle decreases in kidney function. AKI can essentially be split into three types: prerenal AKI, meaning the cause of kidney injury comes from before the kidneys; postrenal AKI, meaning the injury is caused after the kidneys; or intrarenal AKI, meaning the injury happens within the kidneys **(Figure 39.1)**.

## PHYSIOLOGY

Now, the kidneys' job is to regulate what's in the blood, so they might remove waste, or make sure electrolyte levels are steady, or regulate the overall amount of water, and even make hormones; the kidneys do a lot of stuff **(Figure 39.2)**! Blood gets into the kidney through the renal artery, moving into tiny clumps of arterioles called glomeruli, where it's initially filtered, with the filtrate, the stuff filtered out, moving into the renal tubule **(Figure 39.3)**.

Sometimes, fluid or electrolytes can move back from the filtrate into the blood, which is called reabsorption, and sometimes more fluid or electrolytes can move from the blood to the filtrate, which called secretion **(Figure 39.4)**. Along with fluid and electrolytes, waste-containing compounds like urea and creatinine, are also filtered, although some urea is actually reabsorbed back into the blood, whereas only a little bit of creatinine is reabsorbed. In fact, in the blood, the normal ratio of blood urea nitrogen, or BUN, to creatinine is between 5 and 20 to 1, meaning the blood carries 5 to 20 molecules of urea for every one molecule of creatinine **(Figure 39.5)**. This is a pretty good diagnostic for looking at kidney function!

Ultimately, the filtrate is turned into urine and is excreted from the kidney through the ureter, into the bladder, and peed away. Meanwhile, the filtered blood drains into the renal vein **(Figure 39.6)**.

**Figure 39.1**

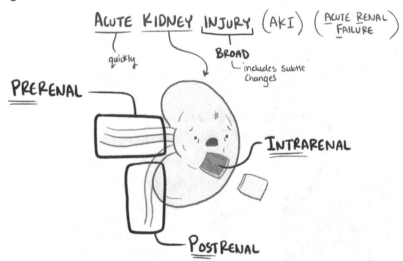

**Figure 39.2**

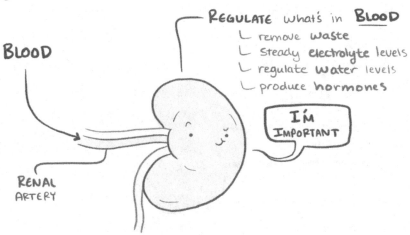

**Figure 39.3**

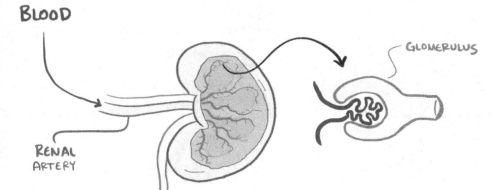

**Figure 39.4**

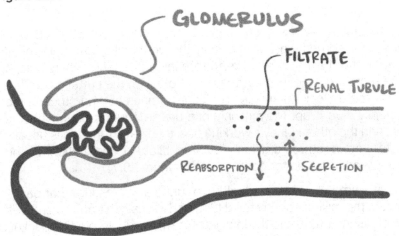

**Figure 39.5**

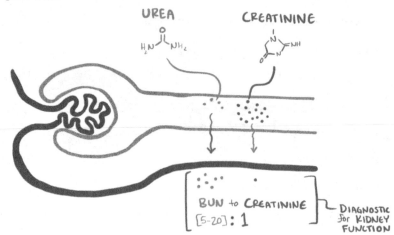

**Figure 39.6**

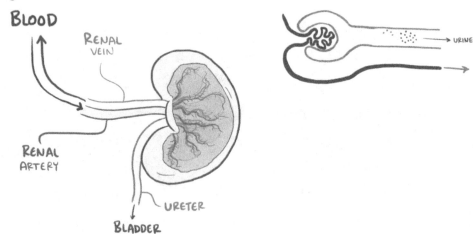

## PATHOLOGY

All right, so with *postrenal* AKI, there's some obstruction to the outflow from the kidneys. Reduced flow can be a result of something compressing the ureter, like intra-abdominal tumors, or compressing the urethra further down, like from benign prostatic hyperplasia, a noncancerous growth of the prostate gland. Both of these sort of pinch the ureter or urethra shut. Also though it could be some blockage inside, like kidney stones getting stuck in the ureter or urethra, which actually plug it up. Now, if only one ureter is obstructed, which is called unilateral obstruction, and the other kidney's working fine, then renal function is usually preserved. If, say, both ureters are obstructed, which is called bilateral obstruction, or the urethra gets blocked, then we've got a recipe for postrenal AKI **(Figure 39.7)**.

Whatever the obstruction is, it ultimately causes a buildup of urine and pressure that backs up into the kidney, all the way to the millions of tiny renal tubules. Normally, filtratration moves fluid from the relatively high pressure arteriole to the low pressure renal tubule, but this backup causes an increase in renal tubule pressure, which reduces the pressure gradient and lowers the amount of fluid that filters across, lowering the glomerular filtration rate, or GFR, which is how much blood the kidneys filter in mL through their glomeruli per minute. This means that less waste products, like urea and creatinine, are filtered *out* of the blood, meaning more stays in the blood. This leaves people with azotemia, or high levels of nitrogen-containing waste compounds in the blood, as well as oliguria, or low levels of urine **(Figure 39.8)**.

**Figure 39.7**

# POSTRENAL AKI

* obstruction to outflow *

    └ COMPRESSION

        • Benign prostatic hyperplasia

  noncancerous   prostate   growth
            gland

        • Intra abdominal tumors

    └ BLOCKAGE

        • Kidney Stones

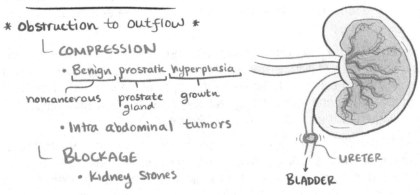

**Figure 39.8**

↓ GLOMERULAR FILTRATION Rate (GFR)

$$\frac{BLOOD\ filtered\ (mL)}{minute}$$

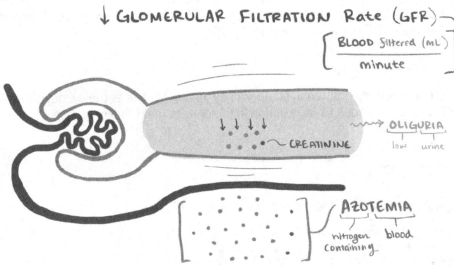

OLIGURIA — low urine

CREATININE

AZOTEMIA — nitrogen containing / blood

**Figure 39.9**

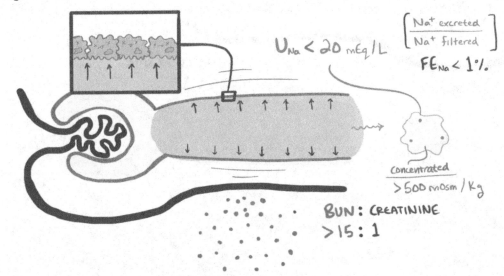

$U_{Na} < 20\ mEq/L$

$$\frac{Na^+\ excreted}{Na^+\ filtered}$$

$FE_{Na} < 1\%$

concentrated
>500 mosm/kg

BUN : CREATININE
>15 : 1

Now, if we follow the stuff that does make it into the tubule, which also includes things like sodium and water, it turns out that the high pressure tubular system essentially forces *more* reabsorption of sodium, water, *and* urea, but not much creatinine because, remember, little to no creatinine gets reabsorbed. Now, this increased urea reabsorption relative to creatinine increases the BUN to creatinine ratio in the blood, typically making it greater than about 15 to 1.

Also, while the tubules aren't functioning normally and reabsorbing appropriately, the urine sodium is typically less than 20 mEq / L, since most of the sodium's being reabsorbed, which means that the fraction of sodium excreted to sodium filtered, or FENa is usually less than 1%. Finally, since most of that water and fluid is being reabsorbed as well, the urine's typically pretty concentrated, usually greater than 500 mOsm / kg **(Figure 39.9)**.

All right, so I say "normally" because, over time, the increased pressure damages the epithelial cells responsible for reabsorption in the tubules. When that happens, less and less urea gets reabsorbed back into the blood and instead stays in the tubule and then gets dumped out into the urine, and this causes the BUN:Cr ratio to fall below 15 to 1. Also, in the same way, less sodium is reabsorbed, so more gets excreted and urine sodium goes above 40 mEq/L. In mild cases, $FE_{Na}$ goes above 1%, but in severe cases it can go above 2%. Finally, just as with the others, less water and fluid being reabsorbed causes the urine to be less concentrated, and urine osmolality falls below 350 mOsm/kg **(Figure 39.10)**.

## SUMMARY

All right, so as a quick recap, postrenal acute kidney injury is where the kidneys aren't functioning at 100%, and this is due to obstruction in the ureters that blocks the flow of urine.

**Figure 39.10**

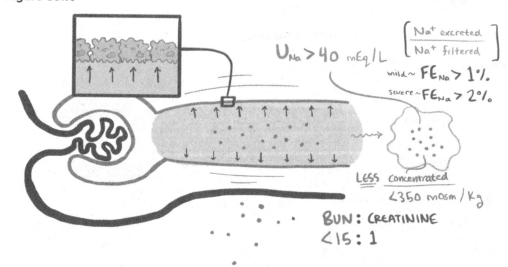

# Poststreptococcal glomerulonephritis

osmosis.org/learn/poststreptococcal_glomerulonephritis

**P**oststreptococcal glomerulonephritis, or PSGN, is where the kidneys' glomeruli, which are where small molecules are first filtered out of the blood and into the urine, become inflamed after an infection by streptococcal bacteria **(Figure 40.1)**.

## PHYSIOLOGY

PSGN usually starts with an infection by strains of group A beta-hemolytic streptococci bacteria with a specific antigen on its surface that lumps it into a group called "group A." This group A streptococci produces an enzyme called streptolysin, and when the bacteria is grown on a petri dish of blood, the enzyme completely lyses red blood cells that are near the bacterial colony, which is called beta-hemolysis. Beta-hemolysis is where they're completely destroyed, as opposed to alpha-hemolysis, where cells aren't actually destroyed, but just damaged or bruised. These strains are considered nephritogenic strains because they carry the M-protein virulence factor, a protein that helps them get around host defenses **(Figure 40.2)**.

**Figure 40.1**

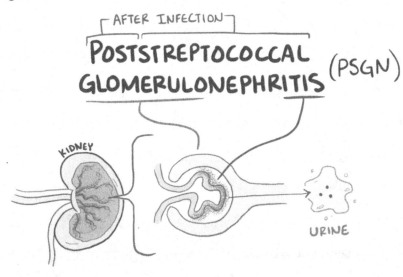

**Figure 40.2**

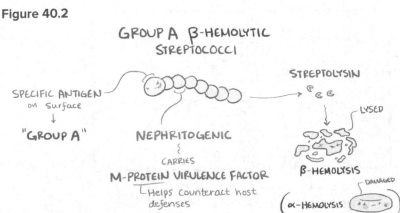

# PATHOLOGY

An infection by a nephritogenic strain of group A beta-hemolytic streptococcus bacteria initiates a type III hypersensitivity reaction, where immune complexes are formed. They're composed of antigens and antibodies, often IgG or IgM, and end up being carried in the bloodstream to the glomerulus and become trapped **(Figure 40.3)**.

Specifically, these deposits end up in the glomerular basement membrane or GBM, and most of the time they're subepithelial, meaning between the epithelial cells, or podocytes, and the basement membrane. It's also possible the antigens from the bacteria are first trapped in the glomeruli, and then the antibodies bind in the glomerulus itself. Either way, these complexes initiate an inflammatory reaction in the glomerulus, which involves activation and deposition of C3 complement, inflammatory cytokines, oxidants, and proteases that all damage the podocytes **(Figure 40.4)**.

This damage ends up allowing larger molecules to filter into the urine, like red blood cells and proteins, which then get into the urine and cause hematuria and proteinuria. Those red blood cells in the urine actually often make it darker or cola-colored; also, there tends to be less urine produced than normal, which called oliguria. These, along with inflammation, are several of the characteristics that make PSGN a nephritic syndrome. Also, as less fluid is excreted into the urine, more's retained by the body, causing peripheral edema as well as periorbital edema, which is fluid buildup around the orbit of the eye **(Figure 40.5)**.

**Figure 40.3**

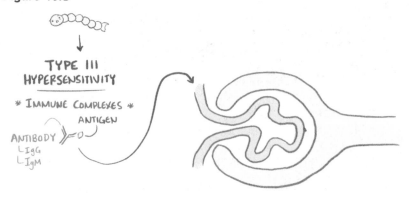

**Figure 40.4**

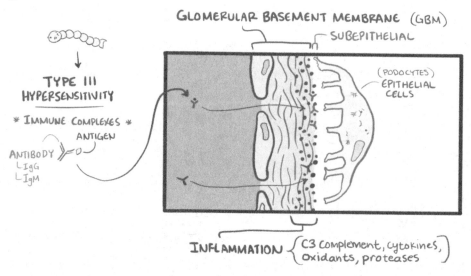

**Figure 40.5**

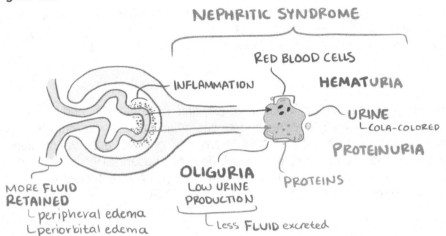

NEPHRITIC SYNDROME

- INFLAMMATION
- RED BLOOD CELLS
- **HEMATURIA**
- URINE
  └ COLA-COLORED
- **PROTEINURIA**
- PROTEINS
- **OLIGURIA** LOW URINE PRODUCTION
  └ Less FLUID excreted
- MORE FLUID **RETAINED**
  └ peripheral edema
  └ periorbital edema

**Figure 40.6**

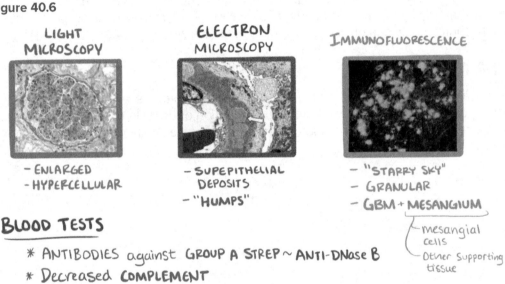

LIGHT MICROSCOPY
- ENLARGED
- HYPERCELLULAR

ELECTRON MICROSCOPY
- SUPEPITHELIAL DEPOSITS
- "HUMPS"

IMMUNOFLUORESCENCE
- "STARRY SKY"
- GRANULAR
- GBM + MESANGIUM
  └ mesangial cells
  └ Other supporting tissue

**BLOOD TESTS**

* ANTIBODIES against GROUP A STREP ~ ANTI-DNase B
* Decreased COMPLEMENT

**Figure 40.7**

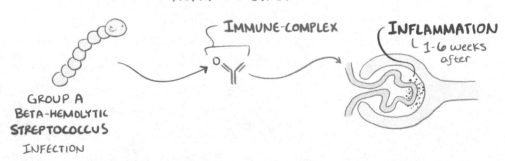

# POSTSTREPTOCOCCAL GLOMERULONEPHRITIS

* NEPHRITIC SYNDROME *

- GROUP A BETA-HEMOLYTIC **STREPTOCOCCUS** INFECTION
- IMMUNE-COMPLEX
- **INFLAMMATION** └ 1-6 weeks after

## SYMPTOMS

Typically, PSGN affects children and follows about six weeks after infections of the skin, called impetigo, or about one to two weeks after infections of the throat, or pharyngitis. Generally, the disease is mild, and it runs its course and spontaneously resolves within a month.

## DIAGNOSIS

Under light microscopy, the glomerulus looks enlarged and hypercellular, and a closer look on electron microscopy shows subepithelial deposits, which appear as "humps". On immunofluorescence, the immune deposits cause a "starry sky" granular appearance along the basement membrane and mesangium, which includes the mesangial cells and other supporting tissue. Blood tests may show antibodies against group A streptococcus, called anti-DNase B, as well as decreased complement levels **(Figure 40.6)**.

## TREATMENT

Since PSGN is generally a mild illness, treatment is usually supportive. A few children, though, progress to renal failure, and about a quarter of adults with PSGN develop rapidly progressive glomerulonephritis, which can quickly lead to renal failure as well.

## SUMMARY

All right, as a quick recap: poststreptococcal glomerulonephritis is a nephritic syndrome involving a group A beta-hemolytic streptococcus infection of the skin or throat that causes immune complex-mediated inflammation of the glomeruli one to six weeks after infection **(Figure 40.7)**.

# Potter sequence

osmosis.org/learn/potter_sequence

Potter sequence is a rare disorder that is sometimes called oligohydramnios sequence, a term that helps define it because *oligo-* means low and *-hydramnios* means amniotic fluid. So, in Potter sequence there's basically very little amniotic fluid, and this makes the uterus a pretty hostile place for the fetus to grow **(Figure 41.1)**.

## PHYSIOLOGY

Typically, around the twentieth week of gestation, the kidneys, ureters, and urethra develop and start producing and excreting urine, which becomes the major source of amniotic fluid **(Figure 41.2)**. Various conditions, like renal agenesis, which is when one or both kidneys are missing, or atresia of the ureter or urethra, which is where those parts of the urinary tract are obstructed, can lead to an inability to produce or excrete urine and therefore lead to oligohydramnios. Other common causes include amniotic rupture, which is the leakage of amniotic fluid, and uteroplacental insufficiency,  which is where there's low blood flow from the placenta, meaning the fetal organs, including the kidneys, see less blood flow, leading to to decreased urine production **(Figure 41.3)**.

**Figure 41.1**

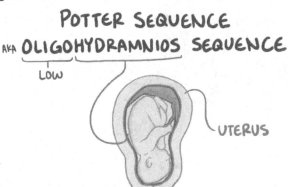

**Figure 41.2**

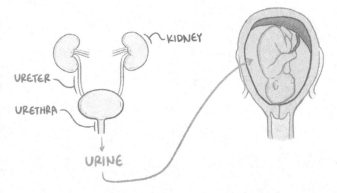

**Figure 41.3**

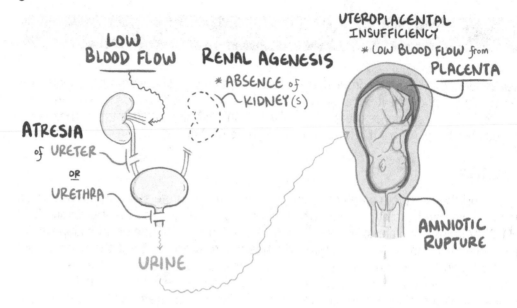

LOW
BLOOD FLOW

RENAL AGENESIS
* ABSENCE of
KIDNEY(S)

UTEROPLACENTAL
INSUFFICIENCY
* LOW BLOOD FLOW from
PLACENTA

ATRESIA
of URETER
OR
URETHRA

URINE

AMNIOTIC
RUPTURE

**Figure 41.4**

DEVELOPMENT of
FETAL LUNGS

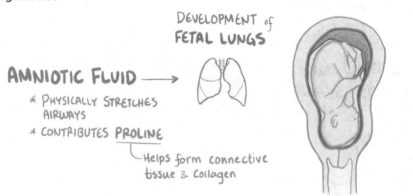

AMNIOTIC FLUID ⟶

* PHYSICALLY STRETCHES
  AIRWAYS
* CONTRIBUTES PROLINE
  └ Helps form connective
    tissue & collagen

**Figure 41.5**

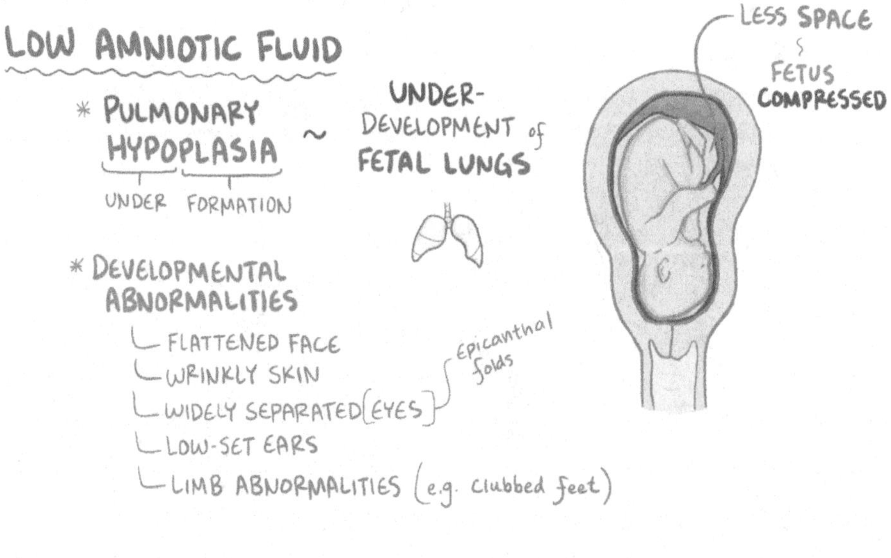

LOW AMNIOTIC FLUID

* PULMONARY        ~   UNDER-
  HYPOPLASIA            DEVELOPMENT of
                        FETAL LUNGS
  UNDER  FORMATION

LESS SPACE
↕
FETUS
COMPRESSED

* DEVELOPMENTAL
  ABNORMALITIES
    └ FLATTENED FACE
    └ WRINKLY SKIN
    └ WIDELY SEPARATED (EYES)      Epicanthal
    └ LOW-SET EARS                 folds
    └ LIMB ABNORMALITIES (e.g. clubbed feet)

# PATHOLOGY

When there's very little amniotic fluid, a couple of things happen as a result. First, amniotic fluid is crucial for the development of the fetal lungs because it both helps the airways physically stretch out and it contributes amino acids like proline, which helps with the formation of connective tissue and collagen in the lung **(Figure 41.4)**.

# SYMPTOMS

With less amniotic fluid, though, there's pulmonary hypoplasia. *Hypo-* means under, and -plasia means formation, so the lungs basically remain underdeveloped. Not only that, with less amniotic fluid, there's less space in the amniotic sac, and so the fetus is literally compressed into a smaller space, causing developmental abnormalities like a flattened face, wrinkly skin, widely separated eyes with epicanthal folds, low-set ears, and limb abnormalities like clubbed feet **(Figure 41.5)**.

# DIAGNOSIS & TREATMENT

Potter sequence usually affects boys since they have a higher rate of urinary tract obstruction anomalies, like posterior urethral valves. Diagnosis of Potter sequence is usually done with ultrasound during the second trimester of pregnancy. Unfortunately, though, by the time this condition is diagnosed, the syndrome is usually very advanced and most cases result in a stillbirth, which is the delivery of a fetus that has already died. When babies do survive, the pulmonary hypoplasia leads to severe respiratory problems which often lead to death shortly after birth.

# SUMMARY

All right, as a quick recap: Potter sequence is an often fatal condition that primarily affects newborn males, and it's caused by oligohydramnios, which is low or absent amniotic fluid. Potter itself is actually a mnemonic, and it stands for **P**ulmonary hypoplasia, **O**ligohydramnios, **T**wisted skin, for the wrinkles, **T**wisted face, **E**xtremity deformities, and **R**enal agenesis **(Figure 41.6)**.

**Figure 41.6**

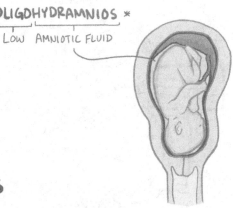

POTTER SEQUENCE
* (MOSTLY) AFFECTS NEWBORN MALES *
* CAUSED BY OLIGOHYDRAMNIOS *
LOW AMNIOTIC FLUID

**P**ULMONARY HYPOPLASIA
**O**LIGOHYDRAMNIOS
**T**WISTED SKIN (WRINKLES)
**T**WISTED FACE
**E**XTREMITY DEFORMITIES
**R**ENAL AGENESIS

# Prerenal acute kidney injury

osmosis.org/learn/prerenal_acute_kidney_injury

**A**cute kidney injury, or AKI, is when the kidney isn't functioning at 100% and this decrease in function develops relatively quickly, typically over a few days. Actually, AKI used to be known as acute renal failure, or ARF, but AKI is a broader term that also includes subtle decreases in kidney function. AKI can essentially be split into three types: prerenal AKI, meaning the cause of kidney injury comes from before the kidneys; postrenal AKI, meaning the injury is caused after the kidneys; or intrarenal AKI, meaning the injury happens within the kidneys **(Figure 42.1)**.

## PHYSIOLOGY

Now, the kidneys' job is to regulate what's in the blood, so they might remove waste, or make sure electrolyte levels are steady, or regulate the overall amount of water, or even make hormones -- the kidneys do a lot of stuff **(Figure 42.2)**! Blood gets into the kidney through the renal artery, entering tiny clumps of arterioles called glomeruli where it's initially filtered, and the filtrate, the stuff filtered out, moves into the renal tubule **(Figure 42.3)**.

Sometimes fluid or electrolytes can move back from the filtrate into the blood, which is called reabsorption, and sometimes more fluid or electrolytes can move from the blood to the fitrate, which is called secretion **(Figure 42.4)**. Along with fluid and electrolytes, though, waste-containing compounds, like urea and creatinine, are also filtered. Some urea is actually *reabsorbed* back into the blood, whereas only a little bit of creatinine is reabsorbed. In fact, in the blood, the normal ratio of blood urea nitrogen, or BUN, to creatinine is between 5 and 20 to 1, meaning the blood carries 5 to 20 molecules of urea for every one molecule of creatinine, and this is a pretty good diagnostic for looking at kidney function **(Figure 42.5)**.

Ultimately, the filtrate is turned into urine and is excreted from the kidney through the ureter, into the bladder, and peed away. Meanwhile, the filtered blood drains into the renal vein **(Figure 42.6)**.

Figure 42.1

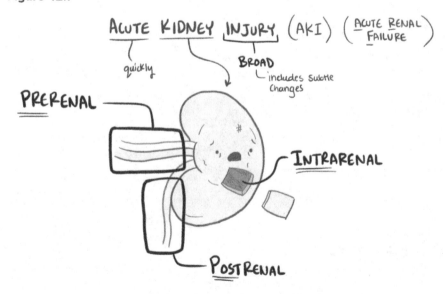

**Figure 42.2**

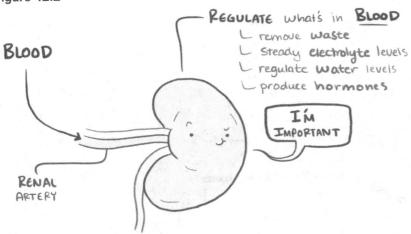

**Figure 42.3**

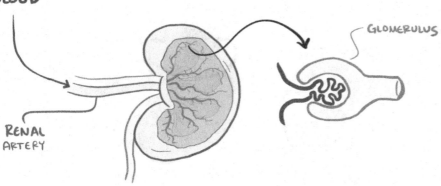

**Figure 42.4**

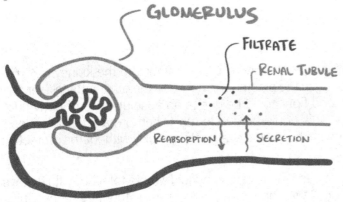

**Figure 42.5**

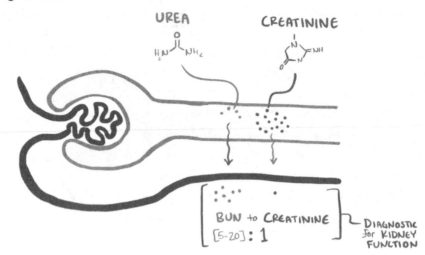

**Figure 42.6**

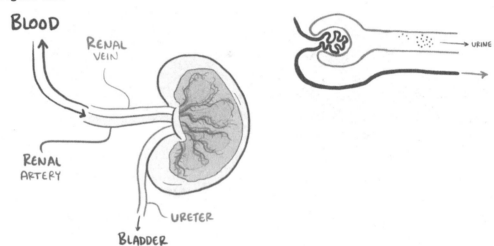

## PATHOLOGY

All right, so prerenal kidney injury is due to a decreased blood flow into the kidneys. You've got your body fluid, with fluid circulating in the plasma as well as all the other intracellular and extracellular fluid, so a decreased blood flow could be due to an absolute loss of body fluid, where fluid actually leaves the body. This could be due to major hemorrhage or blood loss, vomiting, diarrhea, or severe burns, where body fluid evaporates quickly without the protective skin to keep it in **(Figure 42.7)**.

Decreased blood flow could also be due to a *relative* loss of fluid, where total body fluid stays the same. How can that happen, though? Well, one example of this is distributive shock, which is where fluid moves from the blood vessels into the tissues, which keeps the total body fluid volume the same but causes a relative decrease in blood volume. Another example is congestive heart failure, which is where the heart can't pump blood to the tissues, so a portion of blood just pools in the venous side and isn't pumped to the body, meaning less blood is sent to the kidneys. Finally, the issue could be local to the renal artery itself: for example, it could become narrowed, as in renal artery stenosis, or blocked by an embolus, which is a blood clot from somewhere else in the body **(Figure 42.8)**.

**Figure 42.7**

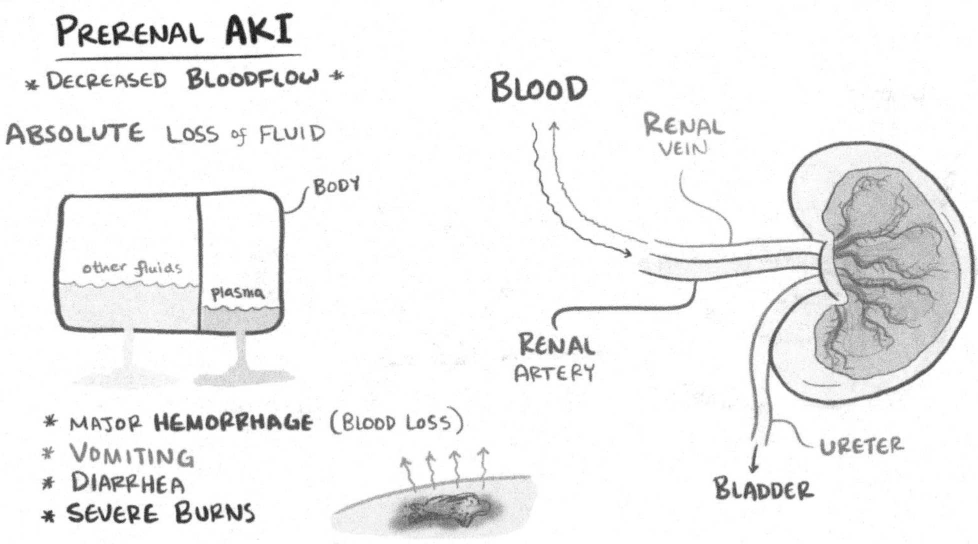

## PRERENAL AKI
### * DECREASED BLOODFLOW *

ABSOLUTE LOSS of FLUID

BODY

other fluids

plasma

* MAJOR **HEMORRHAGE** (BLOOD LOSS)
* VOMITING
* DIARRHEA
* SEVERE BURNS

BLOOD

RENAL VEIN

RENAL ARTERY

URETER

BLADDER

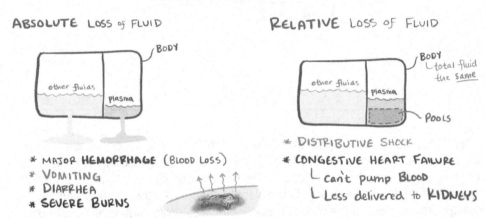

**Figure 42.8**

## PRERENAL AKI
### * DECREASED BLOODFLOW *

ABSOLUTE LOSS of FLUID

BODY

other fluids

plasma

* MAJOR **HEMORRHAGE** (BLOOD LOSS)
* VOMITING
* DIARRHEA
* SEVERE BURNS

RELATIVE LOSS OF FLUID

BODY
└ total fluid the same

other fluids

plasma

POOLS

* DISTRIBUTIVE SHOCK
* CONGESTIVE HEART FAILURE
    └ can't pump BLOOD
    └ Less delivered to **KIDNEYS**

**Figure 42.9**

## PRERENAL AKI
### * DECREASED BLOODFLOW *

EMBOLUS

RENAL ARTERY STENOSIS

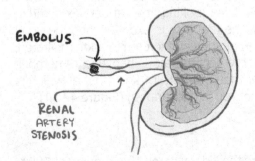

**Figure 42.10**

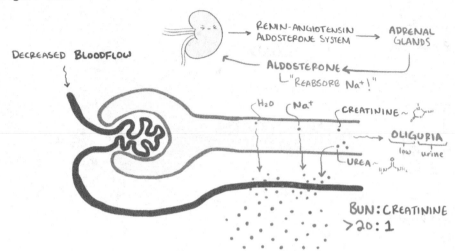

**Figure 42.11**

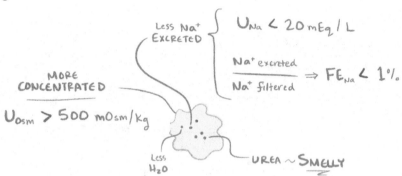

Whatever the case, less blood is going to the kidneys, right? So, less blood is going to the glomeruli, which means less blood is being filtered, so there's a decrease in the glomerular filtration rate, or GFR, which is how much blood, usually in mL, the kidneys filter through their glomeruli per minute. If less blood is being filtered, that means less urea and creatinine are being filtered out, and more stays in the blood. This is called azotemia, high levels of nitrogen-containing compounds in the blood, and will also tend to cause oliguria, an abnormally low amount of urine production. Also, when less blood is being filtered, the kidneys activate the renin-angiotensin system, which causes the adrenal glands to release aldosterone, which tells the kidneys to reabsorb sodium. When sodium is reabsorbed, water gets reabsorbed as well. Water and sodium reabsorption is also tied to urea reabsorption, so in a prerenal situation, urea gets reabsorbed, and so even more urea gets into the blood, resulting in a BUN to creatinine ratio of greater than 20:1 **(Figure 42.10)**. Now, looking at what gets excreted in the urine, more sodium and water being retained means that less is excreted, and the urine sodium is usually less than 20 mEq/L, that the fraction of sodium excreted to sodium filtered, or $FE_{Na}$, is usually less than 1%; finally, that urine is more concentrated—because, remember, less water is excreted, so typically the urine's greater than 500 mOsm/kg—most of which is urea (which is why your pee smells so nitrogen-y when you're dehydrated) **(Figure 42.11)**.

## SUMMARY

All right, to recap: prerenal acute kidney injury is where the kidneys aren't functioning at 100%, and this is due to less blood flowing into the kidneys.

# Rapidly progressive glomerulonephritis

osmosis.org/learn/rapidly_progressive_glomerulonephritis

**C**rescentic glomerulonephritis, which is sometimes called rapidly progressive glomerulonephritis, is a type of nephritic syndrome, meaning it involves inflammation of the kidney's glomeruli. This inflammation ultimately causes a crescent-shaped proliferation of cells in the Bowman's space, and this change leads to renal failure relatively quickly, within weeks to months **(Figure 43.1)**.

## PHYSIOLOGY

The development of crescents in Bowman's space can happen in several ways. In some cases it's idiopathic, meaning there's no identifiable cause. When the cause is identifiable, though, it can be split into several types. Type I is caused by anti-glomerular basement membrane, or GBM, antibodies, antibodies that target the GBM. Type I is associated with Goodpasture syndrome, which also involves pulmonary hemorrhages.

Type II is immune-complex-mediated, meaning caused by immune complexes composed of antigens and antibodies. This might be the case with poststreptococcal glomerulonephritis, systemic lupus erythematosus, IgA nephropathy, and Henoch-Schönlein purpura.

Finally, Type III is known as pauci-immune, meaning little or no anti-GBM antibodies or immune-complex deposits are present. In these cases, often anti-neutrophilic cytoplasmic antibodies or ANCAs are in the blood, which are autoantibodies against the body's own neutrophils. Furthermore, you can break it down into the type of ANCA. C-ANCAs, or cytoplasmic ANCAs, are associated with Wegener granulomatosis. P-ANCAs, or perinuclear ANCAs, on the other hand, are associated with microscopic polyangiitis and Churg-Strauss syndrome, the latter of which can be distinguished by having granulomatous inflammation, which is when immune cells attempt to wall off a substance perceived as foreign, asthma, and eosinophilia **(Figure 43.2)**.

**Figure 43.1**

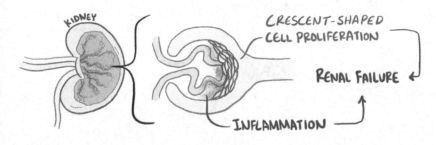

(RAPIDLY PROGRESSIVE) weeks to months
**CRESCENTIC**
GLOMERULONEPHRITIS

\* NEPHRITIC SYNDROME \*

KIDNEY

CRESCENT-SHAPED CELL PROLIFERATION

RENAL FAILURE

INFLAMMATION

**Figure 43.2**

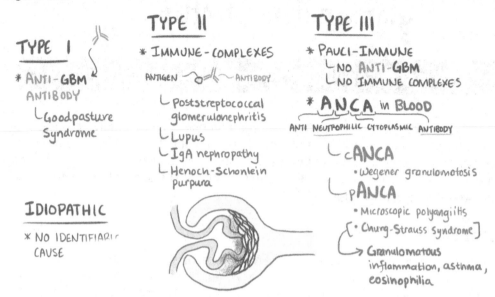

**TYPE I**

* ANTI-GBM ANTIBODY
  └ Goodpasture Syndrome

**IDIOPATHIC**

* NO IDENTIFIABLE CAUSE

**TYPE II**

* IMMUNE-COMPLEXES

ANTIGEN ──○∈ ∋─ ANTIBODY

  └ Poststreptococcal glomerulonephritis
  └ Lupus
  └ IgA nephropathy
  └ Henoch-Schonlein purpura

**TYPE III**

* PAULI-IMMUNE
  └ NO ANTI-GBM
  └ NO IMMUNE COMPLEXES

* ANCA in BLOOD

ANTI NEUTROPHILIC CYTOPLASMIC ANTIBODY

  └ cANCA
    • Wegener granulomatosis
  └ pANCA
    • Microscopic polyangiitis
    [• Churg-Strauss syndrome]
    → Granulomatous inflammation, asthma, eosinophilia

**Figure 43.3**

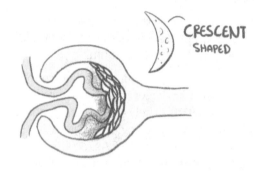

CRESCENT SHAPED

**Figure 43.4**

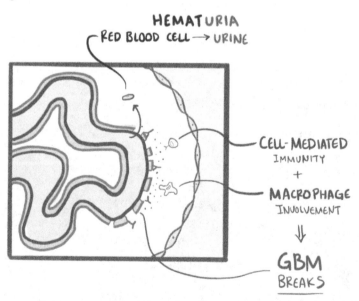

HEMATURIA
RED BLOOD CELL → URINE

CELL-MEDIATED IMMUNITY
+
MACROPHAGE INVOLVEMENT
⇓
GBM BREAKS

**Figure 43.5**

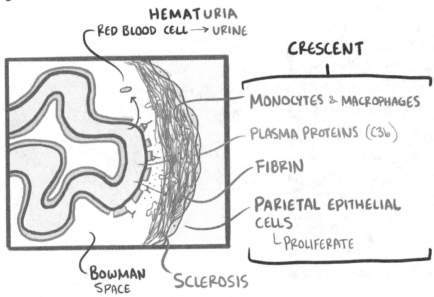

**Figure 43.6**

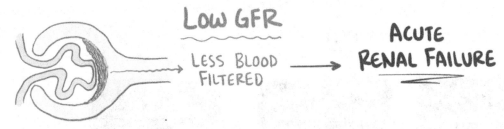

## SYMPTOMS

Whatever the underlying cause is, the common feature is severe glomerular injury and the development of a crescent shape. Typically, as a result of cell-mediated immunity as well as macrophage involvement, the glomerular basement membrane breaks (**Figure 43.3; Figure 43.4**).

This allows stuff circulating in the blood like red blood cells, which can then go on to get into the urine, called hematuria, more inflammatory mediators, plasma proteins, like complement C3b protein, and fibrin to pass through into the Bowman space. Following this flood of stuff, more monocytes and macrophages enter the Bowman space, as well as parietal epithelial cells, which proliferate. The presence of monocytes and macrophages, plasma proteins, fibrin, and parietal epithelial cells lead to the expansion of the normally-thin epithelial layer of cells into a thick, characteristic crescent-moon shape. Over time, this crescent may undergo sclerosis, or scarring, where it's replaced by connective tissue (**Figure 43.5**).

Ultimately, the glomeruli are severely damaged, and the kidneys lose their ability to filter blood effectively, which means the glomerular filtration rate goes down. If left untreated, crescentic glomerulonephritis can quickly lead to acute renal failure (**Figure 43.6**).

**Figure 43.7**

## LIGHT MICROSCOPY

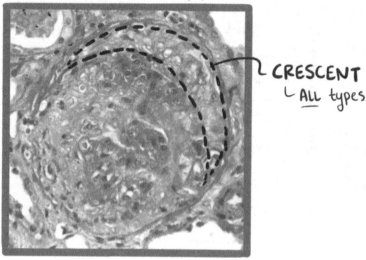

⌐ CRESCENT
  ⌐ ALL types

**Figure 43.8**

## IMMUNOFLUORESCENCE

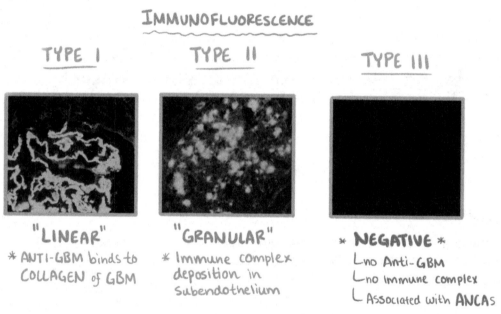

TYPE I          TYPE II          TYPE III

"LINEAR"        "GRANULAR"       * NEGATIVE *
* ANTI-GBM binds to    * Immune complex    ⌐no Anti-GBM
  COLLAGEN of GBM        deposition in       ⌐no Immune complex
                         Subendothelium       ⌐Associated with ANCAS

## DIAGNOSIS

On light microscopy, you'll see the characteristic moon or crescent-shaped glomeruli in all three types **(Figure 43.7)**.

The three types, though, can sometimes be differentiated on immunofluorescence. For Type I, the immunofluorescence pattern will be linear, since antibodies bind to collagen of the glomerular basement membrane. For Type II, the immunofluorescence pattern will be granular as a result of immune complex deposition in the subendothelium. Type III is actually negative on immunofluorescence, since, remember, it's *pauci-immune* and there usually aren't antibodies or immune-complex deposits in the glomeruli; rather, Type III is associated with ANCAs in the blood **(Figure 43.8)**.

## TREATMENT

Crescentic glomerulonephritis most often affects adults in their 50s and their 60s, and typically has a poor prognosis if not treated early. Anticoagulants might be used to reduce fibrin buildup in crescent formation, and plasmapheresis is usually used in combination with immunosuppressants. If the renal failure becomes irreversible, they might need dialysis or a kidney transplant.

## SUMMARY

All right, as a quick recap: crescentic glomerulonephritis is a type of nephritic syndrome that's characterized by epithelial cell proliferation into a thick crescent or moon-shape, which leads to hematuria, decreased glomerular filtration, and can rapidly progress to renal failure **(Figure 43.9)**.

**Figure 43.9**

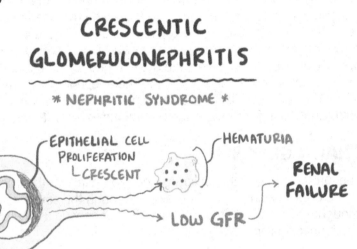

# Renal agenesis

With renal agenesis, *genesis* is the origin or formation of something, the prefix *a* means not, and renal refers to the kidneys, so *renal agenesis* is when the kidneys don't form. Since there are two kidneys, renal agenesis can refer to just one kidney not developing, called unilateral renal agenesis, or URA, or to neither kidney developing, called bilateral renal agenesis, or BRA **(Figure 44.1)**.

## PHYSIOLOGY

During fetal development, a structure called the mesonephric duct is involved in development of urinary and reproductive organs. During the fifth week of gestation, a little guy called the ureteric bud starts pushing its way into another structure called the metanephric blastema. Together, these two little embryologic structures develop into a kidney **(Figure 44.2)**. At about week seven, nephrogenesis, or formation of the kidneys, starts under the influence of that ureteric bud **(Figure 44.3)**. By about twenty weeks, the ureteric bud forms the ureters, renal calyces, collecting ducts, and collecting tubules, while the metanephric blastema develops into the nephron, which includes the epithelial cells and the podocytes of Bowman's capsule. In the third trimester and throughout infancy, the kidneys continue to grow **(Figure 44.4)**.

## UNILATERAL RENAL AGENESIS

With renal agenesis, the ureteric bud fails to induce development of the metanephric blastema, and so either one or both kidneys don't develop. Although the cause of this is not completely known, it's thought that it's a result of a combination of genetic as well as in-utero environmental factors, such as toxins and infections.

## SYMPTOMS

Newborns with unilateral renal agenesis are usually asymptomatic if the other kidney is otherwise healthy. Now that that one kidney's doing all the filtering, though, over time unilateral renal agenesis can lead to hypertrophy, or growth of the kidney, which can increase the risks of hypertension and renal failure later in life **(Figure 44.5)**.

**Figure 44.1**

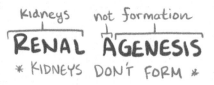

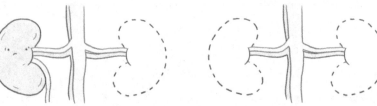

**Figure 44.2**

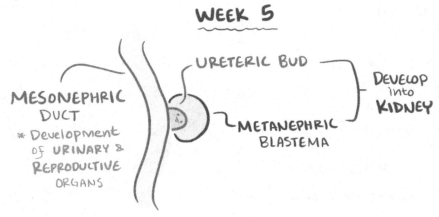

**Figure 44.3**

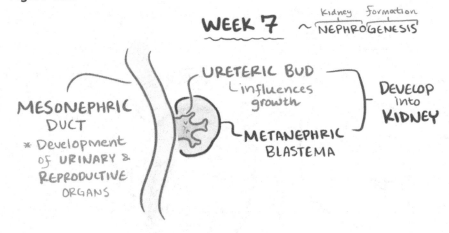

**Figure 44.4**

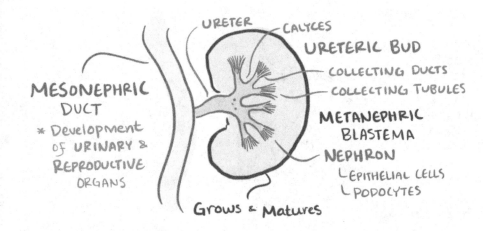

**Figure 44.5**

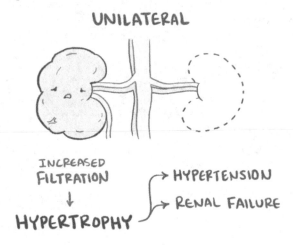

UNILATERAL

INCREASED
FILTRATION
↓
HYPERTROPHY → → HYPERTENSION
→ RENAL FAILURE

**Figure 44.6**

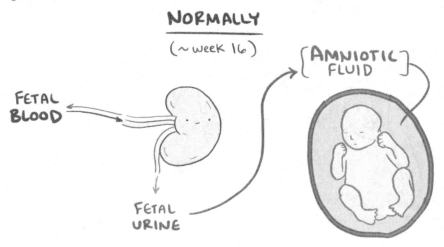

NORMALLY

(~week 16)

FETAL
BLOOD

FETAL
URINE

AMNIOTIC
FLUID

**Figure 44.7**

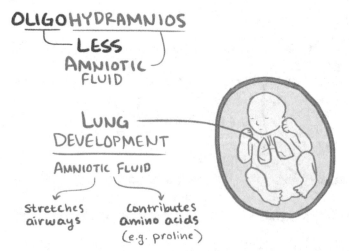

OLIGOHYDRAMNIOS
LESS
AMNIOTIC
FLUID

LUNG
DEVELOPMENT

AMNIOTIC FLUID

Stretches
airways

contributes
amino acids
(e.g. proline)

**Figure 44.8**

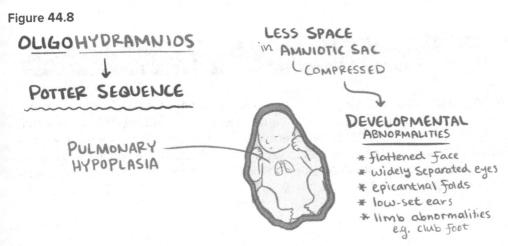

OLIGOHYDRAMNIOS
↓
POTTER SEQUENCE

PULMONARY HYPOPLASIA

LESS SPACE in AMNIOTIC SAC
└ COMPRESSED
↓
DEVELOPMENTAL ABNORMALITIES
* flattened face
* widely separated eyes
* epicanthal folds
* low-set ears
* limb abnormalities
   e.g. club foot

## BILATERAL RENAL AGENESIS

All right, so let's move to bilateral agenesis, which is where there are *no* kidneys. Normally, as the kidneys start to function around week sixteen, they start to filter the fetal blood, which means fetal urine gets produced, some of which contributes to the amniotic fluid that the fetus floats around in **(Figure 44.6)**.

With bilateral renal agenesis—and no kidneys urine isn't produced, so there's less amniotic fluid and the fetus develops oligohydramnios, where *oligo-* means low or less and *-hydramnios* refers to the amount of amniotic fluid **(Figure 44.7)**.

## SYMPTOMS

A couple of things happen as a result of this. First, amniotic fluid is crucial for the development of the fetal lungs, both helping the airways physically stretch out as well as contributing amino acids like proline to help with the formation of mesenchyme and collagen in the lung. So, with less amniotic fluid, the lungs can't develop all the way, which is called pulmonary hypoplasia. Second, with less amniotic fluid, there's less space in the amniotic sac, and so the fetus is literally compressed into a smaller space, which causes developmental abnormalities like a flattened face, widely separated eyes with epicanthal folds, low-set ears, and as limb abnormalities like clubbed feet. Taken together, this set of consequences from oligohydramnios is called Potter sequence, or sometimes Potter syndrome **(Figure 44.8)**.

It's worth mentioning that bilateral renal agenesis isn't the only thing that can cause Potter sequence: it can also be seen with other causes of oligohydramnios, like a blockage in the urinary tract or, occasionally, prolonged rupture of membranes.

## TREATMENT

In general, bilateral renal agenesis is incompatible with life outside the womb, and is therefore usually fatal within the first few days after birth, although, depending on lung development and overall health, some newborns might be put on dialysis until they are strong enough to have a kidney transplant.

## SUMMARY

Okay, so as a super short review: unilateral renal agenesis is where only one kidney develops, and is usually asymptomatic, and bilateral renal agenesis is where neither kidney develops, which results in oligohydramnios and the characteristic features of Potter sequence.

# Renal artery stenosis

osmosis.org/learn/renal_artery_stenosis

**W**ith renal artery stenosis, *stenosis* means narrowing, which refers to a progressive narrowing of the renal artery, which carries blood to the kidney. This means that the blood downstream of the narrowed spot that goes to the kidney is at a lower pressure, which is sensed by the kidney. Since an important role of the kidney is to sense and help the maintain a normal blood pressure, the kidney then tries to raise blood pressure throughout the body **(Figure 45.1)**.

## PHYSIOLOGY

Inside the kidney, there are millions of nephrons, each of which help to filter the blood and then fine-tune the composition of blood by carefully re-absorbing and secreting electrolytes as fluid passes through various parts of the nephron. Blood approaches the nephron via the afferent arteriole. You can remember it as "A" for approach, and then forms a tangle of capillaries called the glomerulus, before exiting via the efferent arteriole, which you can remember as "E" for exit. That efferent arteriole goes on to split into another set of capillaries, the vasa recta, which surround the nephron, and then blood leaves via the venule. So, there are two capillary beds per nephron. Usually we think of it going arteriole - capillary - venule, but in the nephron, it goes arteriole - capillary - arteriole - capillary - and, finally, venule **(Figure 45.2)**.

So, nephrons have the general shape of the letter "U", with the beginning and end portions getting pretty close to each other. The reason that this matters is that over here, lining the inside of the afferent arteriole are endothelial cells. Wrapped around them are juxtaglomerular cells, which are super special smooth muscle cells that contract down like normal smooth muscle cells but also have the ability to release a hormone called renin in response to low blood pressure. Over here, close to the distal convoluted tubule, there is another special group of cells that line the tubule called macula densa cells, which are sodium-chloride-sensing cells that detect the sodium concentration in the tubule **(Figure 45.3)**.

**Figure 45.1**

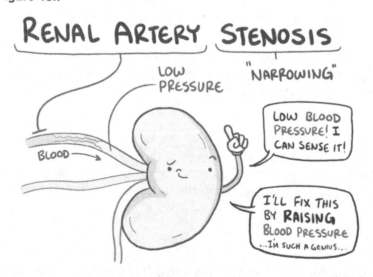

**Figure 45.2**

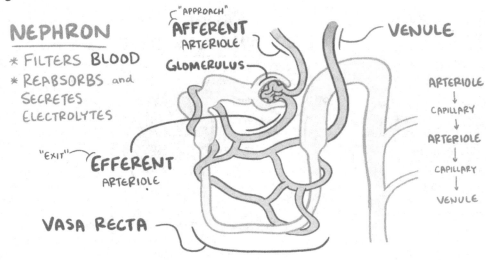

**NEPHRON**
* FILTERS BLOOD
* REABSORBS and SECRETES ELECTROLYTES

"APPROACH"
**AFFERENT** ARTERIOLE
GLOMERULUS

VENULE

ARTERIOLE
↓
CAPILLARY
↓
ARTERIOLE
↓
CAPILLARY
↓
VENULE

"EXIT"
**EFFERENT** ARTERIOLE

**VASA RECTA**

**Figure 45.3**

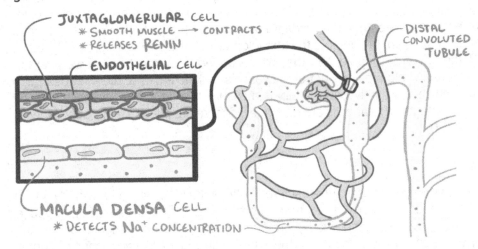

JUXTAGLOMERULAR CELL
* SMOOTH MUSCLE → CONTRACTS
* RELEASES RENIN
ENDOTHELIAL CELL

DISTAL CONVOLUTED TUBULE

MACULA DENSA CELL
* DETECTS Na⁺ CONCENTRATION

**Figure 45.4**

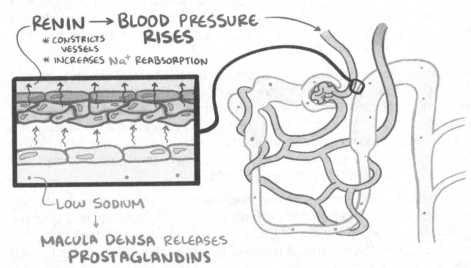

RENIN → BLOOD PRESSURE RISES
* CONSTRICTS VESSELS
* INCREASES Na⁺ REABSORPTION

LOW SODIUM
↓
MACULA DENSA RELEASES PROSTAGLANDINS

**Figure 45.5**

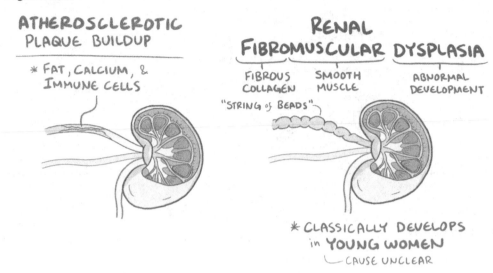

These two clusters of cells work together because if the blood pressure falls, less blood is filtered and less sodium gets into the tubule. This is then detected by the macula densa cells, and they send out a local prostaglandin signal that reaches the juxtaglomerular cells and causes them to release renin. In addition, the juxtaglomerular cells are able to directly sense low pressure in the afferent arteriole, and they also respond to sympathetic nerve fibers to release renin. Now, renin helps to constrict blood vessels and increases sodium reabsorption in the nephrons, which ultimately causes blood pressure to rise. Normally, as the blood pressure rises, the juxtaglomerular cells are no longer triggered to release renin, so balance is restored **(Figure 45.4)**.

## CAUSES

One cause of renal artery stenosis is atherosclerotic plaque buildup, which is where a mix of fat, calcium, and immune cells form a crusty rim on the inside of the artery. Another cause, though, is renal fibromuscular dysplasia, where *fibro-* refers to fibrous collagen connective tissue, *-muscular* refers to smooth muscle in the artery wall, and *-dysplasia* means abnormal development. So, renal fibromuscular dysplasia is when something goes wrong with connective tissue and smooth muscles in the walls of renal artery, resulting in a series of bulges and narrow spots that leaves the artery looking like a "string of beads" instead of a uniform cylinder. Fibromuscular dysplasia classically develops in young women, but the exact underlying cause is still unclear **(Figure 45.5)**.

In both atherosclerosis and renal fibromuscular dysplasia, the renal artery narrows and that causes the blood pressure to stay low in the kidney as well as in all the kidney's nephrons. As a result, the juxtaglomerular cells release renin, which might raise the blood pressure in the body and vessels before the stenosis, but the pressure in the kidney and the afferent arterioles stays low, so they just keep releasing renin. So, renal artery stenosis creates a vicious cycle of high blood pressure, or hypertension, which puts incredible stress on the blood vessels and can contribute to having a stroke or heart attack **(Figure 45.6)**.

Also, since the affected kidney receives less blood than usual, it eventually starts to atrophy, or shrink in size, as the kidney cells die off and get replaced by fibrotic scar tissue. If the renal artery stenosis involves only one of the kidneys, then the other kidney can often pick up the slack, but if both kidneys are affected, then it can lead to acute kidney injury or acute renal failure **(Figure 45.7)**.

**Figure 45.6**

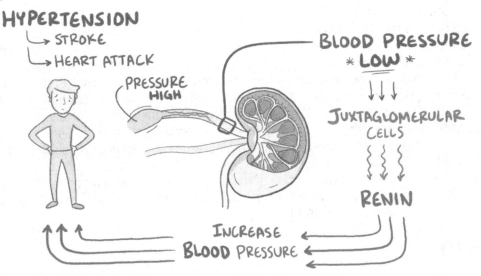

HYPERTENSION
- → STROKE
- → HEART ATTACK

PRESSURE HIGH

BLOOD PRESSURE
\* **LOW** \*
↓↓↓
JUXTAGLOMERULAR CELLS
↓↓↓
RENIN

INCREASE BLOOD PRESSURE

**Figure 45.7**

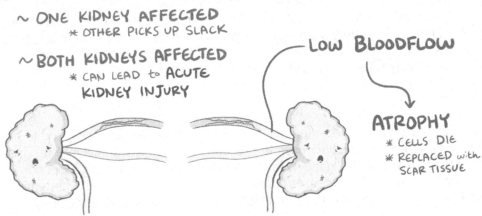

~ ONE KIDNEY AFFECTED
  \* OTHER PICKS UP SLACK

~ BOTH KIDNEYS AFFECTED
  \* CAN LEAD to ACUTE KIDNEY INJURY

LOW BLOODFLOW

ATROPHY
  \* CELLS DIE
  \* REPLACED with SCAR TISSUE

**Figure 45.8**

SYMPTOMS ~ from HYPERTENSION
  \* HEADACHES & BLURRY VISION

DIAGNOSIS
  \* PHYSICAL EXAM → BRUIT ⟩ WHOOSHING SOUND
  \* LAB TESTS ~ SERUM CREATININE & URINALYSIS
  \* IMAGING ~ ULTRASOUND, CT, MRI
        ~ RENAL ARTERIOGRAPHY

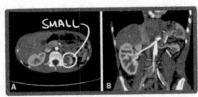

SMALL

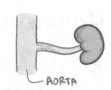

AORTA

## SYMPTOMS & DIAGNOSIS

Symptoms are often a result of the hypertension, which, if it becomes severe, can cause symptoms like headaches and blurry vision. The diagnosis is therefore based on seeing if there's an underlying cause for hypertension. Physical examination might reveal a bruit, which is a whooshing sound heard with a stethoscope over the renal arteries in the abdomen caused by the turbulence of blood flowing through the stenotic part of the renal artery. Basic screening labs like serum creatinine and a urinalysis can help assess kidney function as well, and imaging studies like ultrasound, CT, and MRI can visualize the kidney. For example, in this CT scan of the abdomen, the atrophied kidney is a lot smaller than the healthy one on the other side. Ultimately, since the problem is in the renal artery, a renal arteriography can be done to visualize the renal artery with dye to see if there's evidence of a blockage. Generally, atherosclerosis forms in the beginning portion of the renal artery where it branches from the aorta, whereas fibromuscular dysplasia develops in the middle to far end of the renal artery, which is nearest to the kidney (**Figure 45.8**).

## TREATMENT

Treatment of renal artery stenosis is aimed largely at trying to manage hypertension through using medications, as well as adopting healthy eating and exercising habits. In addition, a surgical procedure called balloon angioplasty can sometimes be used, and this is where a balloon is used to open up the narrowed portions of the renal artery and, in rare cases, a tiny stent is left behind to keep the artery propped open. An alternative option is to simply bypass the stenosis with another artery that is grafted into place. Ultimately, if one kidney becomes atrophied and nonfunctional, it also might be necessary to remove it.

## SUMMARY

All right, as a quick recap: renal artery stenosis is where the artery that carries blood to the kidney becomes more narrow, which reduces the amount of blood that the kidney receives as well as the blood pressure. The kidney senses the low blood pressure and responds by releasing the hormone renin which increases blood pressure, ultimately causing hypertension. Over time, the lack of blood can also cause the affected kidney to atrophy (**Figure 45.9**).

**Figure 45.9**

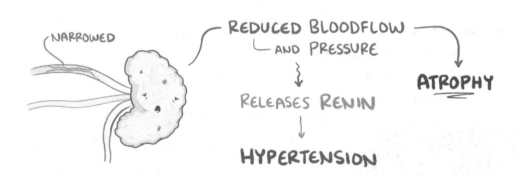

RENAL ARTERY STENOSIS

# Renal cell carcinomas

osmosis.org/learn/renal_cell_carcinomas

R enal cell carcinomas, or RCCs, are the most common type of malignant kidney cancer in adults, generally affecting older men. Unfortunately, RCC is often considered a "silent" cancer because symptoms don't typically get noticed until the tumor has grown pretty large (**Figure 46.1**).

## PHYSIOLOGY

Renal cell carcinomas form from epithelial cells in the proximal convoluted tubule of the kidney; this is the section of the nephron that is usually located in the renal cortex, which is the outer rim of the kidney. The most common type of renal cell carcinoma is composed of polygonal epithelial cells, which have funny angular shapes with at least four sides and are filled with clear cytoplasm full of carbohydrates and lipids. It's those lipids that give the tumors their yellow color (**Figure 46.2**).

At a genetic level, renal cell carcinomas have been linked to mutations on the short arm of chromosome 3, or 3p. An easy way to remember this is that RCC has three letters and it's linked to chromosome 3. One of the main genes involved in renal cell carcinomas is the VHL gene, which codes for the von Hippel-Lindau tumor suppressor protein, or pVHL, which is normally expressed in all tissues. Mutations in pVHL can allow IGF-1, the Type I insulin-like growth factor, pathway to go into overdrive. This does two things. First, there is dysregulated cell growth, and second, it upregulates specific transcription factors called hypoxia-inducible factors. This, in turn, help generate more vascular endothelial growth factor or VEGF, as well as VEGF receptor, leading to growth of new blood vessels, or angiogenesis. Dysregulated cellular growth and angiogenesis are a recipe for tumor formation (**Figure 46.3**).

## PATHOLOGY

Renal cell carcinomas can arise sporadically, or they can be a part of an inherited syndrome. Sporadic tumors are usually solitary tumors in the upper pole of the kidney, and they most often happen among older men that smoke cigarettes. Inherited syndromes, like von Hippel-Lindau disease, can also give rise to renal cell carcinomas, and in this situation, the tumors typically

**Figure 46.1**

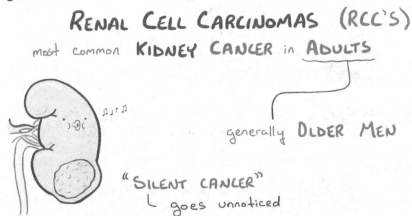

RENAL CELL CARCINOMAS (RCC'S)
most common KIDNEY CANCER in ADULTS

generally OLDER MEN

"SILENT CANCER"
goes unnoticed

**Figure 46.2**

# RENAL CELL CARCINOMAS (RCC'S)
## └ form from EPITHELIAL CELLS

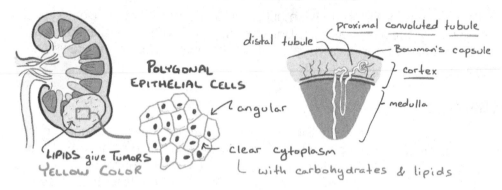

POLYGONAL EPITHELIAL CELLS
→ angular

distal tubule
proximal convoluted tubule
Bowman's capsule
cortex
medulla

LIPIDS give TUMORS YELLOW COLOR

clear cytoplasm
└ with carbohydrates & lipids

**Figure 46.3**

# RENAL CELL CARCINOMAS (RCC'S)

**SPORADICALLY**
* Solitary tumors
* in upper pole of KIDNEY
* OLDER MEN
* SMOKERS

**INHERITED SYNDROMES**
e.g. Von Hippel-Lindau DISEASE
* YOUNGER MEN & WOMEN
* often involves BOTH KIDNEYS
* RARE, autosomal dominant
↓ MUTATION leads to

CYSTS & BENIGN TUMORS
- EYES
- CENTRAL NERVOUS SYSTEM
#1 cause of **DEATH**

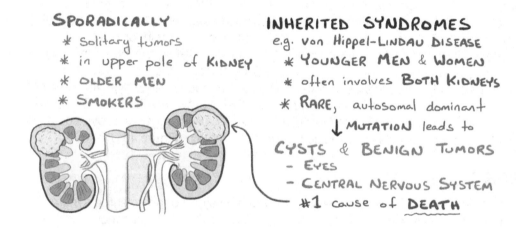

**Figure 46.4**

# RENAL CELL CARCINOMAS (RCC'S)

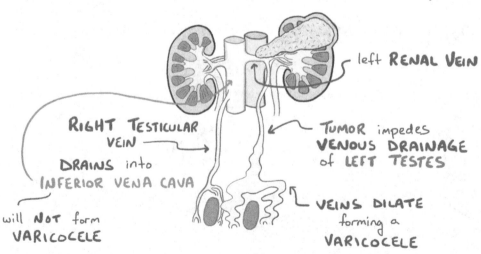

left **RENAL VEIN**

**RIGHT TESTICULAR VEIN**
DRAINS into INFERIOR VENA CAVA

will **NOT** form VARICOCELE

TUMOR impedes **VENOUS DRAINAGE** of **LEFT TESTES**

└ VEINS DILATE forming a VARICOCELE

**Figure 46.5**

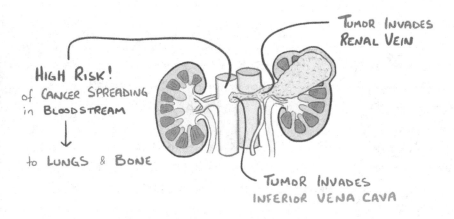

RENAL CELL CARCINOMAS (RCC'S)

TUMOR INVADES
RENAL VEIN

HIGH RISK!
of CANCER SPREADING
in BLOODSTREAM
↓
to LUNGS & BONE

TUMOR INVADES
INFERIOR VENA CAVA

affect younger men and women and often involve both kidneys. Von Hippel Lindau disease is a rare autosomal dominant disorder characterized by a mutation in a tumor suppressor gene that leads to the formation of cysts and benign tumors in various parts of the body like the eye and central nervous system. The number one cause of death in patients with von Hippel-Lindau disease, though, is the development of renal cell carcinomas.

## SYMPTOMS

Individuals with renal cell carcinoma typically have one or more of the following symptoms: hematuria, or red blood cells in the urine, which is most common; a palpable mass in the abdomen or lower back; and pain in the flank or near the hip bone. Since the cancer causes a state of chronic inflammation, other classic symptoms include fever and weight loss. Renal cell carcinoma is also frequently responsible for various paraneoplastic syndromes, which is where the tumor cells generate a hormone that causes its own set of symptoms. For example, these tumors can release the hormone erythropoietin, which increases the production of new red blood cells, and this can lead to polycythemia, or too many red blood cells, which can cause the blood to start sludging or slow down its normal flow. Another paraneoplastic syndrome involves the release of renin, a hormone that is part of the renin-angiotensin-aldosterone system and is involved in raising blood pressure. Some other hormones that renal cell carcinomas are known for releasing include parathyroid hormone-related peptide (or PTHrP), which causes hypercalcemia, and adrenocorticotropic hormone (or ACTH), which increases release of the stress hormone cortisol and can lead to Cushing's syndrome.

In rare cases, a large renal cell carcinoma affecting the left kidney can butt up against the left renal vein, impeding normal venous drainage of the left testes. This leads to dilation of the testicular veins and formation of a varicocele. Since the right testicular vein drains directly into the inferior vena cava, a blockage of the right renal vein by a large tumor doesn't have the same effect **(Figure 46.4)**.

An especially dangerous progression of a renal cell carcinoma is its ability to invade the renal vein, where it literally grow within the vein, eventually reaching the inferior vena cava. This dramatically increases the risk of cancer spreading through the bloodstream with the most likely targets being the lungs since that's the first capillary bed that the tumor cells would reach if they broke free of the growing mass, but also the bones because the tumor cells have an affinity for that tissue **(Figure 46.5)**.

**Figure 46.6**

# RENAL CELL CARCINOMAS (RCC'S)

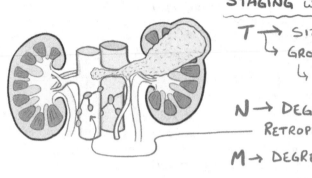

## STAGING with TNM SYSTEM

T →┌→ SIZE of TUMOR
　 └→ GROWN into NEARBY AREAS
　　　↳ e.g. RENAL VEIN

N → DEGREE of SPREAD to
　　　RETROPERITONEAL LYMPH NODES

M → DEGREE of METASTASIS

∅-4 → 4 is most SEVERE

**Figure 46.7**

# RENAL CELL CARCINOMAS (RCC'S)

## TREATMENT

\* RCC's are RESISTANT to
　CHEMOTHERAPY & RADIATION THERAPY

\* if LOCALIZED maybe RESECTION

\* SENSITIVE to IMMUNE SYSTEM
　↳ So, IMMUNOMODULATORY
　AGENTS may be useful
　　　- CHEMOKINES
　　　- ANTIBODIES

\* MOLECULAR TARGETED THERAPIES
　　- VEGF receptor

**Figure 46.8**

# RENAL CELL CARCINOMAS (RCC'S)

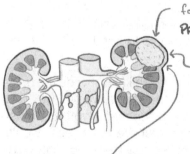

form from EPITHELIAL CELLS of the
PROXIMAL CONVOLUTED TUBULE

Can arise SPORADICALLY or
as part of a GENETIC CONDITION

e.g. VON HIPPEL-LINDAU DISEASE

RESISTANT to CHEMOTHERAPY & RADIATION
& CAUSES PARANEOPLASTIC SYNDROME

# DIAGNOSIS

To determine the risk of renal cell carcinomas, each one is individually staged by the TNM system. 'T' indicates the size of the tumor and whether or not it has grown in nearby areas like, for example, the renal vein. 'N' describes the degree to which the cancer has spread to retroperitoneal lymph nodes. Finally, 'M' indicates the degree to which the cancer has metastasized, or spread to other sites. Each of these categories is ranked from zero to four, with four being the most severe **(Figure 46.6)**.

# TREATMENT

Renal cell carcinomas are stubbornly resistant to both traditional chemotherapy and radiation therapy. So, if the tumor is localized to the kidney, surgical resection may be appropriate. In addition, renal cell carcinomas sometimes regress when they are attacked by the immune system, and they're sensitive to immunomodulatory agents like certain chemokines and monoclonal antibodies. Molecular targeted therapies specifically aimed at inhibiting the VEGF receptor are particularly effective because they reduce tumor vascularization, thereby cutting off the blood supply and killing the tumor **(Figure 46.7)**.

# SUMMARY

All right, as a quick recap: renal cell carcinomas form from epithelial cells in the proximal convoluted tubule of the kidney. These tumors can arise sporadically or as part of a genetic condition like von Hippel-Lindau disease. Renal cell carcinomas can be tricky to treat because they are resistant to traditional chemotherapy and radiation therapy, and they are known to cause paraneoplastic syndromes **(Figure 46.8)**.

# Renal cortical necrosis

osmosis.org/learn/renal__cortical__necrosis

Renal cortical necrosis, sometimes called diffuse cortical necrosis, can be explained by its name. *Renal* refers to the kidneys, *cortical* refers to the outer layer, and *necrosis* refers to tissue death, so renal cortical necrosis describes the outer layer of the kidney dying, usually because of ischemia, a lack of blood flow **(Figure 47.1)**.

## PHYSIOLOGY

Normally, around 20% of the blood leaving the heart goes into the renal arteries and through cortical radial arteries to reach the renal cortex, which is where the glomeruli of the nephrons are located. And that's a lot of blood, especially given that the kidneys are relatively smallish organs when you put them next to the brain and liver **(Figure 47.2)**.

Literally millions of glomeruli in the kidneys work to filter that large volume of blood, and they do so at a rate called the glomerular filtration rate. It's also worth noticing that those cortical radial arteries are end arteries, meaning that they rarely anastomose with adjacent branches, and are, therefore, more susceptible to infarction, since a single blocked artery is all it takes to cause ischemia because the tissue cannot be saved by neighboring arteries. Some causes of reduced blood flow or a complete blockage are thrombi, which are blood clots that fill the blood vessels, and vasospasm, which is the narrowing of the blood vessel **(Figure 47.3)**.

## PATHOLOGY

Interestingly, renal cortical necrosis has been associated with pregnancy complications, like placental abruption, which is when the placental lining is separated from the uterus, prolonged intrauterine fetal death, which is when the fetus dies and then remains dead inside the uterus, and infected abortion, which is when there's an infection of the remnants of the placenta or fetus. All of these are obviously terrible complications, and they relate back to renal cortical necrosis because they can progress to septic shock or disseminated intravascular coagulation, both conditions that can lead to the widespread formation of blood clots.

**Figure 47.1**

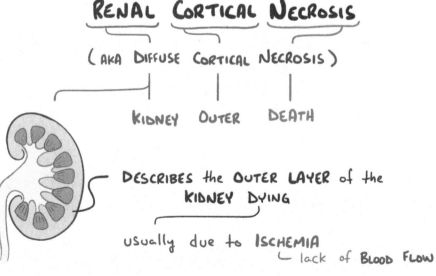

**Figure 47.2**

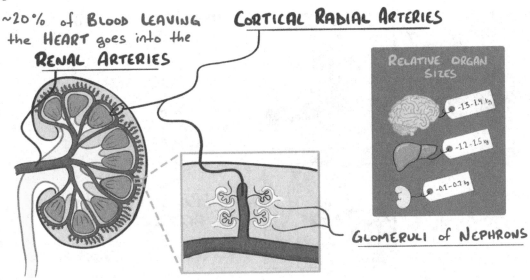

**Figure 47.3**

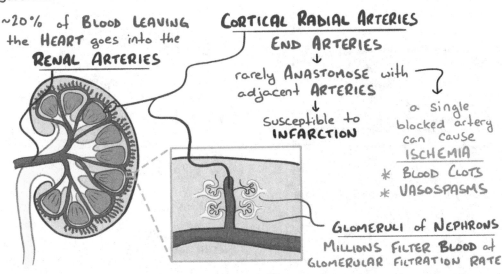

So once there's an obstruction to blood flow, tissue ischemia sets in, and it triggers inflammation in the renal cortex. That inflammation causes fluid to leak into the interstitium of the kidney, which is the space between the cells, and triggers vasoconstriction of the afferent arterioles, which bring blood to the glomeruli of the nephrons. That vasoconstriction reduces the glomerular filtration rate, which is the amount of blood that gets filtered over time **(Figure 47.4)**.

Also, some parts of the nephron that happen to be in the cortex, like the proximal tubule and the thick ascending loop of Henle, need more energy and therefore a bigger supply of blood to carry out their job of reabsorption. Since these cells are very energy-demanding, having a reduced blood supply means that they are the first to start dying and detaching when there's renal ischemia. The dead epithelial cells can clog up the lumen of the nephron and cause an increase in the pressure within that nephron. Since blood likes to move from a high pressure to low pressure space whenever possible, a higher pressure inside the nephron reduces glomerular filtration rate even more **(Figure 47.5)**.

**Figure 47.4**

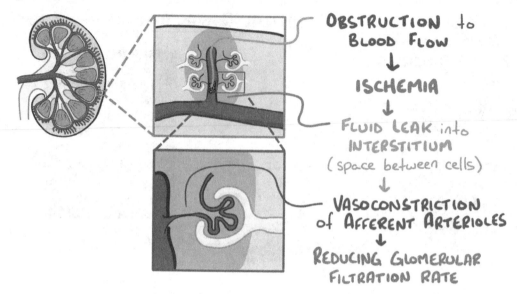

OBSTRUCTION to BLOOD FLOW
↓
ISCHEMIA
↓
FLUID LEAK into INTERSTITIUM
(space between cells)
↓
VASOCONSTRICTION of AFFERENT ARTERIOLES
↓
REDUCING GLOMERULAR FILTRATION RATE

**Figure 47.5**

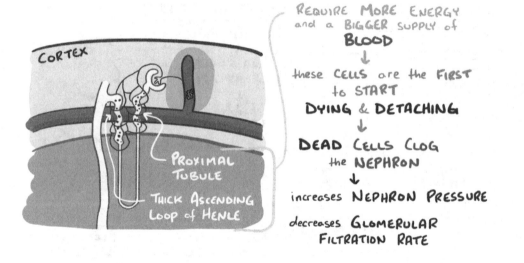

REQUIRE MORE ENERGY and a BIGGER SUPPLY of BLOOD
↓
these CELLS are the FIRST to START DYING & DETACHING
↓
DEAD CELLS CLOG the NEPHRON
↓
increases NEPHRON PRESSURE

decreases GLOMERULAR FILTRATION RATE

**Figure 47.6**

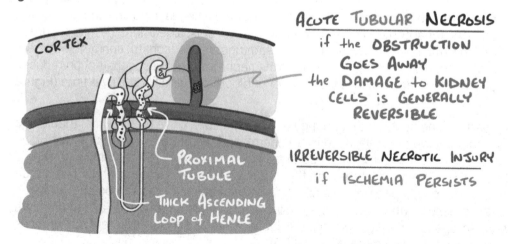

ACUTE TUBULAR NECROSIS
if the OBSTRUCTION GOES AWAY the DAMAGE to KIDNEY CELLS is GENERALLY REVERSIBLE

IRREVERSIBLE NECROTIC INJURY
if ISCHEMIA PERSISTS

**Figure 47.7**

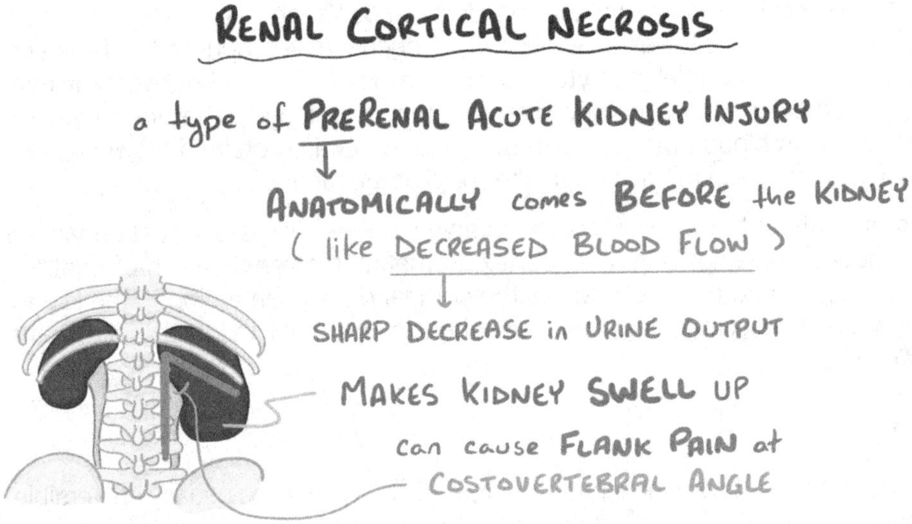

## RENAL CORTICAL NECROSIS

a type of PRERENAL ACUTE KIDNEY INJURY

↓

ANATOMICALLY comes BEFORE the KIDNEY
( like DECREASED BLOOD FLOW )

↓

SHARP DECREASE in URINE OUTPUT

MAKES KIDNEY SWELL UP

can cause FLANK PAIN at
COSTOVERTEBRAL ANGLE

Up to this point, if the obstruction goes away and normal blood flow is recovered, the damage to the kidney cells is generally reversible, and this is also known as acute tubular necrosis. If blood flow isn't recovered, though, and the ischemia persists, then the ischemic damage eventually leads to an irreversible necrotic injury to the renal cortex **(Figure 47.6)**.

Broadly speaking, renal cortical necrosis is a type of prerenal acute kidney injury, which is a category that includes any cause of kidney injury that anatomically comes before the kidneys, like, in this case, a decreased blood flow in this case. The decrease in blood flow leads to one of the main symptoms, which is a sharp decrease in urine output. Renal cortical necrosis makes the kidney swell up and stretches out the renal capsule, and that can cause flank pain at the costovertebral angle **(Figure 47.7)**.

**Figure 47.8**

### DIAGNOSIS

IMAGING STUDIES
    └ e.g. CONTRAST-ENHANCED CT SCANS
    └ SHOW a NON-ENHANCING RENAL CORTEX
    └ SOMETIMES a THIN RIM of CONTRAST
            ENHANCEMENT can OCCUR

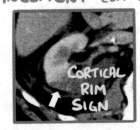

CORTICAL RIM SIGN

## DIAGNOSIS

The diagnosis of renal cortical necrosis is often done through laboratory studies in the blood and urine. The blood typically has an excess of nitrogen waste products, like BUN and creatinine, as well as other serious electrolyte and metabolic imbalances, like hyperkalemia, which is increased potassium levels in blood, and metabolic acidosis. The urine typically shows hematuria, which is blood in the urine, proteinuria, which is protein in the urine, and tubular cell casts, which are dead tubule cells in the mold of the tubule.

Since there is no blood flow to the renal cortex, imaging studies, like a contrast-enhanced CT scan, usually show a nonenhancing renal cortex. Sometimes a very thin rim of contrast enhancement can happen, and this is known as the cortical rim sign.In a biopsy, the kidney cortex might show patchy necrosis and atrophy, whereas the renal medulla looks pretty normal **(Figure 47.8)**.

## TREATMENT

Unfortunately, by the time renal cortical necrosis is treated, the damage is usually irreversible, so the main goal is to increase blood perfusion to the renal cortex. Once kidney function is severely affected, hemodialysis may be needed.

## SUMMARY

All right, as a quick recap: renal cortical necrosis is an irreversible type of prerenal acute kidney injury caused by a sudden drop in blood perfusion to the renal cortex, and it has been associated with pregnancy complications. The reduced blood supply, due in part to the lack of anastomosis among radial end arteries, combined with the relatively high demand for blood in certain parts of the nephron, like the proximal tubule and the thick ascending loop of Henle, causes ischemia to set in **(Figure 47.9)**.

**Figure 47.9**

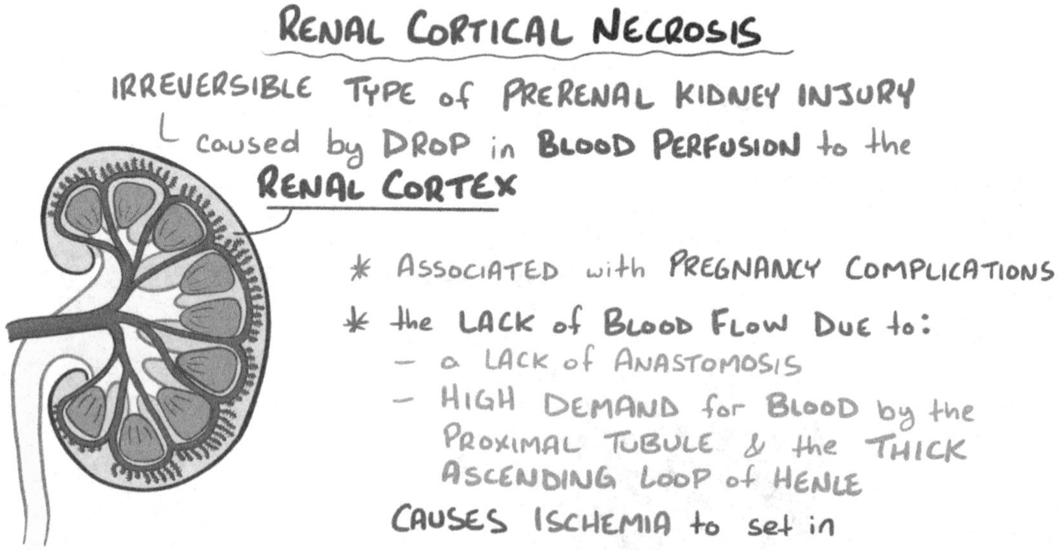

RENAL CORTICAL NECROSIS

IRREVERSIBLE TYPE of PRERENAL KIDNEY INJURY
└ caused by DROP in BLOOD PERFUSION to the RENAL CORTEX

* ASSOCIATED with PREGNANCY COMPLICATIONS
* the LACK of BLOOD FLOW DUE to:
  - a LACK of ANASTOMOSIS
  - HIGH DEMAND for BLOOD by the PROXIMAL TUBULE & the THICK ASCENDING LOOP of HENLE
CAUSES ISCHEMIA to set in

# Renal tubular acidosis

osmosis.org/learn/renal_tubular_acidosis

**W**ith renal tubular acidosis, *renal* refers to the kidney, *tubular* refers to the main tube-portion of the nephron, and *acidosis* refers to increased acidity in blood, which is caused by too many protons. So, renal tubular acidosis, or RTA, is increased blood acidity that happens because the renal tubules can't get rid of protons **(Figure 48.1)**.

## PHYSIOLOGY

The kidneys contain millions of nephrons, each of which has a renal corpuscle and a renal tubule that ends in a collecting duct. The renal corpuscle filters large amounts of solutes that go from the blood into the filtrate and eventually the urine, and the renal tubule and collecting duct are responsible for fine tuning the reabsorption and secretion of solutes, which adjusts the amounts of these that are ultimately retained by or removed from the body. Broadly speaking, renal tubular acidosis can develop in either the proximal convoluted tubule, sometimes called just the proximal tubule, or the distal convoluted tubule, or distal tubule, and the nearby collecting duct **(Figure 48.2)**.

**Figure 48.1**

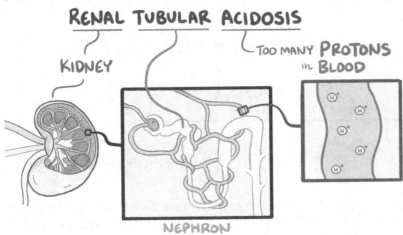

**Figure 48.2**

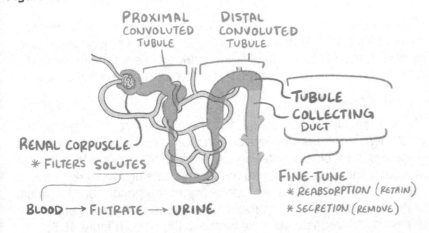

**Figure 48.3**

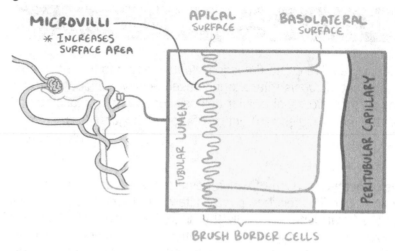

**Figure 48.4**

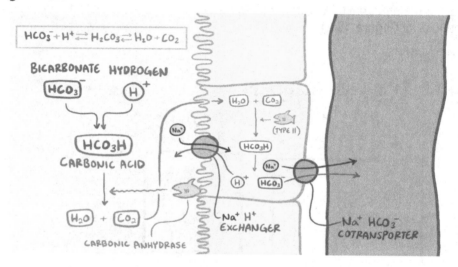

The proximal tubule is lined by brush border cells which have two surfaces. One is the apical surface, which faces the tubular lumen and is lined with microvilli, which are tiny little projections that increase the cell's surface area to help with solute reabsorption. The other is the basolateral surface, which faces the peritubular capillaries that run alongside the nephron **(Figure 48.3)**.

Now, when a molecule of bicarbonate approaches the apical surface of the brush border cell, it binds to hydrogen to form carbonic acid. At that point, an enzyme called carbonic anhydrase Type 4, which lurks in the tubule among the microvilli like a shark, swims along and splits the carbonic acid into water and carbon dioxide **(Figure 48.4)**. The overall equation looks like this:

$$H^+ + HCO_{3^-} <\text{-}> H_2CO_3 <\text{-}> H_2O + CO_2$$

The water and carbon dioxide happily diffuse across the membrane into the cells, where carbonic anhydrase Type 2 then facilitates the reverse reaction, combining them to form carbonic acid, which dissolves into bicarbonate and hydrogen. A sodium bicarbonate cotransporter on the basolateral surface snatches up the bicarbonate and a nearby sodium and shuttles both into the blood. Meanwhile, a sodium-hydrogen exchanger on the apical surface pulls sodium into the cell while pushing hydrogen back into the tubule. So, at the end of the day, there's a movement of bicarbonate from the tubule to the blood **(Figure 48.5)**.

**Figure 48.5**

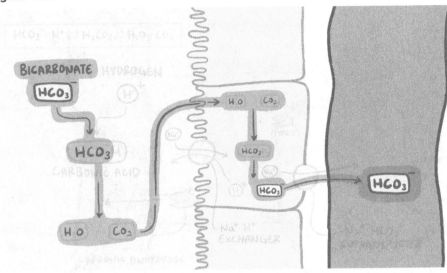

**Figure 48.6**

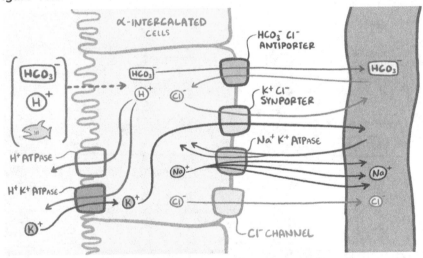

Okay, so now let's shift over to the distal tubule and collecting duct, which we'll talk about together. First off, one type of cell that these are lined with are the alpha-intercalated cells. Like the brush border cells, the alpha intercalated cells move bicarbonate and hydrogen from the tubule into the cell using carbonic anhydrase. The alpha intercalated cells have two major ways to get rid of that hydrogen across the apical surface. First, they have an $H^+$/ATPase, which simply pushes hydrogen into the tubule. Second, they have a hydrogen potassium ATPase ($H^+K^+$ATPase), which pushes hydrogen into the tubule in exchange for potassium **(Figure 48.6)**. With regard to bicarbonate, there is a bicarbonate/chloride antiporter which moves bicarbonate into the blood in exchange for chloride. To prevent chloride from piling up within the cell, there's a potassium/chloride symporter on the basolateral surface that moves both of these ions into the blood. In addition, there's a chloride channel on the basolateral surface that allows chloride to passively move down its concentration gradient into the blood. Finally, it's worth mentioning that, like in all cells, sodium and potassium levels are controlled by Na/K ATPase pumps on the basolateral surface which move two potassium ions into the cell for every three sodium ions they move out of the cell. So overall, there's a net movement of sodium, chloride, and bicarbonate into the blood, while hydrogen is pushed into the tubule **(Figure 48.7)**.

**Figure 48.7**

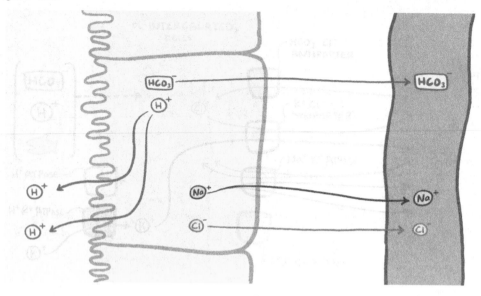

**Figure 48.8**

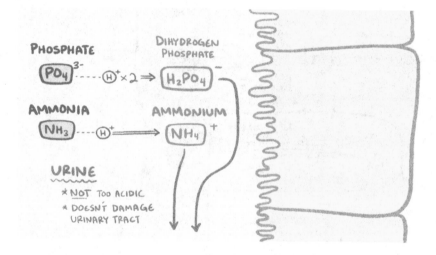

**Figure 48.9**

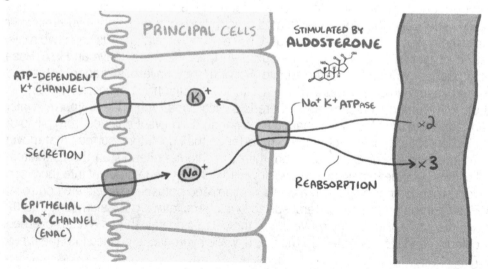

Once it's in the tubule's lumen, hydrogen binds to phosphate or ammonia to form relatively weak acids like dihydrogen phosphate or ammonium, which then get peed out in the urine. This allows protons to be removed without making the urine too acidic, which would damage the cells lining the tubules and the rest of the urinary tract **(Figure 48.8)**.

The other group of cells in the distal tube and collecting duct are the principal cells. They have two pumps on the apical surface, an ATP-dependent potassium channel pump that pushes potassium into the tubule, and an epithelial sodium channel pump called ENaC that pulls sodium into the cell. There's also a Na/K ATPase pump on the basolateral surface that again moves two potassium ions in for every three sodium ions it moves out. All three of these pumps are stimulated by aldosterone, and their combined effect is resorption of sodium and loss of potassium **(Figure 48.9)**.

# RENAL TUBULAR ACIDOSIS TYPE I

In RTA Type I, or distal renal tubular acidosis, the main issue is that alpha intercalated cells of the distal tubule and collecting duct are unable to secrete hydrogen. The buildup of hydrogen in those cells leads to a buildup of hydrogen in the blood, resulting in acidemia. The underlying cause could be a genetic mutation in the $H^+$ATPase pump or the $H^+K^+$ATPase pump of alpha intercalated cells. Alternatively, this could be an acquired defect from a medication like lithium or amphotericin B, both of which can make cells permeable, allowing hydrogen to simply diffuse from the tubule right back into the cell. A less common mechanism of acidemia is a defect in the bicarbonate/chloride antiporter, which causes a decrease in bicarbonate reabsorption, and therefore less bicarbonate in the blood **(Figure 48.10)**.

# RENAL TUBULAR ACIDOSIS TYPE II

In RTA Type II, or proximal renal tubular acidosis, the main issue is that brush border cells of the proximal tubule are unable to reabsorb bicarbonate. As a result, bicarbonate is lost through the urine, meaning that there is nothing to counterbalance the hydrogen ions, and this results in acidemia. One known cause of RTA Type II is a genetic mutation in the sodium bicarbonate cotransporter on the basolateral surface, which makes it less functional. Less movement of bicarbonate out of the cell alters the intracellular bicarbonate concentration, making it more difficult for bicarbonate to get brought across the apical surface into the cell. As a result, less bicarbonate gets reabsorbed by the brush border cells, and more is left behind in the lumen of the tubule. This means that bicarbonate will eventually be lost bicarbonate in the urine, so there will less bicarbonate in the blood, resulting in an acidemia. Unlike in RTA Type II, the distal intercalated cells are still functional and can produce hydrogen ions, and can therefore can generally still acidify the urine **(Figure 48.11)**.

RTA type II can happen independently or can be part of a broader disfunction of the proximal tubular cells that's called Fanconi syndrome. In Fanconi syndrome, in addition to the loss of bicarbonate, there is also phosphaturia, glycosuria, aminoaciduria, uricosuria, and proteinuria, terms that refer to the loss of phosphate, glucose, amino acids, uric acid, and protein in the urine. Fanconi syndrome can be inherited, but it can also be acquired. For example, it can be a side effect of taking certain medications like tetracycline class antibiotics **(Figure 48.12)**.

# RENAL TUBULAR ACIDOSIS TYPE III

In RTA Type III, there are defects in both the distal and proximal tubule, and this is a fairly uncommon situation. The causes of these defects are not well understood, but some cases have been associated with congenital carbonic anhydrase deficiency, and this is because carbonic anhydrases are present in both distal and proximal tubule **(Figure 48.13)**.

Figure 48.10

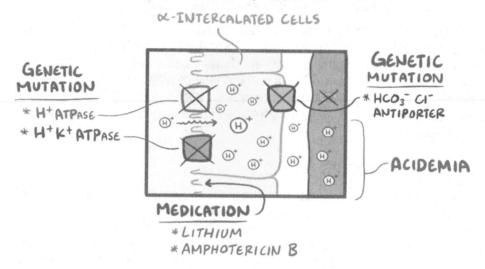

RENAL TUBULAR ACIDOSIS ~ TYPE I

α-INTERCALATED CELLS

GENETIC MUTATION
* H⁺ ATPASE
* H⁺K⁺ ATPASE

GENETIC MUTATION
* HCO₃⁻ Cl⁻ ANTIPORTER

ACIDEMIA

MEDICATION
* LITHIUM
* AMPHOTERICIN B

Figure 48.11

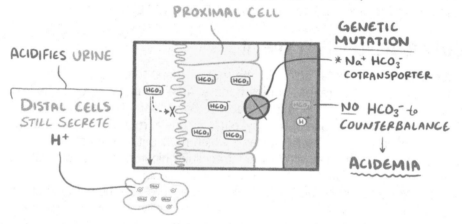

RENAL TUBULAR ACIDOSIS ~ TYPE II

PROXIMAL CELL

ACIDIFIES URINE

DISTAL CELLS STILL SECRETE H⁺

GENETIC MUTATION
* Na⁺ HCO₃⁻ COTRANSPORTER

NO HCO₃⁻ to COUNTERBALANCE

↓

ACIDEMIA

Figure 48.12

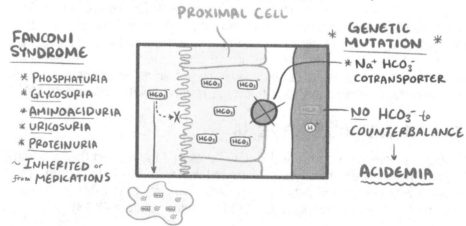

RENAL TUBULAR ACIDOSIS ~ TYPE II

PROXIMAL CELL

FANCONI SYNDROME
* PHOSPHATURIA
* GLYCOSURIA
* AMINOACIDURIA
* URICOSURIA
* PROTEINURIA
~ INHERITED or from MEDICATIONS

* GENETIC MUTATION *
* Na⁺ HCO₃⁻ COTRANSPORTER

NO HCO₃⁻ to COUNTERBALANCE

↓

ACIDEMIA

**Figure 48.13**

## RENAL TUBULAR ACIDOSIS ~ TYPE III
* CONGENITAL CARBONIC ANHYDRASE
  DEFICIENCY (?)

PROXIMAL CELLS        DISTAL CELLS

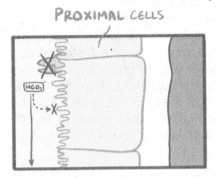 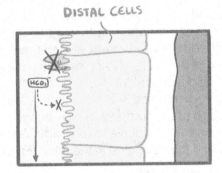

**Figure 48.14**

## RENAL TUBULAR ACIDOSIS ~ TYPE IV
(HYPERKALEMIC ACIDOSIS)
* ALDOSTERONE
  └ DEFICIENCY ~ ADDISON'S DISEASE
  └ RESISTANCE ~ ENAC GENETIC MUTATION

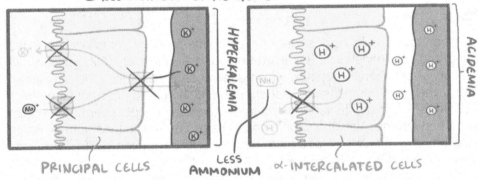

PRINCIPAL CELLS    LESS    α-INTERCALATED CELLS
                 AMMONIUM

**Figure 48.15**

## RENAL TUBULAR ACIDOSIS ~ TYPE IV
(HYPERKALEMIC ACIDOSIS)
* ALDOSTERONE
  └ DEFICIENCY ~ ADDISON'S DISEASE
  └ RESISTANCE ~ ENAC GENETIC MUTATION

* SEVERE HYPOVOLEMIA (LOW FLUID)
  └→ LOW Na⁺ REABSORPTION

* SYSTEMIC LUPUS ERYTHEMATOSUS

* MEDICATIONS
  └ LITHIUM
  └ AMPHOTERICIN B  } → CELLS MORE PERMEABLE

# RENAL TUBULAR ACIDOSIS TYPE IV

Finally, there's RTA Type IV, sometimes called hyperkalemic acidosis, and it's classically due to aldosterone deficiency or aldosterone resistance in the collecting ducts, which would affect both the principal and alpha intercalated cells. Aldosterone has an important role in the regulation of sodium, potassium, and hydrogen levels. An example of aldosterone deficiency is Addison's disease, where the adrenal gland doesn't produce enough of it. An example of aldosterone resistance is a mutation in the epithelial sodium channel (ENaC) that means it doesn't respond well to normal levels of aldosterone. Either way, reduced aldosterone can decrease the function of the $Na^+K^+ATPase$, making sodium levels fall and potassium levels rise in the blood. A reduced effect of aldosterone on the $H^+/ATPase$ in the intercalated cells means that more hydrogen gets retained in the cells and eventually in the blood, causing acidemia. Overall, this causes high potassium, hyperkalemia, and acidemia. Also, since hydrogen usually combines with ammonia in the tubule to form ammonium, with less hydrogen there'll be less ammonium formed and then excreted in the urine **(Figure 48.14)**.

There are some other causes of RTA Type IV as well. One is severe hypovolemia, or low blood fluid, which means less sodium is available for reabsorption in the principal cells. This results in lower sodium levels in the cell, altering the ion exchange between sodium and potassium, resulting in low sodium and high potassium levels in the blood; this hyperkalemia contributes to the acidosis. Other causes of RTA Type IV are systemic lupus and medications like lithium and amphotericin B, which can make the distal tubule and collecting duct cells more permeable to hydrogen ions, allowing these to diffuse into the blood, causing acidosis **(Figure 48.15)**.

## SYMPTOMS

Initially, symptoms of renal tubular acidosis include gastrointestinal problems like decreased appetite, vomiting, and abdominal pain. But, if left untreated, severe metabolic acidosis can lead to vasodilation of peripheral arterioles, which can cause shock. Like other causes of metabolic acidosis, there is a compensatory pattern of breathing called Kussmaul breathing, where a person initially takes rapid shallow breaths that become deeper over time in order to blow off the carbon dioxide. Also, the urine tends to be more alkaline than normal, which means it typically has a pH that's greater than 6. This especially happens in RTA Type I and sometimes in the acute setting for RTA Type II. This high pH causes hypercalciuria, leading to the precipitation of calcium oxalate, which can cause painful kidney stones **(Figure 48.16)**.

**Figure 48.16**

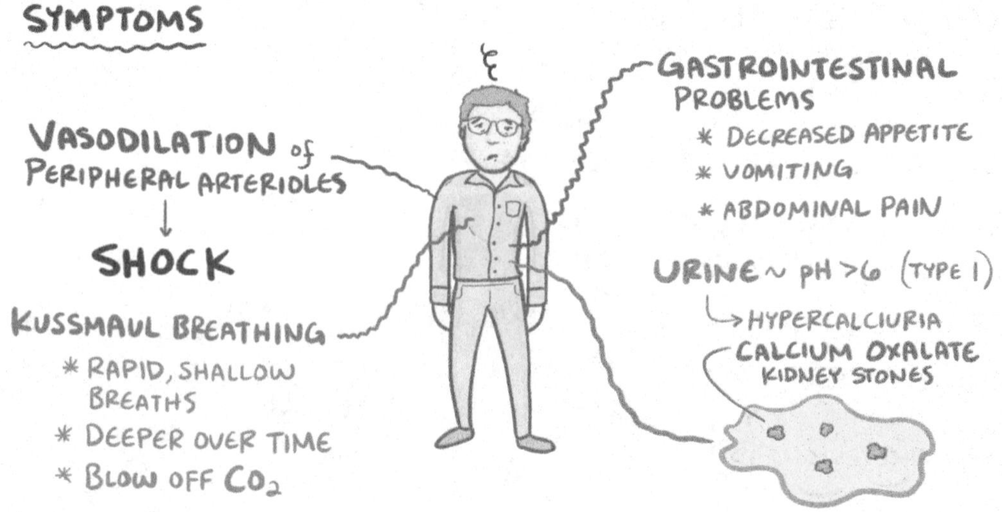

SYMPTOMS

VASODILATION of PERIPHERAL ARTERIOLES
↓
SHOCK

KUSSMAUL BREATHING
* RAPID, SHALLOW BREATHS
* DEEPER OVER TIME
* BLOW OFF $CO_2$

GASTROINTESTINAL PROBLEMS
* DECREASED APPETITE
* VOMITING
* ABDOMINAL PAIN

URINE ~ pH >6 (TYPE I)
↳ HYPERCALCIURIA
CALCIUM OXALATE KIDNEY STONES

# DIAGNOSIS

Renal tubular acidosis is a metabolic acidosis, or a pH below 7.35 and a low bicarbonate level, with a normal anion gap. That means that the difference between measured anions, $Cl^-$ and $HCO_3^-$, and cations, $Na^+$ and $K^+$, is between 8 mEq/L and 12 mEq/L. In addition, blood potassium and urine pH are typically tested to identify the exact type of RTA. Low levels of $HCO_3^-$ in the blood also lead to elevated levels of chloride, so hyperchloremia is a classic finding in RTA.

# TREATMENT

In RTA Types I and II, the main goal of treatment is to replenish bicarbonate and correct hypokalemia with potassium citrate. In RTA Type II, this can be achieved with thiazide diuretics, which cause water loss and increased reabsorption of bicarbonate. For RTA Type IV, the goal is to treat hypoaldosteronism with fludrocortisone or loop diuretics, which increases sodium delivery to the collecting duct and increases potassium hydrogen exchange.

# SUMMARY

All right, as a quick recap: renal tubular acidosis is a condition in which the kidney is unable to secrete acids or reabsorb bicarbonate from the This most commonly results in metabolic acidosis with a normal anion gap. If left untreated, the acidemia can cause peripheral vasodilation and shock **(Figure 48.17)**.

**Figure 48.17**

## RENAL TUBULAR ACIDOSIS

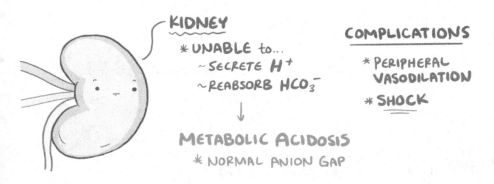

KIDNEY
* UNABLE to...
~ SECRETE $H^+$
~ REABSORB $HCO_3^-$

↓

METABOLIC ACIDOSIS
* NORMAL ANION GAP

COMPLICATIONS
* PERIPHERAL VASODILATION
* SHOCK

# Transitional cell carcinoma

osmosis.org/learn/transitional_cell_carcinoma

The most common form of cancer in the lower urinary tract, or the bladder and the urethra, is transitional cell carcinoma, or TCC, and, to be more specific, urothelial cell carcinoma, or UCC. While this cancer can affect tissues in the upper urinary tract, such as the renal pelvis and the ureter, it most commonly arises in the urothelium of the bladder **(Figure 49.1)**.

## PHYSIOLOGY

The urothelium, or uroepithelium, is a specific type of transitional cell epithelium that lines the inner surface of much of the urinary tract. This tissue is composed of three to seven cell layers, and it forms a tight barrier that holds urine without allowing toxins to move across the epithelium and back into the body. This barrier function is largely accomplished by large umbrella cells that line the inner, or luminal, surface of the urothelium, are held together by high resistance tight junctions, and are lined with a unique protein/lipid complex, called a plaque, along their apical membrane **(Figure 49.2)**.

**Figure 49.1**

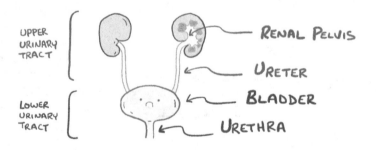

TRANSITIONAL CELL CARCINOMA (TCC)
UROTHELIAL CELL CARCINOMA (UCC)

UPPER URINARY TRACT — RENAL PELVIS — URETER
LOWER URINARY TRACT — BLADDER — URETHRA

**Figure 49.2**

UROTHELIUM or UROEPITHELIUM
└ TRANSITIONAL CELL EPITHELIUM
└ 3 to 7 CELL LAYERS
└ BARRIER LAYER

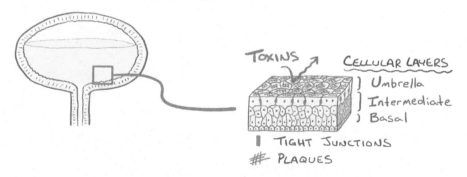

TOXINS   CELLULAR LAYERS
] Umbrella
] Intermediate
] Basal
| TIGHT JUNCTIONS
# PLAQUES

Figure 49.3

# BLADDER
    └ CHANGES SHAPE
    └ REMAINS **IMPERMEABLE**

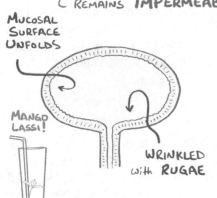

MUCOSAL
SURFACE
UNFOLDS

MANGO
LASSI!

WRINKLED
with RUGAE

# UROTHELIUM
    └ TRANSITIONAL CELL EPITHELIUM
    └ 3 & 7 CELL LAYERS
    └ BARRIER LAYER
    └ CAN STRETCH

TRANSITIONS THROUGH SHAPE

Figure 49.4

# TWO MAIN FORMS of UROTHELIAL CELL CARCINOMAS

### p53 Dependent
  \* Flat Tumor
  \* INVASIVE

### p53 Independent
  \* Less Aggressive
  \* Papillary Tumor

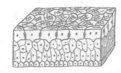

RBCs IN URINE
HEMATURIA

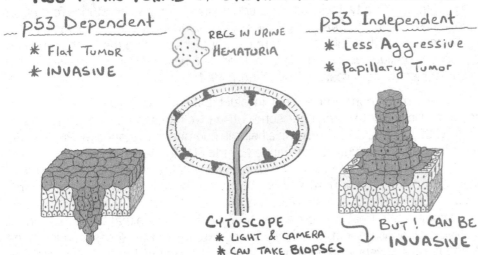

CYTOSCOPE
  \* LIGHT & CAMERA
  \* CAN TAKE BIOPSES

BUT! CAN BE
INVASIVE

Figure 49.5

## UROTHELIAL CELL CARCINOMAS

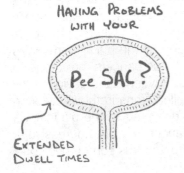

HAVING PROBLEMS
WITH YOUR

Pee SAC?

EXTENDED
DWELL TIMES

RISK FACTORS
└ AGE
└ CARCINOGENS
    \* Phenacetin - a BANNED analgesic
    \* Smoking - #1 risk factor
    \* Analine - rubbers & dyes
    \* Cyclophosphamide - MEDICATION
      - Treats CANCERS and
       AUTOIMMUNE diseases
└ ALCOHOL abuse

Now, when you think about the bladder, it's going to cyclically change shape during the course of its normal function. For example, after you chug a tall mango lassi, your bladder will become completely filled up, only to be emptied again when you rush to the restroom. Therefore, the urothelium has to be able to maintain its impermeable properties during these normal changes in bladder shape. Most of this is allowed by the unfolding of the mucosal surface when the bladder fills up. When the bladder is empty, this surface is highly wrinkled with rugae, which then smooth out as the bladder becomes distended. In addition to this, these umbrella cells of the urothelium have the ability to stretch with an expanding bladder. In fact, the term "transition" in transitional epithelium refers to this ability to go through transitions of shape **(Figure 49.3)**.

## PATHOLOGY

Cancers that affect the urothelium usually arise through two distinct mechanisms. One way for a urothelial cell carcinoma to arise is through a mutation in the tumor suppressor protein p53. Mutations in p53 can allow urothelial cells to start growing horizontally like a flat pancake, some of which begin to invade deeper bladder tissues. The other, less aggressive way for a urothelial cell carcinoma to arise is independent of p53 mutations, and this occurs when finger-like extensions called papillary tumors grow outward from the urothelium. These can can occasionally invade deeper bladder tissues as well. Regardless of the cause of the urothelial cell carcinoma invasion, a telltale sign of the presence of the cancer is the presence of red blood cells in the urine, a typically painless condition known as hematuria. To make a definitive diagnosis, it's possible to look at the inside of the bladder with as cystoscope, which is a thin flexible tube fitted with a light, and a camera that is inserted up the urethra and into the bladder, a procedure called cystoscopy. This tool can also be used to take biopsies, which are used for a subsequent histological analysis **(Figure 49.4)**.

Urothelial cell cancers most commonly occur in older patients, and have been linked to various carcinogens. One way to remember some of the well known causes is the phrase "Having problems with your Pee SAC?" which is a helpful mnemonic: 'P' stands for Phenacetin, which was a common analgesic until it was banned by the FDA in the 80s, in part because of its link to urinary tract cancers. 'S' stands for Smoking, which is the biggest risk factor, giving you yet another reason to not pick up the habit. 'A' stands for Aniline, which is an organic compound used in rubber and dye manufacturing. And 'C' stands for Cyclophosphamide, which is a medication used to treat cancers and autoimmune diseases that has a toxic effect on the bladder. Heavy alcohol use and chronically having extended "dwell times" of urine in the bladder (think about truck drivers who don't pull over very often to use the restroom) are also linked to urothelial cell carcinomas **(Figure 49.5)**.

## TREATMENT

Unfortunately, these cancers can be difficult to treat because they are often multifocal and can recur after treatment. One theory for why this happens is called the field effect, where the entire urothelial 'field' is exposed to a carcinogen, and therefore many of the cells are equally susceptible to tumor formation. Another theory is the implantation theory, where tumor cells detach from one location in the bladder, float through the urine, then implant themselves at another location in the bladder. This could also explain why these cancers are prone to metastasize to nearby structures. If the tumors are localized, non-invasive and obvious they may be able to be resected with the cystoscope in a procedure called Transurethral Resection (TUR). This is often followed up with localized chemotherapy delivered to the bladder via a catheter; this is called a intravesical chemotherapy. If the cancer is more aggressive, a complete removal of the prostate and bladder, or a cysto-prostatectomy, is sometimes done, often in conjunction with chemotherapy **(Figure 49.6)**.

**Figure 49.6**

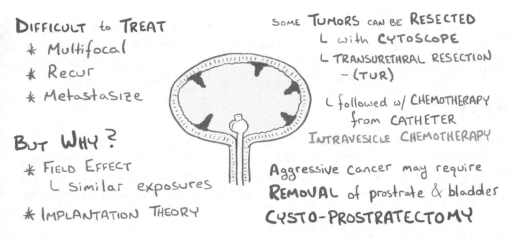

UROTHELIAL CELL CARCINOMAS

DIFFICULT to TREAT
* Multifocal
* Recur
* Metastasize

BUT WHY ?
* FIELD EFFECT
  L similar exposures
* IMPLANTATION THEORY

SOME TUMORS CAN BE RESECTED
L with CYTOSCOPE
L TRANSURETHRAL RESECTION
  - (TUR)
L followed w/ CHEMOTHERAPY
  from CATHETER
INTRAVESICLE CHEMOTHERAPY

Aggressive cancer may require
REMOVAL of prostrate & bladder
CYSTO-PROSTRATECTOMY

## SUMMARY

All right, as a short recap: transitional cell carcinomas are the most common form of cancer in the lower urinary tract. These cancers affect the highly elastic urothelium and are often associated with carcinogens, remembered by Pee SAC (Phenacetin, Smoking, Aniline, and Cyclophosphamide) **(Figure 49.7)**.

**Figure 49.7**

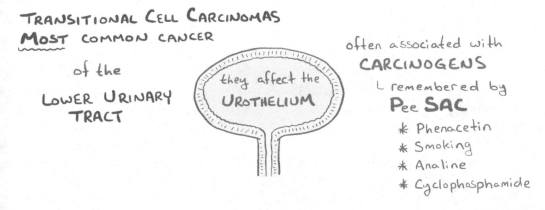

UROTHELIAL CELL CARCINOMAS

TRANSITIONAL CELL CARCINOMAS
MOST COMMON CANCER
   of the
LOWER URINARY
   TRACT

they affect the
UROTHELIUM

often associated with
CARCINOGENS
L remembered by
Pee SAC
* Phenacetin
* Smoking
* Analine
* Cyclophosphamide

# Urinary incontinence

osmosis.org/learn/urinary_incontinence

Urinary incontinence is a problem where the process of urination, also called micturition, happens involuntarily, meaning that a person might urinate unintentionally. Urinary incontinence is particularly problematic because it affects a person's personal hygiene as well as their social life in a way that can be very limiting (Figure 50.1).

## PHYSIOLOGY

Normally, urine is held in the bladder, which receives urine from two ureters coming down from the kidneys; urine then leaves the bladder through the urethra. As urine flows from the kidney, through the ureters, and into the bladder, the bladder starts to expand into the abdomen. The bladder can expand and contract because it's wrapped in a muscular layer called the detrusor muscle, and, within that, lining the bladder itself is a layer of transitional epithelium containing "umbrella cells." These umbrella cells get their name because they physically stretch out as the bladder fills, just like an umbrella opening up in slow-motion. In a grown adult, the bladder can expand to hold about 750 ml. The bladder holds slightly less in women than in men because the uterus takes up space and crowds out the bladder a little bit (Figure 50.2).

**Figure 50.1**

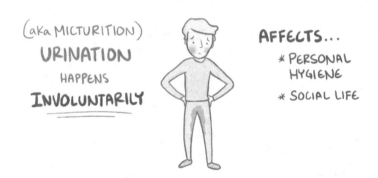

**Figure 50.2**

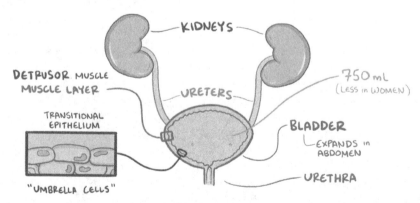

**Figure 50.3**

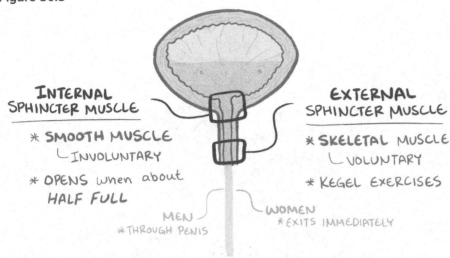

**INTERNAL**
SPHINCTER MUSCLE

* **SMOOTH MUSCLE**
  └ INVOLUNTARY

* **OPENS** when about
  **HALF FULL**

MEN
* THROUGH PENIS

WOMEN
* EXITS IMMEDIATELY

**EXTERNAL**
SPHINCTER MUSCLE

* **SKELETAL MUSCLE**
  └ VOLUNTARY

* **KEGEL EXERCISES**

**Figure 50.4**

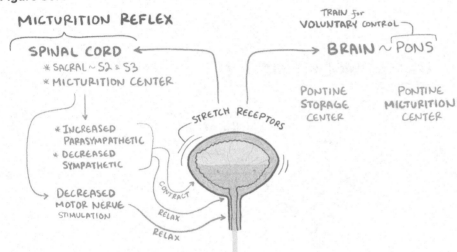

MICTURITION REFLEX

SPINAL CORD
* SACRAL ~ S2 & S3
* MICTURITION CENTER

* INCREASED
  PARASYMPATHETIC
* DECREASED
  SYMPATHETIC

DECREASED
MOTOR NERVE
STIMULATION

CONTRACT
RELAX
RELAX

STRETCH RECEPTORS

TRAIN for
VOLUNTARY CONTROL

BRAIN ~ PONS

PONTINE
STORAGE
CENTER

PONTINE
MICTURITION
CENTER

**Figure 50.5**

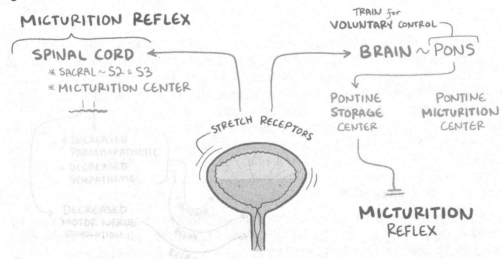

MICTURITION REFLEX

SPINAL CORD
* SACRAL ~ S2 & S3
* MICTURITION CENTER

STRETCH RECEPTORS

TRAIN for
VOLUNTARY CONTROL

BRAIN ~ PONS

PONTINE
STORAGE
CENTER

PONTINE
MICTURITION
CENTER

**MICTURITION**
REFLEX

**Figure 50.6**

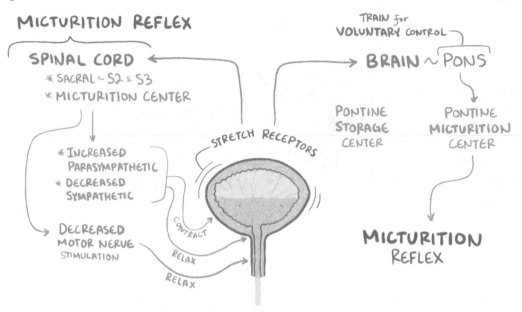

**Figure 50.7**

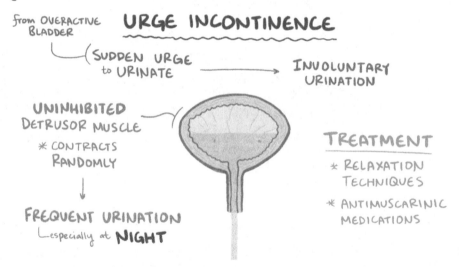

All right, so when the urine is collecting in the bladder, there are basically two "doors" that are shut, holding that urine in. The first door is the internal sphincter muscle, which is made of smooth muscle and is under involuntary control, meaning that it opens and closes automatically. Typically, that internal sphincter muscle opens up when the bladder is about half full. The second door is the external sphincter muscle, and it's made of skeletal muscle and is under voluntary control, meaning that it opens and closes when a person wants it to. This is the reason that it's possible to stop urine midstream by tightening up that muscle, which is called doing kegel exercises. Once urine has passed through the external sphincter muscle, it exits the body. In women the exit is immediate, and in men the urine flows through the penis before it exits **(Figure 50.3)**.

So, when specialized nerves called stretch receptors in the bladder wall sense that the bladder is about half full, they send impulses to the spinal cord, specifically the sacral spinal cord at levels S2 and S3, which known as the micturition center, and the brain, specifically two locations in the pons, the pontine storage center and pontine micturition center. The spinal

**Figure 50.8**

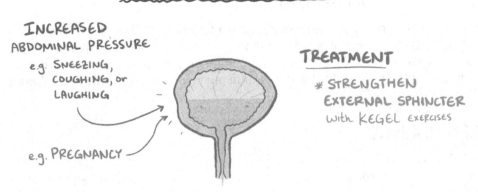

## STRESS INCONTINENCE

INCREASED
ABDOMINAL PRESSURE
   e.g. SNEEZING,
     COUGHING, or
     LAUGHING

e.g. PREGNANCY

TREATMENT
  * STRENGTHEN
   EXTERNAL SPHINCTER
   with KEGEL EXERCISES

**Figure 50.9**

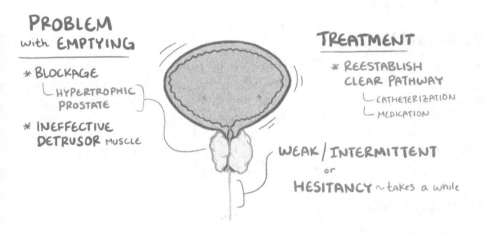

## OVERFLOW INCONTINENCE

PROBLEM
with EMPTYING

* BLOCKAGE
   └ HYPERTROPHIC
     PROSTATE

* INEFFECTIVE
  DETRUSOR muscle

TREATMENT
  * REESTABLISH
   CLEAR PATHWAY
     └ CATHETERIZATION
     └ MEDICATION

WEAK / INTERMITTENT
    or
HESITANCY ~ takes a while

**Figure 50.10**

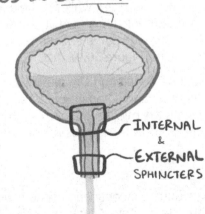

## URINARY INCONTINENCE

URINE INVOLUNTARILY LEAVES the BLADDER

URGE INCONTINENCE
  * OVERACTIVE BLADDER
STRESS INCONTINENCE
  * TOO MUCH PRESSURE
OVERFLOW INCONTINENCE
  * INCOMPLETE EMPTYING

INTERNAL
&
EXTERNAL
SPHINCTERS

cord response is part of the micturition reflex, and it causes an increase in parasympathetic stimulation and decrease in sympathetic stimulation that makes the detrusor muscle contract and the internal sphincter relax. It also decreases motor nerve stimulation to the external sphincter, allowing it to relax as well **(Figure 50.4)**.

At this point, urination would occur at this point if it wasn't for the pons. The pons is the region of the brain that we train to voluntarily control urination. If we want to delay urination, or hold it in, the pontine storage center overrides the micturition reflex, and when we want to urinate, the pontine micturition center allows for the micturition reflex to happen **(Figure 50.5; Figure 50.6)**.

## URGE INCONTINENCE

Now, there are a few types of urinary incontinence. The first is urge incontinence, which is when someone has a sudden urge to urinate because of an "overactive bladder," and that urge is followed immediately by involuntary urination. This is typically due to an uninhibited detrusor muscle that contracts randomly. This usually results in frequent urination, especially at night. To treat urge incontinence, the focus is on decreasing the detrusor muscle activity. Relaxation techniques to relax the bladder as well as antimuscarinic medications can decrease detrusor muscle contractions **(Figure 50.7)**.

## STRESS INCONTINENCE

Stress incontinence is usually due to increased abdominal pressure that overwhelms the sphincter muscles and allows urine to leak out. Think of things that cause exertion, like sneezing, coughing, laughing, or anything that puts pressure on the bladder. This is also relevant during pregnancy when a growing baby puts tremendous pressure on the bladder and causes stress incontinence in some women. The classic finding is urinary leakage with pressure applied to the abdomen. Stress incontinence treatments typically focus on strengthening the external sphincter muscle by doing things like Kegel exercises **(Figure 50.8)**.

## OVERFLOW INCONTINENCE

Another type is overflow incontinence, which is typically caused by some sort of problem with emptying the bladder. This could be due to a blockage in urine flow, like a hypertrophic prostate in men, which presses on the urethra, or an ineffective detrusor muscle. Either way, the bladder doesn't empty properly, and so the bladder fills up and overflows with urine, which then leaks through the sphincters. Typically, this results in a weak or intermittent urinary stream or hesitancy, where it takes a while for the urine to begin to flow because of a blockage in the path. Overflow treatments are aimed at reestablishing a clear pathway for urine flow. For example, that might be through catheterization or medications like alpha-blockers, which can limit prostate enlargement **(Figure 50.9)**.

Finally, there are various conditions like diabetes, bladder cancer, Parkinson's, and multiple sclerosis, as well as procedures such as prostatectomy or hysterectomy that can damage the nerves involved with the micturition reflex, ultimately leading to urinary incontinence. The symptoms and treatment for these problems depend on the exact condition.

## SUMMARY

All right, quick recap: urinary incontinence occurs when urine involuntarily leaves the bladder through the internal and external sphincter muscles. Urge incontinence is due to an overactive bladder, stress incontinence is due to too much pressure for the sphincter muscles to resist, and overflow incontinence is due to incomplete emptying of the bladder **(Figure 50.10)**.

# Vesicoureteral reflux

osmosis.org/learn/vesicoureteral_reflux

**V**esico- refers to the bladder, and *ureteral* refers to the ureter, so vesicoureteral reflux means that urine is refluxing, or getting backed up. Normally, urine flows in one direction: it starts in the kidneys, goes down into the bladder, and, when the bladder is full, urine flows out of the body through the urethra. In vesicoureteral reflux, there is some obstruction in that path which causes pressure to build up, and a current of urine actually pushes backward from the bladder into the ureters and kidneys (**Figure 51.1**).

**Figure 51.1**

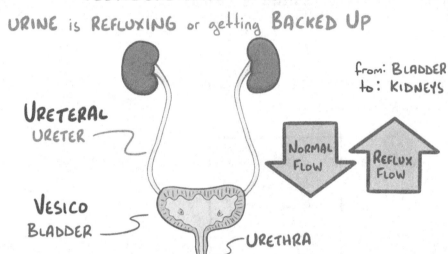

**Figure 51.2**

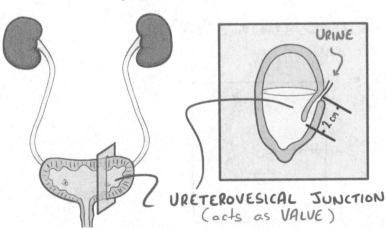

**Figure 51.3**

## PRIMARY VESICOURETERAL REFLUX (VUR)

### ( MOST COMMON )

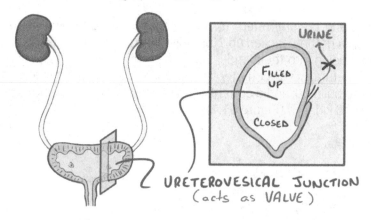

URETEROVESICAL JUNCTION
(acts as VALVE)

**Figure 51.4**

## PRIMARY VESICOURETERAL REFLUX (VUR)

### ( MOST COMMON )

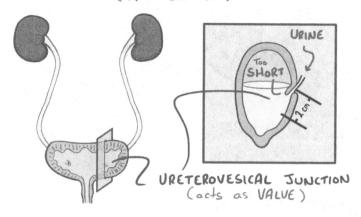

URETEROVESICAL JUNCTION
(acts as VALVE)

**Figure 51.5**

## PRIMARY VESICOURETERAL REFLUX (VUR)

### ( MOST COMMON )

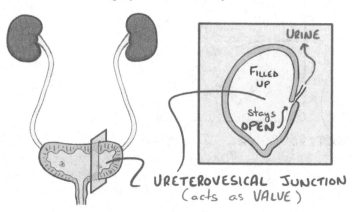

URETEROVESICAL JUNCTION
(acts as VALVE)

Figure 51.6

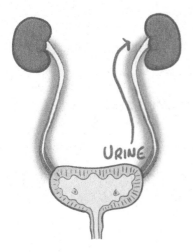

SECONDARY VESICOURETERAL REFLUX (VUR)

OBSTRUCTION ~ increase in pressure

most common
* URINARY TRACT INFECTIONS
   ↳ URETERS SWELL & CLOSE

URINE

Figure 51.7

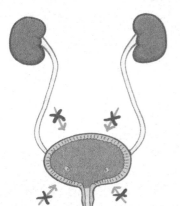

SECONDARY VESICOURETERAL REFLUX (VUR)

OBSTRUCTION ~ increase in pressure

most common
* URINARY TRACT INFECTIONS
   ↳ URETERS SWELL & CLOSE

* POSTERIOR URETHRAL VALVE DISORDER
   — DIAGNOSED in BABIES
   — MEMBRANE forms over URETHRA

* FLACCID NEUROGENIC BLADDER
   ↳ UNABLE to CONTRACT BLADDER

## PRIMARY & SECONDARY VESICOURETERAL REFLUX

There are two types of vesicoureteral reflux, or VUR. Primary vesicoureteral reflux is the most common type and happens when a child is born with a defect at the ureterovesical junction, which is the spot where the ureter enters the bladder and which also acts as a valve preventing urine from pushing back from the bladder into the ureter. Normally, about two centimeters of the ureter sticks into the bladder wall, allowing urine to flow into the bladder, but as the bladder fills up and stretches, it also stretches that section of the ureter and presses it against the top of the bladder, causing the ureter to close shut **(Figure 51.2; Figure 51.3)**.

If the tube isn't long enough though, that small piece of the ureter doesn't stretch very much, and it stays open even when the bladder fills with urine. In that situation, as the bladder pressure builds with more urine, the urine starts to go back up the ureters **(Figure 51.4; Figure 51.5)**.

**Figure 51.8**

# SECONDARY VESICOURETERAL REFLUX (VUR)

OBSTRUCTION ⟿ increase in pressure

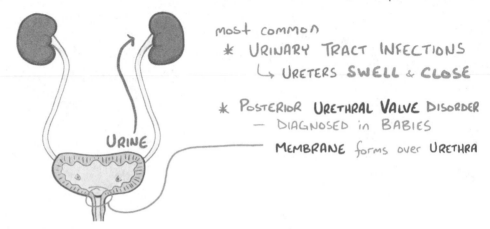

most common
* **URINARY TRACT INFECTIONS**
  ↳ URETERS **SWELL & CLOSE**

* POSTERIOR **URETHRAL VALVE** DISORDER
  — DIAGNOSED in BABIES
  — MEMBRANE forms over URETHRA

URINE

**Figure 51.9**

# GRADES of VESICOURETERAL REFLUX (VUR)
DEPEND on HOW FAR URINE BACKS UP

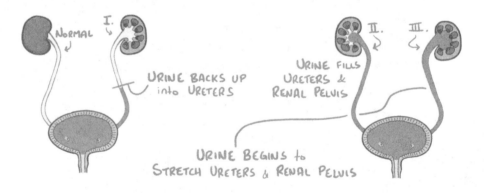

NORMAL

URINE BACKS UP
into URETERS

URINE FILLS
URETERS &
RENAL PELVIS

URINE BEGINS to
STRETCH URETERS & RENAL PELVIS

**Figure 51.10**

# GRADES of VESICOURETERAL REFLUX (VUR)
DEPEND on HOW FAR URINE BACKS UP

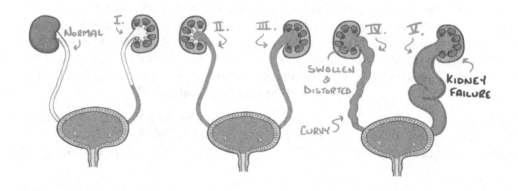

NORMAL

SWOLLEN
&
DISTORTED

CURVY S

KIDNEY
FAILURE

In secondary vesicoureteral reflux, there's an obstruction at some point in the urinary tract that causes an increase in pressure, causing urine to follow the path of least resistance, which often means flowing backward into the ureters or kidneys. Secondary vesicoureteral reflux is most commonly caused by recurrent urinary tract infections, which can cause inflammation in the ureters, making them swell up and close **(Figure 51.6)**.

Another cause that is often diagnosed in babies is called posterior urethral valve disorder, which is when an abnormal membrane develops in the posterior part of the urethra, or the part closest to the bladder, and prevents urine from easily passing from the bladder into the urethra **(Figure 51.7; 51.8)**.

Yet another cause is a flaccid neurogenic bladder, when the bladder is unable to contract to release urine out of the body even when a person is consciously trying to release the urine. This most often results from trauma, disease, or injury to the nervous system.

## CLASSIFICATIONS

Vesicoureteral reflux is usually classified by severity and graded from one through five, depending on how far urine refluxes back up into the urinary tract. Grade I is least severe, and urine only goes up into the ureters. In Grade II, urine fills the entire ureter and the renal pelvis, the center part of the kidney. In Grade III, urine fills and begins to stretch both the ureter and the renal pelvis **(Figure 51.9)**.

In Grade IV, the ureter is so swollen that it begins to get curvy and the renal pelvis and calyces, which are the urine collection ducts, become moderately swollen and distorted. Finally, in Grade V, the most severe classification, urine fills up the ureter, pelvis, and calyces, causing them swell up completely, and this amount of pressure can lead to kidney failure **(Figure 51.10)**.

## SYMPTOMS

Individuals with milder cases show no symptoms. But in severe cases, urine lingers in the urinary tract for so long that there is little flow through the urethra, which allows bacteria to move up the urethra and cause an infection. Chronic vesicoureteral reflux can cause pyelonephritis, or inflammation of the kidney, and renal scarring, or fibrosis, which damages the kidney tissue. The damage can also reduce blood flow to the kidneys, and they can respond by holding on to more fluid to raise the blood pressure, which can ultimately result in hypertension.

## DIAGNOSIS

Vesicoureteral reflux can be diagnosed with an abdominal ultrasound, which can detect blockages in flow of urine and swelling in the ureters or kidneys. Another test, called a voiding cystourethrogram or a VCUG, can show how urine moves through the ureterovesical junction. In a voiding cystourethrogram, a contrast dye is injected into the bladder through a catheter, and X-ray images are taken to see if the dye moves from the bladder up into the ureters and kidneys **(Figure 51.13)**.

A radionuclide cystogram uses a similar procedure as the VCUG, except that it uses a radioactive tracer injected into a blood vessel. The scanner then detects the tracer as it moves from the blood into the kidney and then down through the ureters and into the bladder.

**Figure 51.11**

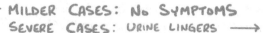
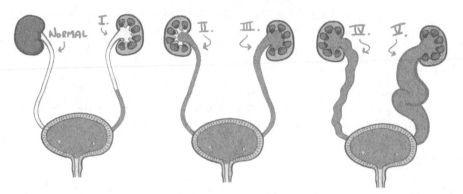

SYMPTOMS

←———————  MILDER CASES: No SYMPTOMS
SEVERE CASES: URINE LINGERS ———→

NORMAL   I.   II.   III.   IV.   V.

**Figure 51.12**

SYMPTOMS

MILDER CASES: No SYMPTOMS
SEVERE CASES: URINE LINGERS
    ↳ causing INFECTION
    ↳ PYELONEPHRITIS
      (INFLAMMATION of KIDNEYS)
      ↳ RENAL SCARRING
         ↓
REDUCES BLOOD FLOW to KIDNEYS
         ↓
INCREASES BLOOD PRESSURE
         ↓
   HYPERTENSION

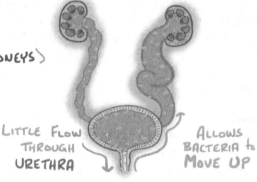

LITTLE FLOW THROUGH URETHRA

ALLOWS BACTERIA to MOVE UP

**Figure 51.13**

DIAGNOSIS

* ABDOMINAL ULTRASOUND
    └ DETECTS BLOCKAGES & SWELLING

* VOIDING CYSTOURETHROGRAM (VCUG)
    └ SHOWS HOW URINE MOVES THROUGH
      the URETEROVESICAL JUNCTION

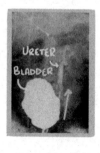

URETER
BLADDER

# TREATMENT

Treatment depends on severity and age because VUR mostly affects young infants and children. As a child grows, the ureter gets longer and the function of the valve improves, so primary vesicoureteral reflux sometimes improves or disappears over time. Some individuals might also need surgery to remove a blockage or to repair the valve at the ureterovesical junction.

# SUMMARY

All right, as a quick recap: vesicoureteral reflux is a condition where pressure in the urinary outflow tract increases and urine gets pushed back up into the ureters or kidneys. Primary vesicoureteral reflux is usually due to a short ureter, while secondary vesicoureteral reflux is usually due to a blockage in the urinary tract. The disease often leads to urinary tract infections that can cause renal inflammation and scarring **(Figure 51.14)**.

**Figure 51.14**

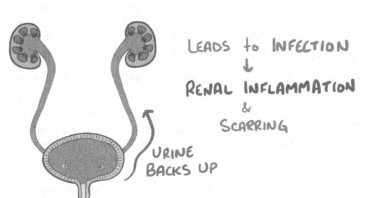

# WAGR syndrome

**W**AGR syndrome stands for Wilms' tumor, aniridia, genitourinary anomalies, and mental retardation, which is now called intellectual disability. WAGR is a genetic disorder that's caused when a part of chromosome 11 is missing or deleted. Not everyone with WAGR has all of the symptoms; for example, only about half of these individuals have Wilms' tumor. On the flip side, some have additional symptoms, too, like progressive kidney failure, growth retardation, small head size, and obesity **(Figure 52.1)**.

## SYMPTOMS

The most specific feature of WAGR syndrome is aniridia, which is the complete or partial absence of the iris, the colored part of the eye. This is an easily noticeable feature and it's present at birth, so it's usually the first thing to raise suspicion of WAGR syndrome. Now, a normal iris controls how much light enters the eye, and it constricts the pupil when there's a lot of light around to keep the vision sharp **(Figure 52.2)**. With aniridia, too much light gets into the eye, which leads to blurry vision and photophobia, which is discomfort when the eyes are exposed to light. Additional eye features in WAGR syndrome can include cataracts, which is a clouded lens, glaucoma, or increased pressure in the eye, and nystagmus, which is abnormal rhythmic eye movement **(Figure 52.3)**.

Wilms' tumor, also called nephroblastoma, is generally a malignant kidney tumor that affects children. Wilms' tumors are composed of metanephric blastema, which is a cell type that's seen in the developing kidney, stromal cells which are part of the connective tissue, and epithelial cells, which self-organize into primitive glomeruli and tubules. Children with Wilms' tumor often develop a large flank mass, as well as hematuria, which is blood in the urine, and hypertension **(Figure 52.4)**.

Now, that hypertension is a result of increased renin secretion, and this either comes from the tumor itself or from healthy kidney tissue that secretes renin because it's physically compressed by the tumor **(Figure 52.5)**.

It's worth noting that Wilms' tumor isn't specific for WAGR syndrome; in fact, it most commonly happens in otherwise-healthy children, and can be a part of other syndromes like Beckwith-Wiedemann syndrome. Fortunately, Wilms' tumor is also treatable and has a fairly high cure rate when it's treated with a combination of chemotherapy, radiation, and nephrectomy, which is removal of the kidney **(Figure 52.6)**.

The most common genital defect in boys with WAGR syndrome is undescended testes, also called cryptorchidism, as well as hypospadias, where the urethra exits the penis on the underside instead of at the tip. The most common genital defect in girls is streak ovaries, which are undeveloped and nonfunctional ovaries that are at an increased risk for developing a tumor called gonadoblastoma. Finally, someone with WAGR syndrome might have ambiguous genitalia, meaning they don't appear to be either clearly male or clearly female **(Figure 52.7)**.

Finally, intellectual disability is present in many but not all people with WAGR syndrome, and WAGR syndrome is also associated with conditions like autism or ADHD, all of which are usually recognized in childhood.

**Figure 52.1**

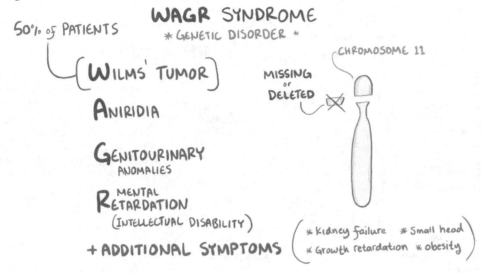

WAGR SYNDROME
* GENETIC DISORDER *

50% of PATIENTS

(WILMS' TUMOR)

ANIRIDIA

GENITOURINARY ANOMALIES

MENTAL RETARDATION (INTELLECTUAL DISABILITY)

+ ADDITIONAL SYMPTOMS

CHROMOSOME 11

MISSING or DELETED

( * Kidney failure   * Small head
  * Growth retardation   * obesity )

**Figure 52.2**

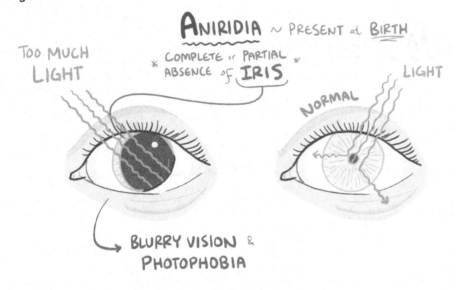

ANIRIDIA ~ PRESENT at BIRTH
* COMPLETE or PARTIAL ABSENCE of IRIS *

TOO MUCH LIGHT

NORMAL

LIGHT

→ BLURRY VISION & PHOTOPHOBIA

**Figure 52.3**

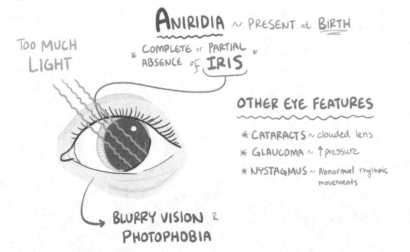

ANIRIDIA ~ PRESENT at BIRTH
* COMPLETE or PARTIAL ABSENCE of IRIS *

TOO MUCH LIGHT

OTHER EYE FEATURES
* CATARACTS ~ clouded lens
* GLAUCOMA ~ ↑ pressure
* NYSTAGMUS ~ Abnormal rhythmic movements

→ BLURRY VISION & PHOTOPHOBIA

**Figure 52.4**

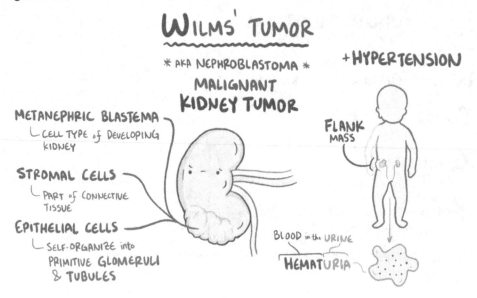

# WILMS' TUMOR
* AKA NEPHROBLASTOMA *
### MALIGNANT KIDNEY TUMOR

+ HYPERTENSION

METANEPHRIC BLASTEMA
└ CELL TYPE of DEVELOPING KIDNEY

STROMAL CELLS
└ PART of CONNECTIVE TISSUE

EPITHELIAL CELLS
└ SELF-ORGANIZE into PRIMITIVE GLOMERULI & TUBULES

FLANK MASS

BLOOD in the URINE
HEMATURIA

**Figure 52.5**

# WILMS' TUMOR

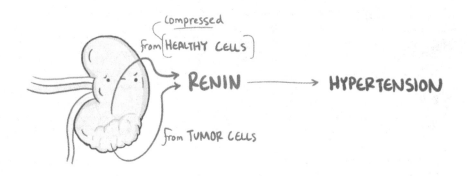

compressed
from HEALTHY CELLS
→ RENIN ——→ HYPERTENSION
from TUMOR CELLS

**Figure 52.6**

# WILMS' TUMOR

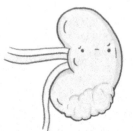

* NOT SPECIFIC for WAGR

* HAPPENS in...
└ OTHERWISE HEALTHY CHILDREN
└ OTHER SYNDROMES
(e.g. BECKWITH-WIEDEMANN SYNDROME)

## TREATMENT

* COMBINATION of CHEMOTHERAPY, RADIATION, & NEPHRECTOMY

# CAUSES

Now, WAGR is a great example of a contiguous gene deletion syndrome. Contiguous means next to each other, so it's caused when two or more genes that are next to each other, along the same chromosome arm are deleted at the same time. In the case of WAGR syndrome, it's a heterozygous deletion of a small part of the short, or p arm, of chromosome 11. There are two particularly important genes within the deleted region: the *PAX6* gene which causes the aniridia, and the *WT1* gene (or the "Wilms' tumor 1" gene) which causes the increased risk of Wilms' tumor as well as the genitourinary abnormalities. If deleting or disrupting a gene results in an increased tumor risk, then it's considered a tumor suppressor gene, so WT1 is an example of a tumor suppressor gene. Finally, the specific gene responsible for intellectual disability in WAGR syndrome is not known. Sometimes, that deletion is also extra large, and includes the gene *BDNF* (which is named for "brain-derived neurotrophic factor"). Deletion of BDNF causes the obesity seen in some patients with WAGR syndrome. This is a phenotype called WAGRO, where 'O' is for obesity. WAGR syndrome is technically autosomal dominant, but it's usually sporadic, meaning that it's caused by a new mutation, rather than being inherited **(Figure 52.8)**.

# DIAGNOSIS

Diagnosis of WAGR syndrome is confirmed using FISH, or fluorescence *in situ* hybridization. This involves a fluorescently labeled probe made of DNA that's complementary to the WAGR region. In a normal cell, the probes can base-pair to both chromosome 11s, so you would expect two bright spots are seen in the microscope when the cell is viewed under fluorescent light. If a WAGR deletion is present, though, one of those WAGR regions is missing, so you'll only a single bright spot **(Figure 52.9)**.

# TREATMENT

There's no single treatment for WAGR syndrome; rather, each problem is addressed individually. For example, for photophobia you might use tinted lenses, or for Wilms' tumor you might use chemotherapy. The most important thing is to have a timely diagnosis of WAGR so that there's adequate medical surveillance, like regular renal ultrasounds and blood pressure checks to look for Wilms' tumor, as well as pelvic ultrasound in women to look for streak ovaries and the subsequent possibility of gonadoblastoma.

**Figure 52.7**

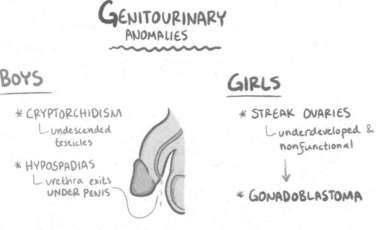

GENITOURINARY ANOMALIES

BOYS
* CRYPTORCHIDISM
  └ undescended testicles
* HYPOSPADIAS
  └ urethra exits UNDER PENIS

GIRLS
* STREAK OVARIES
  └ underdeveloped & nonfunctional
  ↓
* GONADOBLASTOMA

* AMBIGUOUS GENITALIA *

**Figure 52.8**

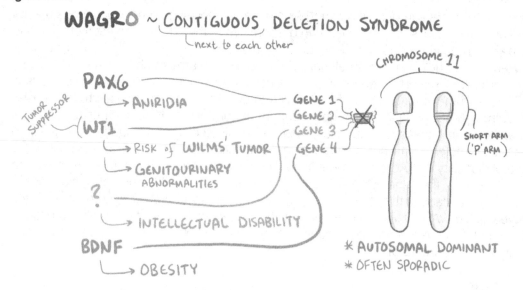

WAGR ~ CONTIGUOUS DELETION SYNDROME
↳ next to each other

PAX6 ——→ ANIRIDIA

TUMOR SUPPRESSOR

(WT1
↳ RISK of WILMS' TUMOR
↳ GENITOURINARY ABNORMALITIES

? ↳ INTELLECTUAL DISABILITY

BDNF
↳ OBESITY

GENE 1
GENE 2
GENE 3
GENE 4

CHROMOSOME 11

SHORT ARM ('P' ARM)

* AUTOSOMAL DOMINANT
* OFTEN SPORADIC

**Figure 52.9**

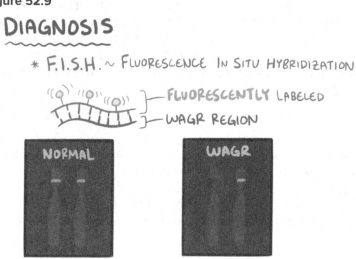

DIAGNOSIS

* F.I.S.H. ~ FLUORESCENCE IN SITU HYBRIDIZATION

— FLUORESCENTLY LABELED
— WAGR REGION

NORMAL          WAGR

## SUMMARY

All right, as a quick recap: WAGR syndrome is a contiguous gene deletion syndrome caused by a deletion of several genes on chromosome 11, including *PAX6* and *WT1*. The result is a risk for Wilms' tumor, aniridia, genitourinary abnormalities, and intellectual disability.

# Wilms' tumor

Wilms' tumor, or nephroblastoma, is a type of kidney tumor composed of metanephric blastemal cells, which are the cells involved in kidney development. It's the most common malignant kidney tumor in children; only rarely is it seen in adults (**Figure 53.1**).

## CAUSES

Wilms' tumor is thought to be caused by mutations in the genes responsible for normal genitourinary development, which includes the kidneys as well as the gonads (**Figure 53.2**). Typically, the genes are located around 11p13, which means chromosome 11, the short arm p, region 1, band 3. One gene critical for normal kidney and gonad development is WT1 (or Wilms' Tumor 1), which is a tumor suppressor gene. Mutations that result in a loss of function of WT1, like deletions, for example, seem to lead to the development of the tumor cells seen with Wilms' tumor (**Figure 53.3**).

**Figure 53.1**

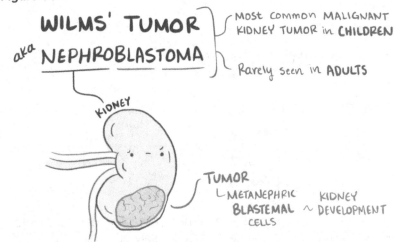

**Figure 53.2**

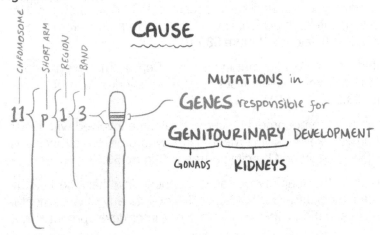

**Figure 53.3**

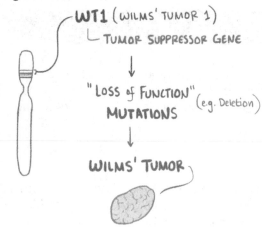

WT1 (WILMS' TUMOR 1)
└ TUMOR SUPPRESSOR GENE

↓

"LOSS of FUNCTION" (e.g. Deletion)
MUTATIONS

↓

WILMS' TUMOR

**Figure 53.4**

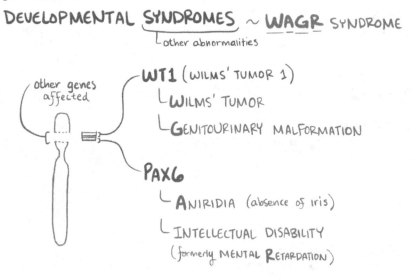

DEVELOPMENTAL SYNDROMES ~ WAGR SYNDROME
└ other abnormalities

other genes affected

WT1 (WILMS' TUMOR 1)
└ WILMS' TUMOR
└ GENITOURINARY MALFORMATION

PAX6
└ ANIRIDIA (absence of iris)
└ INTELLECTUAL DISABILITY
(formerly MENTAL RETARDATION)

Wilms' tumors as a result of WT1 mutations are sometimes part of a developmental syndrome, meaning that other abnormalities are present as well, likely because of deletion or mutation of other genes in addition to WT1. For example, in WAGR syndrome, a mutation in the 11p13 region causes deletion of both WT1 and the PAX6 genes, among others, which leads to **W**ilms' tumor and **G**enitourinary malformations as a result of WT1 deletion, as well as **A**niridia (which is absence of iris) and intellectual disability (which was formerly referred to as mental **R**etardation), as a result of PAX6 deletion **(Figure 53.4)**.

Another syndrome associated with WT1 mutations is Denys-Drash syndrome, which is characterized by Wilms tumor, early-onset nephrotic syndrome, and male pseudohermaphroditism **(Figure 53.5)**.

Another gene, WT2, also located on chromosome 11, seems to also be involved with other Wilms' tumor-containing syndromes, like Beckwith-Wiedemann syndrome, which includes Wilms' tumor, macroglossia, organomegaly, and hemihypertrophy **(Figure 53.6)**.

All that being said, Wilms' tumor, in the majority of cases, happens in otherwise healthy children, and doesn't seem to be associated with WT1 or WT2, or with any developmental syndrome of any kind. So in those situations, the mechanism of tumor development is not well understood.

**Figure 53.5**

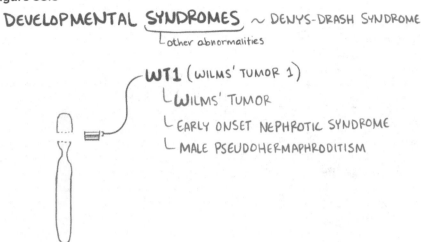

DEVELOPMENTAL SYNDROMES ~ DENYS-DRASH SYNDROME
└ other abnormalities

WT1 (WILMS' TUMOR 1)
└ WILMS' TUMOR
└ EARLY ONSET NEPHROTIC SYNDROME
└ MALE PSEUDOHERMAPHRODITISM

**Figure 53.6**

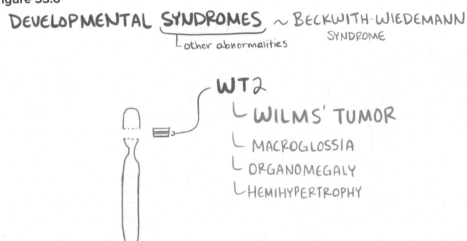

DEVELOPMENTAL SYNDROMES ~ BECKWITH-WIEDEMANN
└ other abnormalities            SYNDROME

WT2
└ WILMS' TUMOR
└ MACROGLOSSIA
└ ORGANOMEGALY
└ HEMIHYPERTROPHY

Regardless of what the exact cause of the tumors are, they're usually composed partly of metanephric blastemal cells, which are cells that give rise to other cells like stromal cells, which are the connective tissue cells, as well as epithelial cells, all of which normally help give rise to structures in the kidney. That being said, in this mass there are usually abortive or partly-developed structures of the nephron, like glomeruli and tubules. A tumor composed of blastemal, stromal, and epithelial cells is called a triphasic blastoma **(Figure 53.7)**.

## SYMPTOMS

Children with Wilms' tumor often present with a flank mass that's large, palpable, and unilateral, and they also sometimes have hematuria, or blood in the urine, as well as hypertension as a result of renin secretion **(Figure 53.8)**.

## TREATMENT

Treatment depends on the extent of spreading of Wilms' tumor, although the overall prognosis is very good, and people with Wilms' tumor often respond well to a combination of nephrectomy, or removal of the kidney, and chemotherapy.

**Figure 53.7**

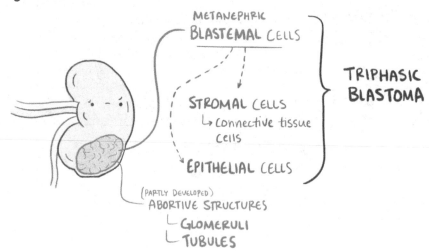

METANEPHRIC
BLASTEMAL CELLS

STROMAL CELLS
→ Connective tissue
cells

EPITHELIAL CELLS

} TRIPHASIC
BLASTOMA

(PARTLY DEVELOPED)
ABORTIVE STRUCTURES
└ GLOMERULI
└ TUBULES

**Figure 53.8**

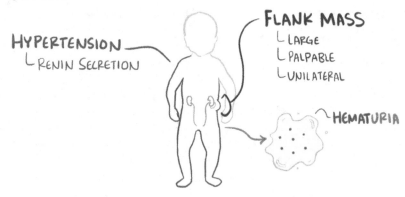

HYPERTENSION
└ RENIN SECRETION

FLANK MASS
└ LARGE
└ PALPABLE
└ UNILATERAL

HEMATURIA

**Figure 53.9**

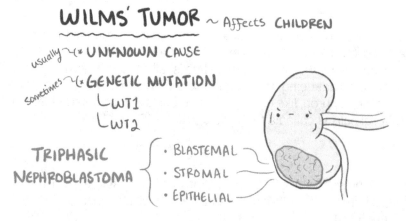

WILMS' TUMOR ~ Affects CHILDREN

usually (* UNKNOWN CAUSE

sometimes (* GENETIC MUTATION
└ WT1
└ WT2

TRIPHASIC
NEPHROBLASTOMA {
• BLASTEMAL
• STROMAL
• EPITHELIAL

## SUMMARY

All right, as a quick recap: Wilms' tumors typically affect children, and usually the cause is unknown, though sometimes it can be caused by gene mutations, specifically WT1 and WT2. The tumor mass, or "triphasic nephroblastoma," is composed of blastema cells, stromal cells, and epithelial cells **(Figure 53.9)**.

# CREDITS

## ACUTE PYELONEPHRITIS

Author: Tanner Marshall, MS

Editor: Rishi Desai, MD, MPH

Illustrator: Tanner Marshall, MS

## ALPORT SYNDROME

Authors: Philip M. Boone, MD, PhD; Thomas M. Schmid, PhD

Editors: Rishi Desai, MD, MPH; Tanner Marshall, MS

Illustrator: Tanner Marshall, MS

## ANGIOMYOLIPOMA

Author: Vincent Waldman, PhD

Editor: Rishi Desai, MD, MPH

Illustrator: Vincent Waldman, PhD

## BLADDER EXSTROPHY

Author: Amanda J. Grieco, PhD

Editor: Rishi Desai, MD, MPH

Illustrator: Tanner Marshall, MS

## CHRONIC KIDNEY DISEASE

Author: Debal Sinharoy, MBBS

Editor: Rishi Desai, MD, MPH

Illustrator: Tanner Marshall, MS

## CHRONIC PYELONEPHRITIS

Author: Tanner Marshall, MS

Editors: Andrea Day, MA; Rishi Desai, MD, MPH

Illustrator: Tanner Marshall, MS

## CYSTITIS (LOWER URINARY TRACT INFECTION)

Author: Tanner Marshall, MS

Editors: Andrea Day, MA; Rishi Desai, MD, MPH; Kyle Slinn, RN, MEd

Illustrator: Tanner Marshall, MS

## DIABETIC NEPHROPATHY

Author: Christa Morris, BA

Editors: Andrea Day, MA; Rishi Desai, MD, MPH

Illustrator: Tanner Marshall, MS

## FOCAL SEGMENTAL GLOMERULOSCLEROSIS

Author: Tanner Marshall, MS

Editors: Andrea Day, MA; Rishi Desai, MD, MPH

Illustrator: Tanner Marshall, MS

## GOODPASTURE SYNDROME

Author: Debal Sinharoy, MBBS

Editors: Andrea Day, MA; Rishi Desai, MD, MPH

Illustrator: Vincent Waldman, PhD

## HEMOLYTIC-UREMIC SYNDROME

Author: Debal Sinharoy, MBBS

Editors: Andrea Day, MA; Rishi Desai, MD, MPH

Illustrator: Vincent Waldman, PhD

## HORSESHOE KIDNEY

Author: Tanner Marshall, MS

Editors: Andrea Day, MA; Rishi Desai, MD, MPH

Illustrator: Tanner Marshall, MS

## HYDRONEPHROSIS

Author:  Maria Fernanda Villarreal, MD

Editors: Andrea Day, MA; Rishi Desai, MD, MPH; Kyle Slinn, RN, MEd

Illustrator: Tanner Marshall, MS

## HYPERCALCEMIA

Author: Maria Fernanda Villarreal, MD

Editors: Andrea Day, MA; Rishi Desai, MD, MPH

Illustrator: Tanner Marshall, MS

## HYPERKALEMIA

Author: Tanner Marshall, MS

Editors: Andrea Day, MA; Rishi Desai, MD, MPH

Illustrator: Tanner Marshall, MS

## HYPERMAGNESEMIA

Author: Debal Sinharoy, MBBS

Editors: Andrea Day, MA; Rishi Desai, MD, MPH

Illustrator: Tanner Marshall, MS

## HYPERNATREMIA

Author: Debal Sinharoy, MBBS

Editors: Andrea Day, MA; Rishi Desai, MD, MPH

Illustrator: Tanner Marshall, MS

## HYPERPHOSPHATEMIA

Author: Charles B. Davis, BS

Editors: Andrea Day, MA; Rishi Desai, MD, MPH

Illustrator: Tanner Marshall, MS

## HYPOCALCEMIA

Author: Maria Fernanda Villarreal, MD

Editors: Andrea Day, MA; Rishi Desai, MD, MPH

Illustrator: Tanner Marshall, MS

## HYPOKALEMIA

Author: Tanner Marshall, MS

Editors: Andrea Day, MA; Rishi Desai, MD, MPH

Illustrator: Tanner Marshall, MS

## HYPOMAGNESEMIA

Author: Debal Sinharoy, MBBS

Editors: Andrea Day, MA; Rishi Desai, MD, MPH

Illustrator: Tanner Marshall, MS

## HYPONATREMIA

Authors: Tanner Marshall, MS; Maria Fernanda Villarreal, MD

Editors: Andrea Day, MA; Rishi Desai, MD, MPH

Illustrator: Tanner Marshall, MS

## HYPOPHOSPHATEMIA

Author: Charles B. Davis, BS

Editors: Andrea Day, MA; Rishi Desai, MD, MPH

Illustrator: Tanner Marshall, MS

## HYPOSPADIAS & EPISPADIAS

Author: Maria Fernanda Villarreal, MD

Editors: Andrea Day, MA; Rishi Desai, MD, MPH; Kyle Slinn, RN, MEd

Illustrator: Tanner Marshall, MS

## IGA NEPHROPATHY (BERGER DISEASE)

Authors: Tanner Marshall, MS; Maureen H. Richards, PhD

Editors: Andrea Day, MA; Rishi Desai, MD, MPH

Illustrator: Tanner Marshall, MS

## INTRARENAL ACUTE KIDNEY INJURY

Author: Tanner Marshall, MS; Thomas R. Shannon, DVM, PhD

Editors: Andrea Day, MA; Rishi Desai, MD, MPH

Illustrator: Tanner Marshall, MS

## LUPUS NEPHRITIS

Author: Debal Sinharoy, MBBS

Editors: Andrea Day, MA; Rishi Desai, MD, MPH

Illustrator: Vincent Waldman, PhD

## MEDULLARY SPONGE KIDNEY

Author: Amanda J. Grieco, PhD

Editors: Andrea Day, MA; Rishi Desai, MD, MPH

Illustrator: Tanner Marshall, MS

## MEMBRANOPROLIFERATIVE GLOMERULONEPHRITIS

Author: Tanner Marshall, MS

Editors: Andrea Day, MA; Rishi Desai, MD, MPH

Illustrator: Tanner Marshall, MS

## MEMBRANOUS GLOMERULONEPHRITIS (MEMBRANOUS NEPHROPATHY)

Author: Tanner Marshall, MS

Editors: Andrea Day, MA; Rishi Desai, MD, MPH

Illustrator: Tanner Marshall, MS

## MINIMAL CHANGE DISEASE

Author: Tanner Marshall, MS

Editors: Andrea Day, MA; Rishi Desai, MD, MPH

Illustrator: Tanner Marshall, MS

## MULTICYSTIC DYSPLASTIC KIDNEY

Author: Tanner Marshall, MS

Editors: Andrea Day, MA; Rishi Desai, MD, MPH

Illustrator: Tanner Marshall, MS

## NEPHROLITHIASIS (KIDNEY STONES)

Author: Tanner Marshall, MS

Editors: Andrea Day, MA; Rishi Desai, MD, MPH

Illustrator: Tanner Marshall, MS

## NEPHRONOPHTHISIS & MEDULLARY CYSTIC KIDNEY DISEASE

Authors: Philip M. Boone, MD, PhD; Thomas R. Shannon, DVM, PhD

Editors: Andrea Day, MA; Rishi Desai, MD, MPH; Tanner Marshall, MS; Kyle Slinn, RN, MEd

Illustrator: Tanner Marshall, MS

## NEUROGENIC BLADDER

Author: Debal Sinharoy, MBBS

Editors: Andrea Day, MA; Rishi Desai, MD, MPH

Illustrator: Tanner Marshall, MS

## NON-UROTHELIAL BLADDER CANCERS

Author: Vincent Waldman, PhD

Editors: Andrea Day, MA; Rishi Desai, MD, MPH

Illustrator: Vincent Waldman, PhD

## POLYCYSTIC KIDNEY DISEASE

Authors: Philip M. Boone, MD, PhD; Thomas R. Shannon, DVM, PhD

Editors: Andrea Day, MA; Rishi Desai, MD, MPH; Tanner Marshall, MS

Illustrator: Tanner Marshall, MS

## POSTERIOR URETHRAL VALVE

Author: Tanner Marshall, MS

Editors: Andrea Day, MA; Rishi Desai, MD, MPH

Illustrator: Tanner Marshall, MS

## POSTRENAL ACUTE KIDNEY INJURY

Author: Rishi Desai, MD, MPH; Tanner Marshall, MS; Thomas Shannon, PhD

Editor: Andrea Day, MA

Illustrator: Tanner Marshall, MS

## POSTSTREPTOCOCCAL GLOMERULONEPHRITIS

Author: Tanner Marshall, MS

Editors: Andrea Day, MA; Rishi Desai, MD, MPH

Illustrator: Tanner Marshall, MS

## POTTER SEQUENCE

Author: Maria Fernanda Villareal, MD

Editors: Rishi Desai, MD, MPH; Kyle Slinn, RN, MEd

Illustrator: Tanner Marshall

## PRERENAL ACUTE KIDNEY INJURY

Authors: Rishi Desai, MD, MPH; Tanner Marshall, MS; Thomas R. Shannon, PhD

Editor: Andrea Day, MA

Illustrator: Tanner Marshall, MS

## RAPIDLY PROGRESSIVE GLOMERULONEPHRITIS

Author: Tanner Marshall, MS

Editors: Andrea Day, MA; Rishi Desai, MD, MPH; Kyle Slinn, RN, MEd

Illustrator: Tanner Marshall, MS

## RENAL AGENESIS

Author: Tanner Marshall, MS

Editors: Andrea Day, MA; Rishi Desai, MD, MPH

Illustrator: Tanner Marshall, MS

## RENAL ARTERY STENOSIS

Author: Charles B. Davis, BS

Editors: Andrea Day, MA; Rishi Desai, MD, MPH; Kyle Slinn, RN, MEd

Illustrator: Tanner Marshall, MS

## RENAL CELL CARCINOMAS

Author: Vincent Waldman, PhD

Editors: Andrea Day, MA; Rishi Desai, MD, MPH

Illustrator: Vincent Waldman, PhD

## RENAL CORTICAL NECROSIS

Author: Maria Fernanda Villarreal, MD

Editors: Andrea Day, MA; Rishi Desai, MD, MPH; Kyle Slinn, RN, MEd

Illustrator: Vincent Waldman, PhD

## RENAL TUBULAR ACIDOSIS

Author: Armando Hasudungan Faigl, BBiomedSc; Maria Fernanda Villarreal, MD

Editors: Andrea Day, MA; Rishi Desai, MD, MPH

Illustrator: Tanner Marshall, MS

## TRANSITIONAL CELL CARCINOMA

Author: Vincent Waldman, PhD

Editors: Andrea Day, MA; Rishi Desai, MD, MPH

Illustrator: Vincent Waldman, PhD

## URINARY INCONTINENCE

Author: Amanda J. Grieco, PhD

Editors: Andrea Day, MA; Rishi Desai, MD, MPH ; Vanita Gaglani, RPT

Illustrator: Tanner Marshall, MS

## VESICOURETERAL REFLUX

Author: Kaityln Harper, MA

Editors: Andrea Day, MA; Rishi Desai, MD, MPH

Illustrator: Vincent Waldman, PhD

## WAGR SYNDROME

Author: Philip M. Boone, MD, PhD

Editors: Andrea Day, MA; Rishi Desai, MD, MPH

Illustrator: Tanner Marshall, MS

**WILMS' TUMOR**

Author: Tanner Marshall, MS

Editors: Andrea Day, MA; Rishi Desai, MD, MPH; Kyle
Slinn, RN, MEd

Illustrator: Tanner Marshall, MS

# SOURCES

## ACUTE PYELONEPHRITIS

Fulop, T. *Acute Pyelonephritis: Practice Essentials, Background, Pathophysiology*. (2017). Retrieved July 28, 2017, from http://emedicine.medscape.com/article/245559-overview?pa=nhLpim80rE8dJNcnqp5krrnogiB4SoAl08gtEirrud50o0W%2Fsdxcl7185DWslt9SlTmkNTBMRnk1C0LdM%2FykynBa6qMPn9v9%2B17kWmU%2BiQA%3D#a3

Kumar, V., Abbas A.K., & Aster, J.C. (2015). *Robbins & Cotran Pathologic Basis of Disease* (9 edition). Philadelphia, PA: Elsevier.

Le, T., Bhushan, V., Sochat, M., & Chavda, Y. (2017). *First Aid for the USMLE Step 1 2017* (27 edition). New York, NY: McGraw-Hill Education / Medical.

Pyelonephritis. (n.d.). In *Wikipedia*. Retrieved July 26, 2017, from https://en.wikipedia.org/wiki/Pyelonephritis

Vesicoureteral reflux. (n.d.). In *Wikipedia*. Retrieved July 21, 2017, from https://en.wikipedia.org/w/index.php?title=Vesicoureteral_reflux&oldid=791560840

Sattar, H.A. (2017). *Fundamentals of Pathology: Medical Course and Step 1 Review* (2017). USA: Pathoma LLC.

## ALPORT SYNDROME

Alport syndrome. (2017, July 28). In *National Center for Biotechnology Information (US)*. Retrieved from https://www.ncbi.nlm.nih.gov/books/NBK22265/

Kashtan, C.E. Alport syndrome and thin basement membrane nephropathy. *GeneReviews* (n.d.). Retrieved July 28, 2017, from https://www.ncbi.nlm.nih.gov/books/NBK1207/

Savige, J. (2014). Alport syndrome: its effects on the glomerular filtration barrier and implications for future treatment. *The Journal of Physiology, 592*(18), 4013–4023. Retrieved July 31, 2017, from https://doi.org/10.1113/jphysiol.2014.274449

## ANGIOMYOLIPOMA

Angiomyolipoma. (n.d.). In *Wikipedia*. Retrieved July 16, 2017, from https://en.wikipedia.org/wiki/Angiomyolipoma

Franz, D. N. (2015). Tuberous sclerosis clinical presentation. In *Medscape*. Retrieved July 18, 2017, from http://emedicine.medscape.com/article/1177711-clinical#b4

Hamartoma. (2017, July 16). In *Wikipedia*. Retrieved from https://en.wikipedia.org/wiki/Hamartoma

Khan, A. N. (2016). Kidney angiomyolipoma imaging. (2017, July 28). In *Medscape*. Retrieved July 28 ,2017, from http://emedicine.medscape.com/article/376848-overview

Le, T., Bhushan, V., Sochat, M., & Chavda, Y. (2017). *First Aid for the USMLE Step 1 2017* (27 edition). New York, NY: McGraw-Hill Education / Medical.

TSC1. (2017, July 16). In *Wikipedia*. Retrieved from https://en.wikipedia.org/wiki/TSC1

TSC2. (2017, July 16). In *Wikipedia*. Retrieved from https://en.wikipedia.org/wiki/TSC2

Tuberous sclerous protein. (2017, July 16). In *Wikipedia*. Retreived from https://en.wikipedia.org/wiki/Tuberous_sclerosis_protein

Sattar, H.A. (2017). *Fundamentals of Pathology: Medical Course and Step 1 Review* (2017). USA: Pathoma LLC.

## BLADDER EXSTROPHY

Borer, J. G. (2017). Clinical manifestations and intial management of infants with bladder exstrophy. In *UpToDate*. Retrieved August 1, 2017, from https://www.uptodate.com/contents/clinical-manifestations-and-initial-management-of-infants-with-bladder-exstrophy?source=search_result&search=bladder%20exstrophy&selectedTitle=1~23

Grady, R. & Mitchell, M. E. (2015). Chapter 58: bladder and cloacal exstrophy. (July 28 2017). In *Clinical Gate*. Retrieved from https://clinicalgate.com/bladder-and-cloacal-exstrophy/

Kumar, V., Abbas A.K., & Aster, J.C. (2015). *Robbins & Cotran Pathologic Basis of Disease* (9 edition). Philadelphia, PA: Elsevier.

Le, T., Bhushan, V., Sochat, M., & Chavda, Y. (2017). *First Aid for the USMLE Step 1 2017* (27 edition). New York, NY: McGraw-Hill Education / Medical.

Moore, K., Persau T.V.N., & Torgia, M.G. (2015). *Before We Are Born: Essentials of Embryology and Birth Defects*, (9 edition). Philadelphia, PA: Elsevier.

Sadler, T.W. (2010). Embryonic origin of ventral body wall defects. *Seminars in Pediatric Surgery, 19*, 209-214. Retrieved July 28, 2017, from http://sci-hub.io/10.1053/j.sempedsurg.2010.03.006

Sattar, H.A. (2017). *Fundamentals of Pathology: Medical Course and Step 1 Review* (2017). USA: Pathoma LLC.

Tortora, G. J. & Derrickson, B. (2014). *Principles of Anatomy and Physiology*. Hoboken, NJ: Wiley.

Yerkes, E. B. (2016). Exstrophy and epispadias. In *Medscape*. Retrieved August 1, 2017, from http://emedicine.medscape.com/article/1014971-overview

## CHRONIC KIDNEY DISEASE

About chronic kidney disease. (2017, February 15). In *National Kidney Foundation*. Retrieved from https://www.kidney.org/atoz/content/about-chronic-kidney-disease

Arora, P. Chronic kidney disease. (2017). In *Medscape*. Retrieved July 28, 2017, from http://emedicine.medscape.com/article/238798-overview#a4

Hyperkalemia bulletin. (n.d.). In *National Kidney Foundation*. Retrieved July 28, 2017, from https://www.kidney.org/sites/default/files/02-10-6785_HBE_Hyperkalemia_Bulletin.pdf

Kidney disease can be treated. (n.d.). In *National Kidney Foundation*. Retrieved July 28, 2017, from https://www.kidney.org/sites/default/files/01-10-7278_HBG_CKD_Stages_Flyer3.pdf

Kasper, D.L., Fauci, A.S. & Hauser S. (2015). *Harrison's Principles of Internal Medicine* (19 edition). New York, NY: McGraw Hill Education / Medical.

Rosenberg, M. (2016). Overview of the management of chronic kidney disease in adults. In *UpToDate*. Retrieved August 1, 2017, from https://www.uptodate.com/contents/overview-of-the-management-of-chronic-kidney-disease-in-adults?source=search_result&search=chronic%20kidney%20disease&selectedTitle=1~150

Sattar, H.A. (2017). *Fundamentals of Pathology: Medical Course and Step 1 Review* (2017). USA: Pathoma LLC.

Webster, A. C., Nagler, E. V., Morton, R. L., & Masson, P. (2017). Chronic kidney disease. *The Lancet, 389*(10075), 1238–1252. Retrieved July 28, 2017, from https://doi.org/10.1016/S0140-6736(16)32064-5

## CHRONIC PYELONEPHRITIS

Kumar, V., Abbas A.K., & Aster, J.C. (2015). *Robbins & Cotran Pathologic Basis of Disease* (9 edition). Philadelphia, PA: Elsevier.

Le, T., Bhushan, V., Sochat, M., & Chavda, Y. (2017). *First Aid for the USMLE Step 1 2017* (27 edition). New York: McGraw-Hill Education / Medical.

Pyelonephritis. (n.d.). In *Wikipedia*. Retrieved July 28, 2017, from https://en.wikipedia.org/wiki/Pyelonephritis

Sattar, H.A. (2017). *Fundamentals of Pathology: Medical Course and Step 1 Review* (2017). USA: Pathoma LLC.

Vesicoureteral reflux. (n.d.). In *Wikipedia*. Retrieved July 28, 2017, from https://en.wikipedia.org/wiki/Angiomyolipoma https://en.wikipedia.org/wiki/Vesicoureteral_reflux

## CYSTITIS (LOWER URINARY TRACT INFECTION)

Brusch, J. L. (2015). Urinary tract infections in diabetes meillitus. In *Medscape*. Retrieved July 28,2017, from http://emedicine.medscape.com/article/2040207-overview

Brusch, J. L. (2015). Urinary tract infection (UTI) and cystitis (bladder infection) in females workup. In *Medscape*. Retrieved July 28, 2017, from http://emedicine.medscape.com/article/233101-workup#c9

Brusch, J. L. (2015). Urinary tract infection (UTI) and cystitis (bladder infection) in females. In *Medscape*. Retrieved July 28, 2015 from http://emedicine.medscape.com/article/233101-overview#a4

Brusch, J. L. (2015). Urinary tract infection (UTI) and cystitis (bladder infection) in females clinical presentation. In *Medscape*. Retrieved July 28, 2017, from http://emedicine.medscape.com/article/233101-clinical

Copstead, L.-E. C., & Banasik, J. L. (2012). *Pathophysiology, 5e* (5 edition). St. Louis, MO: Saunders.

McKance, K.L. & Huethe, S.E. (2014). *Pathophysiology: The Biologic Basis for Disease in Adults and Children* (7 edition). St. Louis, MO: Mosby-Elsevier.

Non-functioning kidney. (n.d.). In *Radiopaedia*. Retrieved July 28, 2017, from http://radiopaedia.org/cases/non-functioning-kidney-1

Sattar, H.A. (2017). *Fundamentals of Pathology: Medical Course and Step 1 Review* (2017). USA: Pathoma LLC.

Unilateral vesicoureteric reflux. (n.d.). In *Radiopaedia*. Retrieved July 28, 2017, from http://radiopaedia.org/cases/unilateral-vesicoureteric-reflux

Urinary tract infection. (n.d.). In *Wikipedia*. Retrieved July 28, 2017, from https://en.wikipedia.org/wiki/Urinary_tract_infection

Urothelial thickening (urinary tract infection). (n.d.).

In *Radiopaedia*. Retrieved July 28, 2017, from http://radiopaedia.org/cases/urothelial-thickening-urinary-tract-infection

## DIABETIC NEPHROPATHY

Agabegi, S.S. & Agabegi E. D. (2016). *Step Up to Medicine* (4 edition). Philadelphia, PA: Lippincott Williams & Wilkins.

Bakris, G. L. (2017). Overview of diabetic nephropathy. In *UpToDate*. Retrieved August 1, 2017, from https://www-uptodate-com.ucsf.idm.oclc.org/contents/overview-of-diabetic-nephropathy?source=search_result&search=diabetic%20nephropathy&selectedTitle=1~150

Bakris, G. L. (2017). Treatment of diabetic nephropathy. In *UpToDate*. Retrieved August 1, 2017, from https://www.uptodate.com/contents/treatment-of-diabetic-nephropathy?source=search_result&search=treatment%20of%20diabetic%20nephropathy&selectedTitle=1~150

Kumar, V., Abbas A.K., & Aster, J.C. (2015). *Robbins & Cotran Pathologic Basis of Disease* (9 edition). Philadelphia, PA: Elsevier.

Le, T., Bhushan, V., Sochat, M., & Chavda, Y. (2017). *First Aid for the USMLE Step 1 2017* (27 edition). New York, NY: McGraw-Hill Education / Medical.

Sattar, H.A. (2017). *Fundamentals of Pathology: Medical Course and Step 1 Review* (2017). USA: Pathoma LLC.

Woredekal Y. & Friedman E. A. (2009) Chapter 54: diabetic nephropathy. *CURRENT Diagnosis & Treatment: Nephrology & Hypertension*. Eds. Edgar V. Lerma, et al. New York, NY: McGraw-Hill, 2009. Retrieved July 31, 2017, from http://accessmedicine.mhmedical.com.ucsf.idm.oclc.org/content.aspx?bookid=372&sectionid=39961197. Accessed March 10, 2017.

## FOCAL SEGMENTAL GLOMERULOSCLEROSIS

Focal segmental glomerulosclerosis. (n.d.). In *Wikipedia*. Retrieved July 28, 2017, from https://en.wikipedia.org/wiki/Focal_segmental_glomerulosclerosis

Kumar, V., Abbas A.K., & Aster, J.C. (2015). *Robbins & Cotran Pathologic Basis of Disease* (9 edition). Philadelphia, PA: Elsevier.

Le, T., Bhushan, V., Sochat, M., & Chavda, Y. (2017). *First Aid for the USMLE Step 1 2017* (27 edition). New York,

NY: McGraw-Hill Education / Medical.

McKance, K.L. & Huethe, S.E. (2014). *Pathophysiology: The Biologic Basis for Disease in Adults and Children* (7 edition). St. Louis, MO: Mosby-Elsevier.

Salifu M. O. (2015). HIV-associated nephropathy. In *Medscape*. Retrieved July 28, 2017, from http://emedicine.medscape.com/article/246031-overview#a3

Sattar, H.A. (2017). *Fundamentals of Pathology: Medical Course and Step 1 Review* (2017). USA: Pathoma LLC.

Sreepada, T. K. R. (2016). Focal segmental glomerulosclerosis. In *Medscape*. Retrieved July 28, 2017, from http://emedicine.medscape.com/article/245915-overview#a5

## GOODPASTURE SYNDROME

Borza, D.-B., Neilson, E. G., & Hudson, B. G. (2003). Pathogenesis of Goodpasture syndrome: a molecular perspective. *Seminars in Nephrology, 23*(6), 522–531. Retrieved July 28, 2017, from https://www.ncbi.nlm.nih.gov/pubmed/14631560

Goodpasture syndrome. (n.d.). In *National Institutes of Health*. Retrieved July 28, 2017, from https://rarediseases.info.nih.gov/diseases/2551/goodpasture-syndrome

Alenzi, F. Q., Salem, M. L., Alenazi, F. A., & Wyse, R. K. (2012). Cellular and molecular aspects of Goodpasture syndrome. *Iranian Journal of Kidney Diseases, 6*(1), 1–8. Retrieved July 28, 2017, from https://www.ncbi.nlm.nih.gov/pubmed/22218111

Kasper, D. L., Fauci, A. S., Hauser, S., Longo, D., Jameson, J. L., & Loscalzo, J. (2015). *Harrison's Principles of Internal Medicine* (19 edition). New York, NY: McGraw-Hill Education / Medical.

Kumar, V., Abbas A.K., & Aster, J.C. (2015). *Robbins & Cotran Pathologic Basis of Disease* (9 edition). Philadelphia, PA: Elsevier.

Le, T., Bhushan, V., Sochat, M., & Chavda, Y. (2017). *First Aid for the USMLE Step 1 2017* (27 edition). New York, NY: McGraw-Hill Education / Medical.

Sattar, H.A. (2017). *Fundamentals of Pathology: Medical Course and Step 1 Review* (2017). USA: Pathoma LLC.

## HEMOLYTIC-UREMIC SYNDROME

Kasper, D. L., Fauci, A. S., Hauser, S., Longo, D., Jameson, J. L., & Loscalzo, J. (2015). *Harrison's Principles of*

*Internal Medicine* (19 edition). New York, NY: McGraw-Hill Education / Medical.

Kumar, V., Abbas A.K., & Aster, J.C. (2015). *Robbins & Cotran Pathologic Basis of Disease* (9 edition). Philadelphia, PA: Elsevier.

Le, T., Bhushan, V., Sochat, M., & Chavda, Y. (2017). *First Aid for the USMLE Step 1 2017* (27 edition). New York, NY: McGraw-Hill Education / Medical.

Mead, P. S., & Griffin, P. M. (1998). Escherichia coli O157:H7. *The Lancet, 352*(9135), 1207–1212. Retrieved July 28, 2017, from https://doi.org/10.1016/S0140-6736(98)01267-7

Niaudet, P. (2017). Overview of hemolytic uremic syndrome in children. In *UpToDate*. Retrieved August 1, 2017, from https://www.uptodate.com/contents/overview-of-hemolytic-uremic-syndrome-in-children?source=search_result&search=hemolytic%20uremic%20syndrome&selectedTitle=1~150

Sattar, H.A. (2017). *Fundamentals of Pathology: Medical Course and Step 1 Review* (2017). USA: Pathoma LLC.

Zoja, C., Buelli, S., & Morigi, M. (2010). Shiga toxin-associated hemolytic uremic syndrome: pathophysiology of endothelial dysfunction. *Pediatric Nephrology, 25*(11), 2231–2240. Retrieved July 28, 2017, from https://doi.org/10.1007/s00467-010-1522-1

## HORSESHOE KIDNEY

Allen, R. C. (2016). Horseshoe kidney: practice essentials, epidemiology, etiology. In *Medscape*. Retrieved July 28, 2017, from http://emedicine.medscape.com/article/441510-overview#a7 http://emedicine.medscape.com/article/441510-overview#a7

Allen, Robert C. (2016). Horseshoe kidney treatment: management. In *Medscape*. Retrieved July 28, 2017, from http://emedicine.medscape.com/article/441510-treatment#d11

Eisendrath, D. N., Phifer, F. M. & Culver, H. B. (1925). Horseshoe kidney. *Annals of Surgery 82*(5): 735-764. Retrieved July 28, 2017, from https://www.ncbi.nlm.nih.gov/pmc/articles/PMC1400255/

Horseshoe kidney. (n.d.). In *Radiopaedia*. Retrieved July 28, 2017, from http://radiopaedia.org/articles/horseshoe-kidney

Horseshoe kidney. (n.d.). In *Wikipedia*. Retrieved July 28, 2017, from https://en.wikipedia.org/wiki/Horseshoe_kidney

Kidney development. (n.d.). In *Wikipedia*. Retrieved July 28, 2017, from https://en.wikipedia.org/wiki/Kidney_development

Le, T., Bhushan, V., Sochat, M., & Chavda, Y. (2017). *First Aid for the USMLE Step 1 2017* (27 edition). New York, NY: McGraw-Hill Education / Medical.

Natsis, K., Piagkou, M., Skotsimara, A. & Skandalakis, P. (2013). Horseshoe kidney: a review of anatomy and pathology. *Surgical and Radiologic Anatomy: SRA, 36*(6), 517–526. Retrieved July 28, 2017, from https://doi.org/10.1007/s00276-013-1229-7

Sattar, H.A. (2017). *Fundamentals of Pathology: Medical Course and Step 1 Review* (2017). USA: Pathoma LLC.

## HYDRONEPHROSIS

Goljan, E. F. (2013). *Rapid Review Pathology* (4 edition). Milton, ON: Elsevier Canada.

Hydronephrosis. (n.d.). In *Radiopaedia*. Retrieved July 28, 2017, from https://radiopaedia.org/articles/hydronephrosis

Hydronephrosis. (n.d.). In *Wikipedia*. Retrieved July 28, 2017, from https://en.wikipedia.org/wiki/Hydronephrosis

Obstructive uropathy and urolithiasis on ultrasound. (n.d.). In *Radiopaedia*. Retrieved July 28, 2017, from https://radiopaedia.org/cases/25562/

Le, T., Bhushan, V., Sochat, M., & Chavda, Y. (2017). *First Aid for the USMLE Step 1 2017* (27 edition). New York, NY: McGraw-Hill Education / Medical.

Mergener, K., Weinerth, J. L., & Baillie, J. (1997). Dietl's crisis: a syndrome of episodic abdominal pain of urologic origin that may present to a gastroenterologist. *The American Journal of Gastroenterology, 92*(12), 2289–2291. Retrieved July 28, 2017, from https://www.ncbi.nlm.nih.gov/pubmed/9399772

Mollard, P., Deasy, B., & Mathon, C. (1972). [Primary idiopathic megaureters. Pathogenesis and treatment. (91 patients-113 ureters)]. *Annales D'urologie, 6*(1), 45–55. Retrieved July 28, 2017, from https://www.ncbi.nlm.nih.gov/pubmed/5012702

Sattar, H.A. (2017). *Fundamentals of Pathology: Medical Course and Step 1 Review* (2017). USA: Pathoma LLC.

Stephens, F. D., & Gupta, D. (1994). Pathogenesis of the prune belly syndrome. *The Journal of Urology, 152*(6 Pt 2), 2328–2331.

Wein, A.J., Kavoussi, L. R., Novick, A. C., Partin, A.W. & Peters, C.A. (2007). *Campbell-Walsh Urology* (9 edition).

Philadelphia, PA: Saunders.

## HYPERCALCEMIA

Agus, Z.S. (2011). Relation between total and ionized serum and calcium concentration. In *Curso Enarm*. Retrieved July 28, 2017, from http://cursoenarm.net/UPTODATE/contents/mobipreview.htm?1/31/1534?source=see_link#H404378

Armstrong, C. M. & Cota, G. (1991). Calcium ion as a cofactor in Na channel gating. In *National Center for Biotechnology Information*. Retrieved July 28, 2017, from https://www.ncbi.nlm.nih.gov/pmc/articles/PMC52119/?page=3

Barrett, K. E., Barman, S.M, Boitano, S., Brooks, H.L. (2015). Hormonal control of calcium & phosphate metabolism & the physiology of bone. *Ganong's Review of Medical Physiology* (25 edition). New York, NY: McGraw-Hill.

Costanzo, L. S. (2017). *Physiology* (6 edition). Philadelphia, PA: Elsevier.

Goldfarb, Stanley. (2009). Chapter 6: Disorders of calcium balance: hypercalcemia & hypocalcemia. *CURRENT Diagnosis & Treatment: Nephrology & Hypertension*. Edgar V. Lerma, Jeffrey S. Berns & Allen R. Nissenson (Eds). New York, NY: McGraw-Hill. Retrieved July 28, 2017, from http://accessmedicine.mhmedical.com/content.aspx?bookid=372&sectionid=39961141

Goltzman, D. Etiology of hypocalcemia in adults. (n.d.). In *Curso Enarm*. Retrieved July 28, 2017, from http://cursoenarm.net/UPTODATE/contents/mobipreview.htm?8/53/9040

Kasper, D. L., Fauci, A. S., Hauser, S., Longo, D., Jameson, J. L., & Loscalzo, J. (2015). *Harrison's Principles of Internal Medicine* (19 edition). New York, NY: McGraw-Hill Education / Medical.

Le, T., Bhushan, V., Sochat, M., & Chavda, Y. (2017). *First Aid for the USMLE Step 1 2017* (27 edition). New York, NY: McGraw-Hill Education / Medical.

Levine, M.A. Hypocalcemia and hypercalcemia: a board review. (n.d.). In *Cleveland Clinic*. Retrieved July 28, 2017, from http://www.clevelandclinicmeded.com/live/courses/ann/EndoReview/osyllabus/SatOct3/0900LevineHyperandHypoCalcemia.pdf

Sattar, H.A. (2017). *Fundamentals of Pathology: Medical Course and Step 1 Review* (2017). USA: Pathoma LLC.

Skugor, M. Hypocalcemia. (n.d.). In *Cleveland Clinic*. Retrieved July 28, 2017, from http://www.clevelandclinicmeded.com/medicalpubs/diseasemanagement/endocrinology/hypocalcemia/

Yu, A. S. L. & Stubbs, J. R. (2016). Relation between total and ionized serum calcium concentrations. In *UpToDate*. Retrieved July 28, 2017, from https://goo.gl/6SHKa1

## HYPERKALEMIA

Copstead, L.-E. C., & Banasik, J. L. (2012). *Pathophysiology* (5 edition). St. Louis, MO: Saunders.

Costanzo, L. S. (2017). *Physiology* (6 edition). Philadelphia, PA: Elsevier.

Hyperkalemia. (n.d.). In *Wikipedia*. Retrieved July 28, 2017, from https://en.wikipedia.org/wiki/Hyperkalemia

Le, T., Bhushan, V., Sochat, M., & Chavda, Y. (2017). *First Aid for the USMLE Step 1 2017* (27 edition). New York, NY: McGraw-Hill Education / Medical.

Moratinos, J. & Reverte, M. (1993). Effects of catecholamines on plasma potassium: the role of alpha- and beta-adrenoceptors. In *National Center for Biotechnology Information*. Retrieved July 31, 2017, from https://www.ncbi.nlm.nih.gov/pubmed/8388847

Palmer, B. F. (2010). A physiologic-based approach to the evaluation of a patient with hyperkalemia. *Am J Kidney Dis. 2010, 26*(3), 387-393. Retrieved August 1, 2017, from http://www.medscape.com/viewarticle/730660_3

## HYPERMAGNESEMIA

Baaij, J. H. F. de, Hoenderop, J. G. J., & Bindels, R. J. M. (2015). Magnesium in man: implications for health and disease. *Physiological Reviews, 95*(1), 1–46. Retrieved July 31, 017 from https://doi.org/10.1152/physrev.00012.2014https://academic.oup.com/ckj/article/5/Suppl_1/i3/447534/Magnesium-basics#6699635

Fulop, T. (2015). Hypermagnesemia. In *Medscape*. Retrieved July 31, 2017, from http://emedicine.medscape.com/article/246489-overview#a4

Hall, J. & Premji, A. (2015). *Toronto Notes 2015*. Toronto, Canada: University of Toronto Press.

Kasper, D. L., Fauci, A. S., Hauser, S., Longo, D., Jameson, J. L., & Loscalzo, J. (2015). *Harrison's Principles of Internal Medicine* (19 edition). New York, NY: McGraw-Hill Education / Medical.

Riccardi, D. & Brown, E. M. (2010). Physiology and pathophysiology of the calcium-sensing receptor in the kidney. *American Journal of Physiology - Renal Physiology, 298*(3), F485–F499. Retrieved July 31, 2017, from https://www.ncbi.nlm.nih.gov/pmc/articles/PMC2838589/

Romani, A. M. P. (2011). Cellular magnesium homeostasis. *Archives of Biochemistry and Biophysics, 512*(1), 1–23. Retrieved July 31, 2017, from https://doi.org/10.1016/j.abb.2011.05.010

## HYPERNATREMIA

Kasper, D. L., Fauci, A. S., Hauser, S., Longo, D., Jameson, J. L., & Loscalzo, J. (2015). *Harrison's Principles of Internal Medicine* (19 edition). New York, NY: McGraw-Hill Education / Medical.

Le, T., Bhushan, V., Sochat, M., & Chavda, Y. (2017). *First Aid for the USMLE Step 1 2017* (27 edition). New York, NY: McGraw-Hill Education / Medical.

Merali, Z. & Woodfine, J. (2016). *Toronto Notes 2016.* Toronto, Canada: University of Toronto Press.

Sterns, R. H. (2015). Etiology and evaluation of hypernatremia in adults. In *UpToDate*. Retrieved August 1, 2017, from https://www.uptodate.com/contents/etiology-and-evaluation-of-hypernatremia-in-adults?source=search_result&search=hypernatremia&selectedTitle=2~150

## HYPERPHOSPHATEMIA

Collins, J. F. (2016). *Molecular, Genetic, and Nutritional Aspects of Major and Trace Minerals.* Gainesville, FL: Academic Press.

Costanzo, L. S. (2017). *Physiology* (6 edition). Philadelphia, PA: Elsevier.

Han, P., Trinidad, B. J., & Shi, J. (2015). Hypocalcemia-induced seizure: demystifying the calcium paradox. *ASN NEURO, 7*(2). Retrieved July 31, 2017, from https://doi.org/10.1177/1759091415578050

Le, T., Bhushan, V., Sochat, M., & Chavda, Y. (2017). *First Aid for the USMLE Step 1 2017* (27 edition). New York, NY: McGraw-Hill Education / Medical.

Lederer, E. Hyperphosphatemia: practice essentials, background, pathophysiology. (2017). In *Medscape*. Retrieved July 31, 2017, from http://emedicine.medscape.com/article/241185-overview

Lewis III, J. L.Hyperphosphatemia (n.d.). In *Merck Manuals*. Retrieved July 28 2017, from http://www.merckmanuals.com/professional/endocrine-and-metabolic-disorders/electrolyte-disorders/hyperphosphatemia

Lewis III, J. L. Hyperphosphatemia (high level of phosphate in the blood). (n.d.). In *Merck Manuals*. Retrieved July 28 2017, from https://www.merckmanuals.com/home/hormonal-and-metabolic-disorders/electrolyte-balance/hyperphosphatemia-high-level-of-phosphate-in-the-blood

Lewis III, J. L. Overview of phosphate's role in the body. (n.d.). In *Merck Manuals*. Retrieved July 28 2017, from http://www.merckmanuals.com/home/hormonal-and-metabolic-disorders/electrolyte-balance/overview-of-phosphate-s-role-in-the-body

Stubbs, J. R. & Yu, A. S. L. (2015). Overview of the causes and treatment of hyperphosphatemia. In *UpToDate*. Retrieved July 31, 2017, from https://www.uptodate.com/contents/overview-of-the-causes-and-treatment-of-hyperphosphatemia

Takeda, E., Taketani, Y., Sawada, N., Sato, T., & Yamamoto, H. (2004). The regulation and function of phosphate in the human body. *BioFactors, 21*(1–4), 345–355. Retrieved July 31, 2017, from https://doi.org/10.1002/biof.552210167

Nguyen, T. Q., Maalouf, N. M., Sakhaee, K., & Moe, O. W. (2011). Comparison of insulin action on glucose versus potassium uptake in humans. *Clinical Journal of the American Society of Nephrology : CJASN, 6*(7), 1533–1539. Retrieved July 31, 2017, from https://doi.org/10.2215/CJN.00750111

## HYPOCALCEMIA

Agus, Z.S. (2011). Relation between total and ionized serum and calcium concentrations. In *Curso Enarm*. Retrieved July 28, 2017, from http://cursoenarm.net/UPTODATE/contents/mobipreview.htm?1/31/1534?source=see_link#H404378Goldfarb, S. Chapter 6: disorders of calcium balance: hypercalcemia & hypocalcemia." *CURRENT Diagnosis & Treatment: Nephrology & Hypertension.* Eds. Edgar V. Lerma, et al. New York, NY: McGraw-Hill, 2009.

Armstrong, C. M. & Cota, G. (1991). Calcium ion as a cofactor in Na channel gating. (2017, July 28). In *National Center for Biotechnology Information*. Retrieved from https://www.ncbi.nlm.nih.gov/pmc/articles/PMC52119/?page=3

Barrett, K. E., Barman, S.M, Boitano, S., Brooks, H.L. (2015). Hormonal control of calcium & phosphate metabolism & the physiology of bone. *Ganong's Review* of Medical Physiology (25 edition). New York, NY: McGraw-Hill.

Costanzo, L. S. (2017). Physiology (6 edition). Philadelphia, PA: Elsevier.

Goltzman, D. (2011). Etiology of hypocalcemia in adults. In Curso Enarm. Retrieved July 31, 2017, from http://cursoenarm.net/UPTODATE/contents/mobipreview.htm?8/53/9040

Kasper, D. L., Fauci, A. S., Hauser, S., Longo, D., Jameson, J. L., & Loscalzo, J. (2015). Harrison's Principles of Internal Medicine (19 edition). New York, NY: McGraw-Hill Education / Medical.

Le, T., Bhushan, V., Sochat, M., & Chavda, Y. (2017). First Aid for the USMLE Step 1 2017 (27 edition). New York, NY: McGraw-Hill Education / Medical.

Levine, M.A. Hypocalcemia and hypercalcemia: a board review. (n.d.). In Cleveland Clinic. Retrieved July 28, 2017, from http://www.clevelandclinicmeded.com/live/courses/ann/EndoReview/osyllabus/SatOct3/0900LevineHyperandHypoCalcemia.pdf

Sattar, H.A. (2017). Fundamentals of Pathology: Medical Course and Step 1 Review (2017). USA: Pathoma LLC.

Skugor, M. (2014). Hypocalcemia. In Cleveland Clinic. Retrieved July 31, 2017, from http://www.clevelandclinicmeded.com/medicalpubs/diseasemanagement/endocrinology/hypocalcemia/

Yu, A. S. L. & Stubbs, J. R. (2016). Relation between total and ionized serum calcium concentrations. In UpToDate. Retrieved July 28, 2017, from https://goo.gl/6SHKa1

## HYPOKALEMIA

Costanzo, L. S. (2017). Physiology (6 edition). Philadelphia, PA: Elsevier.

Le, T., Bhushan, V., Sochat, M., & Chavda, Y. (2017). First Aid for the USMLE Step 1 2017 (27 edition). New York, NY: McGraw-Hill Education / Medical.

Hypokalemia. (n.d.). In Wikipedia. Retrieved July 28, 2017, from https://en.wikipedia.org/wiki/Hypokalemia

Moratinos, J. & Reverte, M. (1993). Effects of catecholamines on plasma potassium: the role of alpha- and beta-adrenoceptors. In National Center for Biotechnology Information. Retrieved July 31, 2017, from https://www.ncbi.nlm.nih.gov/pubmed/8388847Copstead, L.-E. C., & Banasik, J. L. (2012). Pathophysiology, 5e (5 edition). St. Louis, MO: Saunders.

Mount, D. B. (2016). Causes of hypokalemia in adults. In UpToDate. Retrieved July 28 2017, from https://www.uptodate.com/contents/causes-of-hypokalemia-in-adults#H17666515

## HYPOMAGNESEMIA

Baaij, J. H. F. de, Hoenderop, J. G. J., & Bindels, R. J. M. (2015). Magnesium in man: implications for health and disease. Physiological Reviews, 95(1), 1–46. Retrieved July 31, 017 from https://doi.org/10.1152/physrev.00012.2014https://academic.oup.com/ckj/article/5/Suppl_1/i3/447534/Magnesium-basics#6699635

Fulop, T. (2015). Hypermagnesemia. In Medscape. Retrieved July 31, 2017, from http://emedicine.medscape.com/article/246489-overview#a4

Hall, J. & Premji, A. (2015). Toronto Notes 2015. Toronto, Canada: University of Toronto Press.

Jahnen-Dechent, W., & Ketteler, M. (2012). Magnesium basics. Clinical Kidney Journal, 5(Suppl. 1), i3–i14. Retrieved July 31, 2017, from https://doi.org/10.1093/ndtplus/sfr163 https://academic.oup.com/ckj/article/5/Suppl_1/i3/447534/Magnesium-basics#6699635

Kasper, D. L., Fauci, A. S., Hauser, S., Longo, D., Jameson, J. L., & Loscalzo, J. (2015). Harrison's Principles of Internal Medicine (19 edition). New York: McGraw-Hill Education / Medical.

Riccardi, D. & Brown, E. M. (2010). Physiology and pathophysiology of the calcium-sensing receptor in the kidney. American Journal of Physiology - Renal Physiology, 298(3), F485–F499. Retrieved July 31, 2017, from https://www.ncbi.nlm.nih.gov/pmc/articles/PMC2838589/

Romani, A. M. P. (2011). Cellular magnesium homeostasis. Archives of Biochemistry and Biophysics, 512(1), 1–23. Retrieved July 31, 2017, from https://doi.org/10.1016/j.abb.2011.05.010

## HYPONATREMIA

Le, T., Bhushan, V., Sochat, M., & Chavda, Y. (2017). First Aid for the USMLE Step 1 2017 (27 edition). New York, NY: McGraw-Hill Education / Medical.

Sattar, H.A. (2017). Fundamentals of Pathology: Medical Course and Step 1 Review (2017). USA: Pathoma LLC.

Sterns, R. H. Causes of hyponatremia. (2017, July 28). In Curso Enarm. Retrieved from http://cursoenarm.net/

UPTODATE/contents/mobipreview.htm?9/59/10160

Spasovski G., Vanholder R., Allolio B., et al. Clinical practice guideline on diagnosis and treatment of hyponatraemia. *Eur J Endocrinol, 2014 170*(3): G1-G47.

Sterns, R. H., Hix, J. K. & Silver, S.M. Management of hyponatremia in the ICU. *Chest, 2013 144*(2): 672-679.


## HYPOPHOSPHATEMIA

Costanzo, L. S. (2017). *Physiology* (6 edition). Philadelphia, PA: Elsevier.

Hypophosphatemia. (n.d.). In *Wikipedia*. Retrieved July 28, 2017, from https://en.wikipedia.org/wiki/Hypophosphatemia

Le, T., Bhushan, V., Sochat, M., & Chavda, Y. (2017). *First Aid for the USMLE Step 1 2017* (27 edition). New York, NY: McGraw-Hill Education / Medical.

Lederer, E. Hypophosphatemia: practice essentials, background, pathophysiology. (2017). In *Medscape*. Retrieved July 31, 2017, from http://emedicine.medscape.com/article/242280-overview

Lewis III, J. L.Hypophosphatemia (n.d.). In *Merck Manuals*. Retrieved July 28 2017, from http://www.merckmanuals.com/professional/endocrine-and-metabolic-disorders/electrolyte-disorders/hypophosphatemia

Lewis III, J. L. Overview of phosphate's role in the body. (n.d.). In *Merck Manuals*. Retrieved July 28 2017, from http://www.merckmanuals.com/home/hormonal-and-metabolic-disorders/electrolyte-balance/overview-of-phosphate-s-role-in-the-body

Takeda, E., Taketani, Y., Sawada, N., Sato, T., & Yamamoto, H. (2004). The regulation and function of phosphate in the human body. *BioFactors, 21*(1–4), 345–355. Retrieved July 31, 2017, from https://doi.org/10.1002/biof.552210167


## HYPOSPADIAS & EPISPADIAS

Barlogie, B., Jagannath, S., Dixon, D. O., Cheson, B., Smallwood, L., Hendrickson, A. & Alexanian, R. (1990). High-dose melphalan and granulocyte-macrophage colony-stimulating factor for refractory multiple myeloma. *Blood, 76*(4), 677–680. Retrieved July 31, 2017, from https://www.ncbi.nlm.nih.gov/pubmed/2200536

Differentiated stage of the male genitalia. (2017, July 28). In Embryology.ch. Retrieved from http://www.embryology.ch/anglais/ugenital/genitexterne02.html

Dudek, R. W. (2014). *BRS Embryology* (6 edition). Baltimore, MD: Lippincott Williams & Wilkins.

Epispadias. (n.d.). In *Wikipedia*. Retrieved July 28, 2017, from https://en.wikipedia.org/wiki/Epispadias

Goljan, E. F. (2013). *Rapid Review Pathology* (4 edition) Milton, ON: Elsevier Canada.

Hypospadias. (n.d.). In *Wikipedia*. Retrieved July 28, 2017, from https://en.wikipedia.org/wiki/Hypospadias

Le, T., Bhushan, V., Sochat, M., & Chavda, Y. (2017). *First Aid for the USMLE Step 1 2017* (27 edition). New York, NY: McGraw-Hill Education / Medical.

Mollard, P., Basset, T., & Mure, P. Y. (1997). Female epispadias. *The Journal of Urology 158*(4), 1543–1546. Retrieved July 31, 2017, from https://doi.org/10.1016/S0022-5347(01)64276-9

Orkiszewski, M. (2012). A standardized classification of hypospadias. *Journal of Pediatric Urology, 8*(4), 410–414. Retrieved July 31, 2017, from https://doi.org/10.1016/j.jpurol.2011.08.011

Sattar, H.A. (2017). *Fundamentals of Pathology: Medical Course and Step 1 Review* (2017). USA: Pathoma LLC.

Sadler, T. W. (2015). *Langman: Embriologia Medica*. Philadelphia, PA: Lippincott Williams & Wilkins.

*USMLE Step 1 Lecture Notes 2015*. (2015). Kaplan Lecture Notes 2015. Fort Lauderdale, FL: Kaplan.


## IGA NEPHROPATHY (BERGER DISEASE)

Allen, A. C., Bailey, E. M., Barratt, J., Buck, K. S., & Feehally, J. (n.d.). Analysis of IgA1 O-glycans in IgA nephropathy by fluorophore-assisted carbohydrate electrophoresis. *Journal of the American Society of Nephrology*. Retrieved July 31, 2017, from http://jasn.asnjournals.org

Brake, M. IgA nephropathy: background, pathophysiology, epidemiology. (2017). In *Medscape*. Retrieved July 31, 2017, from from http://emedicine.medscape.com/article/239927-overview#a5

Brake, M. IgA nephropathy: treatment & management. (2017). In *Medscape*. Retrieved July 31, 2017, from http://emedicine.medscape.com/article/239927-treatment

Copstead, L.-E. C., & Banasik, J. L. (2012). *Pathophysiology* (5 edition). St. Louis, MO: Saunders.

Henoch-Schönlein purpura. (July 28 2017). In

Wikipedia. Retrieved from https://en.wikipedia.org/wiki/Henoch%E2%80%93Sch%C3%B6nlein_purpura

IgA nephropathy (2017, July 31). In *National Institutes of Diabetes and Digestive Kidney Diseases*. Retrieved from https://www.niddk.nih.gov/health-information/health-topics/kidney-disease/iga-nephropathy/Pages/facts.aspx#10

IgA nephropathy. (n.d.). In *Wikipedia*. Retrieved July 28, 2017, from https://en.wikipedia.org/wiki/IgA_nephropathy

Lau, K. K., Suzuki H., Novak J. & Wyatt, R.J. (2009). Pathogenesis of Henoch-Schönlein purpura nephritis. *Pediatr. Nephrol.* Retrieved July 31 2017, from https://openi.nlm.nih.gov/detailedresult.php?img=PMC2778786_467_2009_1230_Fig1_HTML&req=4

Macpherson, A. J., McCoy, K. D., Johansen, F.-E., & Brandtzaeg, P. (2008). The immune geography of IgA induction and function. *Mucosal Immunology*, 1(1), 11–22. Retrieved July 31, 2017, from https://doi.org/10.1038/mi.2007.6

McKance, K.L. & Huethe, S.E. (2014). *Pathophysiology: The Biologic Basis for Disease in Adults and Children* (7 edition). St. Louis, MO: Mosby-Elsevier.

Roos, A. & van Kooten, C. (2007). Underglycosylation of IgA in IgA nephropathy: More than a diagnostic marker? In *PubMed*. Retrieved July 31, 2017, from https://www.researchgate.net/publication/6309540_Underglycosylation_of_IgA_in_IgA_nephropathy_More_than_a_diagnostic_marker

Sattar, H.A. (2017). *Fundamentals of Pathology: Medical Course and Step 1 Review* (2017). USA: Pathoma LLC.

van den Wall Bake, A. W., Daha, M. R., Radl, J., Haaijman, J. J., Van der Ark, A., Valentijn, R. M., & Van Es, L. A. (1988). The bone marrow as production site of the IgA deposited in the kidneys of patients with IgA nephropathy. *Clinical and Experimental Immunology*, 72(2), 321–325. Retrieved July 31, 2017, from http://www.ncbi.nlm.nih.gov/pmc/articles/PMC1541534/

## INTRARENAL ACUTE KIDNEY INJURY

Acute kidney injury. (2017, July 28) In *Wikipedia*. Retrieved from https://en.wikipedia.org/wiki/Acute_kidney_injury

Kumar, V., Abbas A.K., & Aster, J.C. (2015). *Robbins & Cotran Pathologic Basis of Disease* (9 edition). Philadelphia, PA: Elsevier.

Le, T., Bhushan, V., Sochat, M., & Chavda, Y. (2017). *First Aid for the USMLE Step 1 2017* (27 edition). New York, NY: McGraw-Hill Education / Medical.

Sattar, H.A. (2017). *Fundamentals of Pathology: Medical Course and Step 1 Review* (2017). USA: Pathoma LLC.

## LUPUS NEPHRITIS

Bishop, L. & Rovin, B. (2016). Grand rounds: lupus nephritis with Dr. Rovin. *Louisville Lectures Medical Lecture Series*. Retrieved August 1, 2017, from http://www.louisvillelectures.org/imblog/2016/1/29/t0sr0816mckfk14g4xkd8u0crylonh

Goljan, E. F. (2013). *Rapid Review Pathology* (4 edition) Milton, ON: Elsevier Canada.

Kumar, V., Abbas A.K., & Aster, J.C. *Robbins & Cotran Pathologic Basis of Disease* (9 edition). Philadelphia, PA: Elsevier.

Le, T., Bhushan, V., Sochat, M., & Chavda, Y. (2017). *First Aid for the USMLE Step 1 2017* (27 edition). New York, NY: McGraw-Hill Education / Medical.

Sattar, H.A. (2017). *Fundamentals of Pathology: Medical Course and Step 1 Review* (2017). USA: Pathoma LLC.

## MEDULLARY SPONGE KIDNEY

Borofsky, M. (2017). The diagnostic dilemma of medullary sponge kidney. In The University of Chicago. Retrieved July 31, 2017, from http://kidneystones.uchicago.edu/the-diagnostic-dilemma-of-medullary-sponge-kidney/

Evan A.P., Worchester E.M., Williams Jr. J.C., Sommer A.J., Lingeman J.E., Phillips C.L., Coe F.L. (2015). Biopsy proven medullary sponge kidney: clinical findings, histopathology, and role of osteogenesis in stone and plaque formation. *The Anatomical Record, 298*, 865-877. Retrieved July 31, 2017, from http://sci-hub.io/10.1002/ar.23105

Gambaro G., Danza F.M., Fabris A. (2013). Medullary sponge kidney. *Current Opinion Nephrol Hypertens, 22*(4), 421-6. Retrieved July 31, 2017, from http://sci-hub.io/10.1097/MNH.0b013e3283622b86

Ghosh, A. K. (2016). Medullary sponge kidney: practice essentials, pathophysiology and etiology, epidemiology. In *Medscape*. Retrieved August 1, 2017, from http://emedicine.medscape.com/article/242886-overview

Kass-Iliyya A., Young J.G. (2016). Medullary

sponge kidney: a treatment conundrum. *Journal of Clinical Urology*, 1-8. Retrieved July 31, 2017, from https://www.researchgate.net/profile/Antoine_Kass-Iliyya2/publication/296196718_Medullary_sponge_kidney_A_treatment_conundrum/links/56d3621f08aeb52500d186e6.pdf

Kumar, V., Abbas A.K., & Aster, J.C. *Robbins & Cotran Pathologic Basis of Disease* (9 edition). Philadelphia, PA: Elsevier.

Medullary sponge kidney. (n.d.). In *Radiopaedia*. Retrieved July 28, 2017, from https://radiopaedia.org/articles/medullary-sponge-kidney

Medullary sponge kidney: what is medullary sponge kidney? (2017, July 31). In *National Institute of Diabetes and Digestive and Kidney Diseases. Retrieved from https://www.niddk.nih.gov/health-information/kidney-disease/children/medullary-sponge-kidney*

Mezzabot F., Cristofaro R., Ceol M., Del Prete D., Priante G., Familiari A., Fabris A., D'Angelo A., Gambaro G., Anglani F. (2015). Spontaneous calcification process in primary renal cells from a medullary sponge kidney patient harboring a GDNF mutation. *J. Cell Mol. Med., 19*(4); 889-902. Retrieved July 31, 2017, from http://sci-hub.io/10.1111/jcmm.12514

Pfau A., Knauf F. (2016). Update on nephrolithiasis: core curriculum. *Am J Kidney Dis, 68*(6); 973-985. Retrieved July 31, 2017, from http://www.ajkd.org/article/S0272-6386(16)30254-2/fulltext#sec4

Ross M.H., Pawlina W. (2011). *Histology: A Text and Atlas* (6 edition). Philadelphia, PA: Lippincott Williams & Wilkins.

Tortora G.J., Derrickson B. (2014). *Principles of Anatomy & Physiology* (14 edition). Hoboken, NJ: Wiley.

What is medullary sponge kidney? (2017, July 28). In Kidney Stoners. Retrieved from http://www.kidneystoners.org/information/what_is_medullary_sponge_kidney/

## MEMBRANOPROLIFERATIVE GLOMERULONEPHRITIS

Alchi, B. & Jayne, D. (2010). Membranoproliferative glomerulonephritis. *Pediatr Nephrol 25*(8), 1409-1418. Retrieved August 1, 2017, from http://www.ncbi.nlm.nih.gov/pmc/articles/PMC2887509/

Appel, G. B., Cook, H. T., Hageman, G., Jennette, J. C., Kashgarian, M., Kirschfink, M., & Zipfel, P. F. (2005). Membranoproliferative glomerulonephritis type II (dense deposit disease): an update. *Journal of the American Society of Nephrology, 16*(5), 1392–1403. Retrieved August 1, 2017, from https://doi.org/10.1681/ASN.2005010078 http://jasn.asnjournals.org/content/16/5/1392.full

Corchado, J. C. & Smith, R. J. H. (2011). Dense deposit disease/membranoproliferative glomerulonephritis type II. *GeneReviews* (n.d.). Retrieved August 1, 2017, from http://www.ncbi.nlm.nih.gov/books/NBK1425/

Kathuria, P. (2016). Membranoproliferative glomerulonephritis: background, pathophysiology, etiology. In *Medscape*. Retrieved August 1, 2017, from http://emedicine.medscape.com/article/240056-overview#a3

Membranoproliferative glomerulonephritis. (n.d.). In Wikipedia. *Retrieved* August 1, 2017, from https://en.wikipedia.org/wiki/Membranoproliferative_glomerulonephritis

## MEMBRANOUS GLOMERULONEPHRITIS (MEMBRANOUS NEPHROPATHY)

Kumar, V., Abbas A.K., & Aster, J.C. *Robbins & Cotran Pathologic Basis of Disease* (9 edition). Philadelphia, PA: Elsevier.

Mansur, A. (2016). Membranous glomerulonephritis. In *Medscape*. Retrieved July 31, 2017, from http://emedicine.medscape.com/article/239799-overview?pa=Sef54Rn6mTA4jk5HNSClghG3o6sN2eBexCl%2BVyBZ3V3HWve%2BMlqC%2BTw3XB%2FeJDcSIG%2BadLhcsY9Ybn4LOmdWLON5lPYw%2FtQ7Z8WOOzpssmw%3D#a5

Membranous glomerulonephritis. (n.d.). In *Wikipedia*. Retrieved July 28, 2017, from https://en.wikipedia.org/wiki/Membranous_glomerulonephritis

Sattar, H.A. (2017). *Fundamentals of Pathology: Medical Course and Step 1 Review* (2017). USA: Pathoma LLC.

## MINIMAL CHANGE DISEASE

Kumar, V., Abbas A.K., & Aster, J.C. *Robbins & Cotran Pathologic Basis of Disease* (9 edition). Philadelphia, PA: Elsevier.

Le, T., Bhushan, V., Sochat, M., & Chavda, Y. (2017). *First Aid for the USMLE Step 1 2017* (27 edition). New York, NY: McGraw-Hill Education / Medical.

Mansur, A. (2017). Minimal-change disease. In *Medscape*. Retrieved July 31, 2017, from http://emedicine.medscape.com/article/243348-overview#a5

Menzel, S., & Moeller, M. J. (2011). Role of the podocyte

in proteinuria. *Pediatric Nephrology (Berlin, Germany)*, *26*(10), 1775–1780. Retrieved July 31, 2017, from https://doi.org/10.1007/s00467-010-1725-5

Minimal change disease. (n.d.). In *Wikipedia*. Retrieved July 28, 2017, from https://en.wikipedia.org/wiki/Minimal_change_disease#Names

Nephrotic syndrome. (n.d.). In *Wikipedia*. Retrieved July 28, 2017, from https://en.wikipedia.org/wiki/Nephrotic_syndrome

Sattar, H.A. (2017). *Fundamentals of Pathology: Medical Course and Step 1 Review* (2017). USA: Pathoma LLC.

## MULTICYSTIC DYSPLASTIC KIDNEY

Multicystic dysplastic kidney. (n.d.). In *Wikipedia*. Retrieved July 28, 2017, from https://en.wikipedia.org/wiki/Multicystic_dysplastic_kidney

Swlatecka-Urban, A. (2016). Multicystic renal dysplasia. In *Medscape*. Retrieved July 31, 2017, from http://emedicine.medscape.com/article/982560-overview#a5

What causes kidney dysplasia? (n.d.). In National Institute of Diabetes and Digestive and Kidney Diseases. Retrieved July 31,2017, from https://www.niddk.nih.gov/health-information/health-topics/kidney-disease/kidney-dysplasia/Pages/facts.aspx#causes

## NEPHROLITHIASIS (KIDNEY STONES)

Becker, M. A. (2017). Uric acid balance. In *UpToDate*. Retrieved July 31, 2017, from http://www.uptodate.com/contents/uric-acid-balance

Copstead, L.-E. C., & Banasik, J. L. (2012). *Pathophysiology* (5 edition). St. Louis, MO: Saunders.

Dave, C. (2016) Nephrolithiasis: practice essentials, background, anatomy. In *Medscape*. Retrieved July 31, 2017, from http://emedicine.medscape.com/article/437096-overview#a4 http://emedicine.medscape.com/article/437096-overview#a4

Fathallah-Shaykh, S. (2017). Uric acid stones: background, pathophysiology, epidemiology. In *Medscape*. Retrieved July 31, 2017, from http://emedicine.medscape.com/article/983759-overview#a5

Hyperuricosura. (n.d.). In *Wikipedia*. Retrieved July 28, 2017, from https://en.wikipedia.org/wiki/Hyperuricosuria

Jackstone calculus. (n.d.). In *Radiopaedia*. Retrieved July 28, 2017, from https://radiopaedia.org/articles/jackstone-calculus

Meng, M. (2016) Struvite and staghorn calculi. In *Medscape*. Retrieved July 31, 2017, from http://emedicine.medscape.com/article/439127-overview#a8

Mid-ureteric calculus. (n.d.). In *Radiopaedia*. Retrieved July 28, 2017, from https://radiopaedia.org/cases/mid-ureteric-calculus

Purine. (n.d.). In *Wikipedia*. Retrieved July 28, 2017, from https://en.wikipedia.org/wiki/Purine

Sattar, H.A. (2017). *Fundamentals of Pathology: Medical Course and Step 1 Review* (2017). USA: Pathoma LLC.

Struvite. (n.d.). In *Wikipedia*. Retrieved July 28, 2017, from https://en.wikipedia.org/wiki/Struvite

## NEPHRONOPHTHISIS & MEDULLARY CYSTIC KIDNEY DISEASE

Medullary cystic kidney disease 1; MCKD1. (2017, August 1). In OMIM. Retrieved from http://www.omim.org/entry/174000

Medullary cystic kidney disease 2; MCKD2. (n.d.). In *OMIM*. Retrieved August 1, 2017, from http://www.omim.org/entry/603860

Nephronophthisis 1; NPHP1. ( (n.d.). In *OMIM*. Retrieved August 1, 2017, from http://www.omim.org/entry/256100

Renal medulla. (July 28 2017). In *Wikipedia*. Retrieved from https://en.wikipedia.org/wiki/Renal_medulla

Hildebrandt, F., & Zhou, W. (2007). Nephronophthisis-associated ciliopathies. *Journal of the American Society of Nephrology: JASN*, *18*(6), 1855–1871. Retrieved July 31, 2017, from https://doi.org/10.1681/ASN.2006121344

Scolari, F., & Ghiggeri, G. M. (2003). Nephronophthisis-medullary cystic kidney disease: from bedside to bench and back again. *Saudi Journal of Kidney Diseases and Transplantation: An Official Publication of the Saudi Center for Organ Transplantation, Saudi Arabia*, *14*(3), 316–327. Retrieved July 31, 2017, from https://www.ncbi.nlm.nih.gov/pubmed/17657103

## NEUROGENIC BLADDER

Gill, B. C. (2017). Neurogenic bladder. In *Medscape*. Retrieved July 31, 2017, from http://emedicine.medscape.com/article/453539-overview#a7

Hall, J. E. (2015). *Guyton and Hall Textbook of Medical Physiology*. St. Louis, MO: Saunders.

Kalsi, V. & Fowler, C. J. Therapy insight: bladder

dysfunction associated with multiple sclerosis. *Nat Clin Pract Urol., 2005, 2*(10), 492-501. Retrieved August 1, 2017, from http://www.medscape.com/viewarticle/515091_2

Kasper, D. L., Fauci, A. S., Hauser, S., Longo, D., Jameson, J. L., & Loscalzo, J. (2015). *Harrison's Principles of Internal Medicine* (19 edition). New York, NY: McGraw-Hill Education / Medical.

khanacademymedicine. (2014). Urination | Renal system physiology | NCLEX-RN | Khan Academy. Retrieved July 31, 2017, from https://www.youtube.com/watch?v=rheO1tVyB0U

khanacademymedicine. (2014). Urination | Renal system physiology | NCLEX-RN | Khan Academy. Retrieved July 31, 2017, from https://www.youtube.com/watch?v=rheO1tVyB0U

## NON-UROTHELIAL BLADDER CANCERS

Dadhania, V., Czerniak, B., & Guo, C. C. (2015). Adenocarcinoma of the urinary bladder. *American Journal of Clinical and Experimental Urology, 3*(2), 51–63. Retrieved July 31, 2017, from http://www.ncbi.nlm.nih.gov/pmc/articles/PMC4539107/

Idrees, M. T. (2013). Pathologic findings in squamous cell bladder carcinoma: overview of squamous cell carcinoma, gross findings in squamous cell carcinoma, microscopic findings in squamous cell carcinoma. Retrieved July 31, 2017, from http://emedicine.medscape.com/article/1951756-overview#showall

Steinberg, G. D. (2017). Bladder cancer: practice essentials, background, anatomy. In *Medscape*. Retrieved July 31, 2017, from http://emedicine.medscape.com/article/438262-overview#a5

Squamous metaplasia. (n.d.). In *Wikipedia*. Retrieved July 28, 2017, from https://en.wikipedia.org/wiki/Squamous_metaplasia

## POLYCYSTIC KIDNEY DISEASE

Harris, P. C. & Torres, V. E. Polycystic kidney disease, autosomal dominant. *GeneReviews* (n.d.). Retrieved July 31, 2017, from https://www.ncbi.nlm.nih.gov/books/NBK1246/

Le, T., Bhushan, V., Sochat, M., & Chavda, Y. (2017). *First Aid for the USMLE Step 1 2017* (27 edition). New York, NY: McGraw-Hill Education / Medical.

Rimoin, D., Pyeritz, R. & Korf, B. *Principles and Practice of Medical Genetics* (2013). Los Angeles, CA: Academic Press.

Sattar, H.A. (2017). *Fundamentals of Pathology: Medical Course and Step 1 Review* (2017). USA: Pathoma LLC.

Sweeney, William E. & Avner, E. D. Polycystic kidney disease, autosomal recessive. *GeneReviews* (n.d.). Retrieved July 31, 2017, from https://www.ncbi.nlm.nih.gov/books/NBK1326/

Wills, E. S., Roepman, R., & Drenth, J. P. H. (2014). Polycystic liver disease: ductal plate malformation and the primary cilium. *Trends in Molecular Medicine, 20*(5), 261–270. Retrieved July 31, 2017, from https://doi.org/10.1016/j.molmed.2014.01.003

## POSTERIOR URETHRAL VALVE

Bomalaski, M. B. Posterior urethral valves. In *Medscape*. Retrieved July 31, 2017, from http://emedicine.medscape.com/article/1016086-overview?pa=fa902AsmJwEvozbz3%2BM0yHKyKZssu2TBFJAiPu3kyyEknSzbiicvliAf1usolus4yVMyaBe652rmShYeirmn2iwhCTQqz25Ki1mL6i64Z7Vg%3D#a5

Bomalaski, M. B. (2016). Posterior urethral valves treatment & management. In *Medscape*. Retrieved July 31, 2017, from http://emedicine.medscape.com/article/1016086-treatment

Holmes, N. (2016). Clinical presentation and diagnosis of posterior urethral valves. In *UpToDate*. Retrieved July 31, 2017, from https://www.uptodate.com/contents/clinical-presentation-and-diagnosis-of-posterior-urethral-valves?source=search_result&search=posterior%20urethral%20valves&selectedTitle=1~32

Posterior urethral valve. (n.d.). In *Wikipedia*. Retrieved July 28, 2017, from https://en.wikipedia.org/wiki/Posterior_urethral_valve

Posterior urethral valves. (n.d.). In *Radiopaedia*. Retrieved July 28, 2017, from https://radiopaedia.org/articles/posterior-urethral-valves

Potter sequence. (n.d.). In *Wikipedia*. Retrieved July 28, 2017, from https://en.wikipedia.org/wiki/Potter_sequence

Schenkman, N. S. (2016). Male urethra anatomy. In *Medscape*. Retrieved July 31, 2017, from http://emedicine.medscape.com/article/1972482-overview

## POSTRENAL ACUTE KIDNEY INJURY

Acute kidney injury. (July 28 2017). In *Wikipedia*.

Retrieved from https://en.wikipedia.org/wiki/Acute_kidney_injury

Kumar, V., Abbas A.K., & Aster, J.C. *Robbins & Cotran Pathologic Basis of Disease* (9 edition). Philadelphia, PA: Elsevier.

Le, T., Bhushan, V., Sochat, M., & Chavda, Y. (2017). *First Aid for the USMLE Step 1 2017* (27 edition). New York, NY: McGraw-Hill Education / Medical.

Sattar, H.A. (2017). *Fundamentals of Pathology: Medical Course and Step 1 Review* (2017). USA: Pathoma LLC.


## POSTSTREPTOCOCCAL GLOMERULONEPHRITIS

Copstead, L.-E. C., & Banasik, J. L. (2012). *Pathophysiology* (5 edition). St. Louis, MO: Saunders.

Le, T., Bhushan, V., Sochat, M., & Chavda, Y. (2017). *First Aid for the USMLE Step 1 2017* (27 edition). New York, NY: McGraw-Hill Education / Medical.

McKance, K.L. & Huethe, S.E. (2014). *Pathophysiology: The Biologic Basis for Disease in Adults and Children* (7 edition). St. Louis, MO: Mosby-Elsevier.

Sattar, H.A. (2017). *Fundamentals of Pathology: Medical Course and Step 1 Review* (2017). USA: Pathoma LLC.


## POTTER SEQUENCE

Le, T., Bhushan, V., Sochat, M., & Chavda, Y. (2017). *First Aid for the USMLE Step 1 2017* (27 edition). New York, NY: McGraw-Hill Education / Medical.

Potter sequence. (n.d.). In *Wikipedia*. Retrieved July 28, 2017, from https://en.wikipedia.org/wiki/Potter_sequence

Potter sequence. (n.d.). In *Radiopaedia*. Retrieved July 28, 2017, from https://radiopaedia.org/articles/potter-sequence

Sattar, H.A. (2017). *Fundamentals of Pathology: Medical Course and Step 1 Review* (2017). USA: Pathoma LLC.

Shastry, S. M., Kolte, S. S., & Sanagapati, P. R. (2012). Potter's Sequence. *Journal of Clinical Neonatology*, 1(3), 157–159. Retrieved July 28, 2017, from https://www.ncbi.nlm.nih.gov/pmc/articles/PMC3762025/


## PRERENAL ACUTE KIDNEY INJURY

Acute kidney injury. (n.d.). In *Wikipedia*. Retrieved July 28, 2017, from https://en.wikipedia.org/wiki/Acute_kidney_injury

Kumar, V., Abbas A.K., & Aster, J.C. *Robbins & Cotran Pathologic Basis of Disease* (9 edition). Philadelphia, PA: Elsevier.

Le, T., Bhushan, V., Sochat, M., & Chavda, Y. (2017). *First Aid for the USMLE Step 1 2017* (27 edition). New York, NY: McGraw-Hill Education / Medical.

Sattar, H.A. (2017). *Fundamentals of Pathology: Medical Course and Step 1 Review* (2017). USA: Pathoma LLC.


## RAPIDLY PROGRESSIVE GLOMERULONEPHRITIS

Copstead, L.-E. C., & Banasik, J. L. (2012). *Pathophysiology* (5 edition). St. Louis, MO: Saunders.Le, T., Bhushan, V., Sochat, M., & Chavda, Y. (2017). *First Aid for the USMLE Step 1 2017* (27 edition). New York, NY: McGraw-Hill Education / Medical.

McKance, K.L. & Huethe, S.E. (2014). *Pathophysiology: The Biologic Basis for Disease in Adults and Children* (7 edition). St. Louis, MO: Mosby-Elsevier.

Sattar, H.A. (2017). *Fundamentals of Pathology: Medical Course and Step 1 Review* (2017). USA: Pathoma LLC.


## RENAL AGENESIS

Chin, T. W. (2014). Pediatric pulmonary hypoplasia. In *Medscape*. Retrieved July 31, 2017, from http://emedicine.medscape.com/article/1005696-overview#a5

Gill, P.S. & Rosenblum, N. D. (2006). Control of murine kidney development by Sonic hedgehog and its GLI effectors. *Cell Cycle, 5*(13): 1426-1430. Retrieved July 31, 2017 from http://www.tandfonline.com/doi/pdf/10.4161/cc.5.13.2928

Gupta, S. (2015). Potter syndrome. In *Medscape*. Retrieved July 31, 2017, from http://emedicine.medscape.com/article/983477-overview#a5

Le, T., Bhushan, V., Sochat, M., & Chavda, Y. (2017). *First Aid for the USMLE Step 1 2017* (27 edition). New York, NY: McGraw-Hill Education / Medical.

Nigam, S. K., & Shah, M. M. (n.d.). How does the ureteric bud branch? In *Journal of the American Society of Nephrology*. Retrieved July 31, 2017, from https://doi.org/10.1681/ASN.2008020132

Potter sequence. (n.d.). In *Wikipedia*. Retrieved July 28, 2017, from https://en.wikipedia.org/wiki/Potter_sequence

Renal agenesis. (n.d.). In *Wikipedia*. Retrieved July 28, 2017, from https://en.wikipedia.org/wiki/Renal_agenesis

Sattar, H.A. (2017). *Fundamentals of Pathology: Medical Course and Step 1 Review* (2017). USA: Pathoma LLC.

Yalavarthy, R. & Parikh, C. R. (2003). Congenital renal agenesis: a review. *Saudi Journal of Kidney Diseases and Transplantation, 13*(3): 336-341. Retrieved July 31, 2017, from http://www.sjkdt.org/article.asp?issn=1319-2442;year=2003;volume=14;issue=3;spage=336;epage=341;aulast=Yalavarthy

## RENAL ARTERY STENOSIS

Kumar, V., Abbas A.K., & Aster, J.C. *Robbins & Cotran Pathologic Basis of Disease* (9 edition). Philadelphia, PA: Elsevier.

Lee, J. J., Pai, K. S., Shin, J. I. & Park, S. J. (2014). Renovascular hypertension treated by renal artery embolization. *Yonsei Med. J.* Retrieved July 31, 2017, from https://openi.nlm.nih.gov/detailedresult.php?img=PMC3874892_ymj-55-273-g001&query=renal+artery+stenosis&it=xg&req=4&npos=55

Olin, J. W., Gornik, H. L., Bacharach, J. M., Biller, J., Fine, L. J., Gray, B. H. & Stanley, J. C. (2014). Fibromuscular dysplasia: state of the science and critical unanswered questions: a scientific statement from the American Heart Association. *Circulation, 129*(9), 1048-1078. Retrieved July 31, 2017, from http://circ.ahajournals.org/content/early/2014/02/18/01.cir.0000442577.96802.8c

Sattar, H.A. (2017). *Fundamentals of Pathology: Medical Course and Step 1 Review* (2017). USA: Pathoma LLC.

Spinowitz, B. S. (2016). Renal artery stenosis: practice essentials, pathophysiology, etiology. In *Medscape*. Retrieved July 31, 2017, from http://emedicine.medscape.com/article/245023-overview

Textor, S. (2017). Treatment of unilateral atherosclerotic renal artery stenosis. In *UpToDate*. Retrieved July 31, 2017, from https://www.uptodate.com/contents/treatment-of-unilateral-atherosclerotic-renal-artery-stenosis?source=see_link

## RENAL CELL CARCINOMAS

Le, T., Bhushan, V., Sochat, M., & Chavda, Y. (2017). *First Aid for the USMLE Step 1 2017* (27 edition). New York, NY: McGraw-Hill Education / Medical.

Sattar, H.A. (2017). *Fundamentals of Pathology: Medical Course and Step 1 Review* (2017). USA: Pathoma LLC.

## RENAL CORTICAL NECROSIS

Acute tubular necrosis vs. renal cortical necrosis. (1959). *New England Journal of Medicine, 261*(4), 206-206. Retrieved July 31, 2017, from http://www.nejm.org/doi/pdf/10.1056/NEJM195907232610421

Bonventre, J. V. & Yang, L. (2011). Cellular pathophysiology of ischemic acute kidney injury. *J Clin Invest*, 121(11):4210-4221. Retrieved July 31, 2017, from https://www.ncbi.nlm.nih.gov/pmc/articles/PMC3204829/

Eaton, D. C. & Pooler, J. P. (2013). *Vander's Renal Physiology* (8 edition). New York, NY: McGraw-Hill.

Goljan, E. F. (2013). *Rapid Review Pathology* (4 edition). Milton, ON: Elsevier Canada.

Le, T., Bhushan, V., Sochat, M., & Chavda, Y. (2017). *First Aid for the USMLE Step 1 2017* (27 edition). New York, NY: McGraw-Hill Education / Medical.

Renal cortical necrosis. (n.d.). In *WikiVisually*. Retrieved July 28, 2017, from http://www.wikivisually.com/wiki/Renal_cortical_necrosis

Sattar, H.A. (2017). *Fundamentals of Pathology: Medical Course and Step 1 Review* (2017). USA: Pathoma LLC.

## RENAL TUBULAR ACIDOSIS

Blood cleaning by the kidneys. (n.d.). In *IvyRose Holistic*. Retrieved July 28, 2017, from http://www.ivyroses.com/HumanBody/Urinary/Urinary_System_Kidneys_Actions.php

Galla, H.J. H., Kurtz, I., Kraut, J. A., Lipschik, G. Y. & Macrae, J. P. (2009). Chapter 5. acid–base disorders. *CURRENT Diagnosis & Treatment: Nephrology & Hypertension*. Eds. Edgar V. Lerma, et al. New York, NY: McGraw-Hill. Retrieved July 31, 2017, from http://accessmedicine.mhmedical.com.ezp-prod1.hul.harvard.edu/content.aspx?bookid=372&sectionid=39961140

Goljan, E. F. (2013). *Rapid Review Pathology* (4 edition). Milton, ON: Elsevier Canada.

Le, T., Bhushan, V., Sochat, M., & Chavda, Y. (2017). *First Aid for the USMLE Step 1 2017* (27 edition). New York, NY: McGraw-Hill Education / Medical.

Nephrology On-Demand. (2011). 10-minute Rounds: Renal Tubular Acidoses (The purpose of Ammonia). Retrieved July 31, 2017, from https://www.youtube.com/watch?v=1o3P_0_88cl

Nephron, parts, and histology. (n.d.). In *Boundless*. Retrieved July 28, 2017, from https://www.boundless.

com/physiology/textbooks/boundless-anatomy-and-physiology-textbook/urinary-system-25/the-kidneys-239/nephron-parts-and-histology-1170-2287

Purkerson, J. M. & Schwartz, G. J. (2007). The role of carbonic anhydrases in renal physiology. In *Kidney International*. Retrieved July 31, 2017, from http://www.kidney-international.org/article/S0085-2538(15)52330-2/pdf

Renal tubular acidosis. (n.d.). In *Wikipedia*. Retrieved July 28, 2017, from https://en.wikipedia.org/wiki/Renal_tubular_acidosis

Sattar, H.A. (2017). *Fundamentals of Pathology: Medical Course and Step 1 Review* (2017). USA: Pathoma LLC.

Stern, S. D. C., Cifu A. S. & Atkorn, D. (2014). Acid-base abnormalities. *Symptom to Diagnosis: An Evidence-Based Guide* (3 edition). New York, NY: McGraw-Hill. Retrieved July 31, 2017, from http://accessmedicine.mhmedical.com.ezp-prod1.hul.harvard.edu/content.aspx?bookid=1088&sectionid=61696804

## TRANSITIONAL CELL CARCINOMA

Bladder cancer: diagnosis. (2017). In *Mayo Clinic*. Retrieved July 31, 2017, from http://www.mayoclinic.org/diseases-conditions/bladder-cancer/basics/tests-diagnosis/con-20027606

Le, T., Bhushan, V., Sochat, M., & Chavda, Y. (2017). *First Aid for the USMLE Step 1 2017* (27 edition). New York, NY: McGraw-Hill Education / Medical.

Renal pelvis, uterer, bladder, and other urinary equivlalent terms, definitions, tables and illustrations. (n.d.). In National Cancer Institute. Retrieved July 31, 2017, from http://seer.cancer.gov/tools/mphrules/2007/urinary/terms_defs.pdf

Sattar, H.A. (2017). *Fundamentals of Pathology: Medical Course and Step 1 Review* (2017). USA: Pathoma LLC.

Steinberg, G. D. (2017). Bladder cancer: practice essentials, background, anatomy. In *Medscape*. Retrieved July 31, 2017, from http://emedicine.medscape.com/article/438262-overview

Transitional cell carcinoma. (n.d.). In *Wikipedia*. Retrieved July 28, 2017, from https://en.wikipedia.org/wiki/Transitional_cell_carcinoma

## URINARY INCONTINENCE

Marieb, E. N. & Hoehn, K. N. (2014). *Human Anatomy & Physiology* (10 edition). London, UK: Pearson.

Patient education: urinary incontinence. (2017, August 1). In *UpToDate*. Retrieved from https://www.uptodate.com/contents/urinary-incontinence-the-basics?source=search_result&search=urinary%20incontinence&selectedTitle=19~150

Urinary incontinence. (2015). In *Clinical Gate*. Retrieved July 31, 2017, from http://clinicalgate.com/urinary-incontinence/

Sattar, H.A. (2017). *Fundamentals of Pathology: Medical Course and Step 1 Review* (2017). USA: Pathoma LLC.

Tortora, G. J. & Derrickson, B. (2014). *Principles of Anatomy and Physiology*. Hoboken, NJ: Wiley.

## VESICOURETERAL REFLUX

Nelson, C. P. (2016). Pediatric vesicoureteral reflux. In *Medscape*. Retrieved July 31, 2017, from http://emedicine.medscape.com/article/1016439-overview

Posterior urethral valves symptoms & causes. (n.d.). In *Boston's Children's Hospital*. Retrieved July 31, 2017, from http://www.childrenshospital.org/conditions-and-treatments/conditions/posterior-urethral-valves/symptoms-and-causes

Sattar, H.A. (2017). *Fundamentals of Pathology: Medical Course and Step 1 Review* (2017). USA: Pathoma LLC.

Vesicoureteral reflux: definition. (2014). In *Mayo Clinic*. Retrieved July 31, 2017, from http://www.mayoclinic.org/diseases-conditions/vesicoureteral-reflux/basics/definition/con-20031544

Vesicoureteral reflux. (n.d.). In *Wikipedia*. Retrieved July 28, 2017, from https://en.wikipedia.org/wiki/Vesicoureteral_reflux

## WAGR SYNDROME

Fischbach, B. V., Trout, K. L., Lewis, J., Luis, C. A. & Sika, M. (2005). WAGR syndrome: a clinical review of 54 cases. *Pediatrics* 116(4), 984-988. Retrieved July 31, 2017, from https://www.ncbi.nlm.nih.gov/pubmed/16199712

Kumar, V., Abbas A.K., & Aster, J.C. *Robbins & Cotran Pathologic Basis of Disease* (9 edition). Philadelphia, PA: Elsevier.

Le, T., Bhushan, V., Sochat, M., & Chavda, Y. (2017). *First Aid for the USMLE Step 1 2017* (27 edition). New York, NY: McGraw-Hill Education / Medical.

Learning about WAGR syndrome. (n.d.). hIn *National*

*Human Genome Research Institute*. Retrieved July 28, 2017, from https://www.genome.gov/26023527/

Sattar, H.A. (2017). *Fundamentals of Pathology: Medical Course and Step 1 Review* (2017). USA: Pathoma LLC.

WAGR syndrome. (n.d.). In *National Library of Medicine*. Retrieved July 28, 2017 from https://ghr.nlm.nih.gov/condition/wagr-syndrome

WAGR syndrome. (n.d.). In *Wikipedia*. Retrieved July 28, 2017, from https://en.wikipedia.org/wiki/WAGR_syndrome

## WILMS' TUMOR

Kumar, V., Abbas A.K., & Aster, J.C. *Robbins & Cotran Pathologic Basis of Disease* (9 edition). Philadelphia, PA: Elsevier.

Le, T., Bhushan, V., Sochat, M., & Chavda, Y. (2017). *First Aid for the USMLE Step 1 2017* (27 edition). New York, NY: McGraw-Hill Education / Medical.

Paulino, A. C. Wilms' tumor. (2017, July 28). In *Medscape*. Retrieved from http://emedicine.medscape.com/article/989398-overview#a5

Sattar, H.A. (2017). *Fundamentals of Pathology: Medical Course and Step 1 Review* (2017). USA: Pathoma LLC.

WAGR syndrome. (2017, July 28). In *National Institutes of Health*. Retrieved from https://ghr.nlm.nih.gov/condition/wagr-syndrome

Wilms' tumor. (n.d.). In *Wikipedia*. Retrieved July 28, 2017, from https://en.wikipedia.org/wiki/Wilms_tumor

# INDEX

Numbers in red indicate the term is
defined on those pages.

## A

acidosis  94
acute kidney injury  **171–178, 244–
    248, 256–260**
acute pyelonephritis  **15–19**, 41
acute renal failure  171. *See* acute kidney
    injury
adenocarcinomas. *See* non-urothelial
    bladder cancer
ADHD  310
ADPKD. *See* polycystic kidney disease
adrenal insufficiency.
    *See* hypoaldosteronism
afferent arteriole  **52**
AKI. *See* acute kidney injury
alcoholism  142
aldosterone  99, 133, 260
alpha-hemolysis  **249**
Alport syndrome  **20–25**
aminoacyl-tRNA  **70**
aneurysm  28
Angiomyolipomas  **26–29**
aniridia  **310**
antenatal hydronephrosis  **80**
anterior lenticonus  **22**
apoptosis  **85**, 123
ARF. *See* acute renal failure; *See* acute
    kidney injury
ascending cholangitis  239
atherosclerosis  272
atypical hemolytic uremic syndrome
    **72**
autism  310
autosomal dominant PKD.
    *See* polycystic kidney disease
azotemia  175, **246**, 260

## B

bacteremia  17
Beckwith-Wiedemann syndrome  310,
    316
benign prostatic hyperplasia  **42**
Berger disease. *See* IgA nephropathy
beta-hemolysis  **249**
bilateral renal agenesis. *See* renal
    agenesis
Bladder exstrophy  **30–33**
bladder outlet obstruction  15

blood urea nitrogen  244, 256
BRA. *See* renal agenesis
BUN. *See* blood urea nitrogen

## C

catecholamines  94, 131
Cell lysis  95
cervical carcinoma  **42**
chlamydia trachomatis  **49**
cholangiocytes  239
chordee  **161**
chronic kidney disease  116
chronic pyelonephritis  19, 41, **41–44**
Churg-Strauss syndrome  261
Chvostek's sign  **120**, 127, 142
citrobacter  **46**
cloaca  **30**
cloacal membrane  30
collagen  **20**, 22, 24, 25, 63, 269
collagen Type IV. *See* collagen
colloid casts  43
congenital obstructive posterior
    urethral membrane  **240**
COPUM. *See* congenital obstructive
    posterior urethral membrane
corticomedullary junction  218
creatinine  244, 256
crescentic glomerulonephritis  **261–
    265**
cryptorchidism  **161**
cystitis  **45**

## D

Denys-Drash syndrome  316
detrusor muscle  221
D- hemolytic uremic syndrome.
    *See* atypical hemolytic uremic
    syndrome
diabetes mellitus  47, 140, 177, 223
diabetes type I  52
diabetes type II  52
diabetic ketoacidosis  120
diabetic nephropathy  **52–56**
diapedesis  **47**
diarrhea-positive hemolytic syndrome
    68
diffuse cortical necrosis. *See* renal
    cortical necrosis
DiGeorge syndrome  125
d positive hemolytic syndrome,.
    *See* diarrhea-positive hemolytic
    syndrome

## E

E. coli  15, 46, 68
ectoderm  30
edema  59, 181
efferent arteriole  **52**
embolization  **29**
Enterobacter  15, 46
Enterococcus  46
enterohemorrhagic E. coli  68
epispadias  30, **158–163**
esophageal varices  237
euvolemic hyponatremia.
    *See* hyponatremia

## F

false hypocalcemia  **125**
false hyponatremia. *See* hyponatremia
Fanconi syndrome  **153**
fenestrated capillary endothelium  20
fibrocystin  237
fibromuscular dysplasia  272
filtrate  **52**
flaccid neurogenic bladder  307
focal glomerular sclerosis. *See* focal
    segmental glomerulosclerosis
focal segmental glomerulosclerosis
    **57–61**
FSGS. *See* focal segmental
    glomerulosclerosis

## G

Gb3-receptor  70
GBM. *See* glomerular basement
    membrane
Gitelman syndrome  140
glaucoma  **310**
globotriaosylceramide  70
glomerular basement membrane  20
glomerular capillary  20
glomerular filtration rate  **54**
glomerulonephritis  177
glomerulus  20, 52
glycosaminoglycans  91, **129**
glycosuria  52
Goodpasture syndrome  22, **62–67**,
    261
granulomatous tissue  **43**
gross hematuria  **20**

## H

hamartomas  **26**
hematuria  **66**, 181, 250, **263**, 296
hemolytic anemia  72